Neuronal Control of Locomotion

Neuronal Control of Locomotion
From Mollusc to Man

G. N. ORLOVSKY, T. G. DELIAGINA, and S. GRILLNER
Nobel Institute for Neurophysiology,
Department of Neuroscience, Karolinska Institute,
S-17177 Stockholm, Sweden

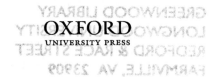

OXFORD
UNIVERSITY PRESS

*This book has been printed digitally and produced in a standard specification
in order to ensure its continuing availability*

OXFORD
UNIVERSITY PRESS

Great Clarendon Street, Oxford OX2 6DP

Oxford University Press is a department of the University of Oxford.
It furthers the University's objective of excellence in research, scholarship,
and education by publishing worldwide in

Oxford New York

Auckland Bangkok Buenos Aires Cape Town Chennai
Dar es Salaam Delhi Hong Kong Istanbul Karachi Kolkata
Kuala Lumpur Madrid Melbourne Mexico City Mumbai Nairobi
São Paulo Shanghai Taipei Tokyo Toronto

Oxford is a registered trade mark of Oxford University Press
in the UK and in certain other countries

Published in the United States
by Oxford University Press Inc., New York

© G. N. Orlovsky, T. G. Deliagina, and S. Grillner, 1999

The moral rights of the authors have been asserted

Database right Oxford University Press (maker)

Reprinted 2003

ISBN 0 19 852405 6

Preface

The ability to locomote, that is move actively in space, is characteristic of the animal kingdom. The evolution of the nervous system was, to a large extent, related to the evolution of locomotion. Numerous motor centres in the brain cooperate while controlling locomotion. All sensory systems are involved in supplying the motor centres with the necessary information.

The extreme importance of locomotion for any living being has stimulated studies of the neural mechanisms responsible for the locomotor control in different species, from lower animals to humans. As a result of these studies, a description of the control system at a functional level has been obtained for different species, and the distribution of functions between different subdivisions within the central nervous system (CNS) has been characterized. In some species, such as molluscs, leech, tadpole, and lamprey, the neuronal mechanisms for locomotor control have been analysed at the network and cellular level. In general, the investigation of locomotor control is one of the most developed areas of motor physiology.

An important strategy in these studies is the comparative analysis of the locomotor mechanisms in phylogenetically remote species. Such an analysis helps in revealing basic principles in the organization and operation of these mechanisms. Animals with simpler nervous system can also be used as 'biological models' for studying the locomotor control mechanisms at the cellular and network level, since such a study is difficult to perform in more complex animals such as mammals.

The major aim of the present book is to integrate our knowledge of the organization and operation of the locomotor control system in different species, both invertebrate and vertebrate. This is needed to combine the efforts of experts in different specific fields (motor physiology of invertebrates and vertebrates, sensory physiology, modelling, etc.), and to supply them with the knowledge and ideas available in adjacent areas.

The authors of this book have the advantage that each of them, during their scientific career, has worked on different, distantly related species, but addressed similar problems related to the control of locomotion. This is why we think that we can provide valuable information to the scientific community, and critically evaluate the state of the art in the whole area. For the readers of this book, even if they are experts on some specific aspects of motor physiology, this integrated view may be useful.

The book consists of four parts. Part 1 considers the neuronal networks for the control of locomotion in invertebrates. A few species have been chosen, in which the analysis of the networks is advanced and the basic principles of locomotor coordination can be illustrated. Part 2 considers the neuronal locomotor mechanisms in lower vertebrates to make a bridge to higher vertebrates. Part 3 is the central one; it is mainly devoted to the locomotor control system of the cat, the favourite object for this kind of study for half a century. In Part 4, the main findings and ideas, derived from the simpler systems, are considered in relation to

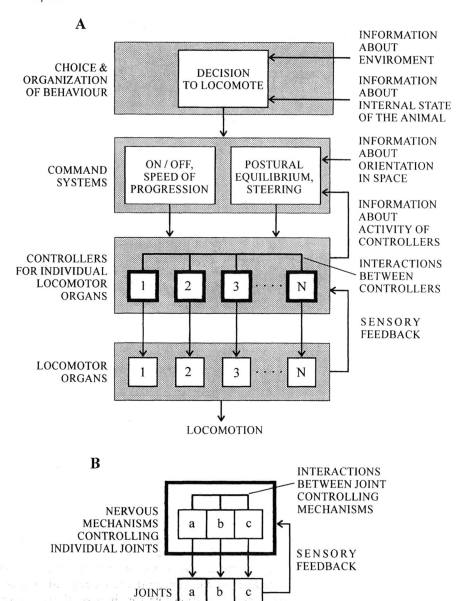

Fig. 0.1 A: Basic components and functional organization of the generalized system for the control of locomotion. The system has a hierarchical structure. The decision to locomote is made by a system responsible for behavioural choice, on the basis of information about environment and about the internal state of the animal. When decision is made, two command systems come into operation: one of them is responsible for activation of the controllers for individual locomotor organs—legs, wings, trunk segments, etc. (on/off function and regulation of the speed of progression). The other one, driven by signals about orientation of the animal in space and about activity of the locomotor organs and their controllers, determines the posture of the animal and the direction of progression. The controllers determine the motor patterns of the locomotor organs. Activities of individual controllers are coordinated due to their mutual interactions. Afferent signals from mechanoreceptors located in the locomotor organs provide sensory feedback promoting

the human locomotor system. Out of the scope of this book are the problems not directly related to operative neuronal locomotor control, such as biomechanical, ethological, and ontogenetical aspects of locomotion, as well as pathophysiology and plasticity of the locomotor control mechanisms.

In this book we wish to show that despite the enormous diversity in the structure of the locomotor organs and the CNS in different species, locomotor control is based on a few fundamental principles which can be traced from mollusc to man. Figure 1A shows the basic functional organization of a generalized system for the control of locomotion. The system has a multilevel, hierarchical structure. Locomotion is caused by the activity of locomotor organs (legs, wings, fins, trunk, etc.), which generate a propulsive force moving the animal forward, and also serve to support the animal, for maintaining the necessary posture, etc. Each of the locomotor organs is driven by a special nervous mechanism, the controller. Usually, the activity of locomotor organs is rhythmical, as for example in stepping legs, and this rhythm is generated by the individual controllers. The activities of the different locomotor organs are coordinated, that is they have a common rhythm and maintain definite phase relations with each other. This coordination is achieved due to the interactions between the individual controllers. In many animals, the locomotor organ consists of a number of segments connected by joints (like a leg or the trunk of a fish). The corresponding controllers can in these cases typically be viewed as a number of separate but connected nervous mechanisms, each generating movements of one individual segment around a particular joint. These mechanisms interact with each other, resulting in coordination of movements of individual joints of the locomotor organ (Fig. 1B).

The activity of locomotor organs can be modified and adapted to the environmental conditions. This is achieved due to the sensory feedback supplying the individual controllers with information about the current state of the locomotor organs and their interaction with the external medium (ground, water, etc.). Thus, an individual controller represents a control system with a closed feedback loop. Interruption of the feedback usually results in considerable distortions of the motor pattern or, in some cases, even in a complete disappearance of the coordinated motor activity. In most species, however, some essential features of the pattern may persist. The nervous mechanism generating the motor pattern under open loop conditions is termed the central pattern generator.

There are two main command systems. One is responsible for the activation and inactivation of a set of controllers (on/off function) and for regulation of the speed of progression. Another system is responsible for the spatial orientation of the locomoting animal, that is for the control of its posture and direction of progression (steering). This system receives information about the animal's orientation in space via sensory inputs of different modalities (visual, vestibular,

---

adaptation of movements to external conditions. B: The controller for an individual organ may contain separate but connected nervous mechanisms responsible for movements at different joints. This scheme is based on the ideas formulated by Bässler (1986), Grillner (1975, 1981, 1997), Grillner *et al.* (1995), Orlovsky and Shik (1976), Rossignol (1996), Shik and Orlovsky (1976), Stein (1977b, 1978), and Pearson (1993).

somatosensory). It also receives information about the activity of individual controllers. On the bases of this information, the system modifies the activity of controllers and thus affects the movement of locomotor organs, which results in a change of the spatial orientation of the animal.

On top of the locomotor control system is the nervous mechanism making the decision to locomote. This mechanism represents a part of the system responsible for the choice of behaviour and for overall planning of the locomotor activity, it operates on the basis of information about the environment and information about the internal state of the animal. When a decision to locomote is made, the animal assumes an adequate posture, selects the necessary direction of progression, and starts to locomote.

This functional organization of the locomotor control system can be found in animals belonging to very remote branches of the evolutionary tree, from molluscs to man, and exhibiting very different forms of locomotion (walking, swimming, flying, crawling). In higher animals, however, some new nervous mechanisms for the locomotor control have been evolved, which supplement the basic system shown in Fig. 0.1.

Though the basic functional organization of the locomotor control system is similar in different species, a remarkable diversity is observed in the concrete solutions for each of the functional blocks (controllers for locomotor organs, system of their interaction, command systems, etc.). This diversity is related to the diversity in the structure and function of the locomotor organs (see for example Gray 1968) and to the diversity in the structure of CNS observed in the animal kingdom. In the following chapters, we shall consider the systems for the control of locomotion in 13 different species, from mollusc to man. We hope that this consideration will allow the reader to see both the common features of the locomotor control mechanisms in different species, and the remarkable inventiveness of evolution when creating various neuronal networks.

ACKNOWLEDGEMENTS

The authors are grateful to Dr Fredrik Ullén and Prof. Ansgar Büschges for numerous valuable comments on the manuscript.

Full details and bibliographic references to all material reproduced are to be found in the figure legends and in the reference section.

The following are thanked for permission to reproduce or reprint copyright material: Academic Press, Inc., Orlando, Florida 32887–6777, USA, for material from *Behavioral and neural biology* used in Fig. 2.3; Acta Physiologica Scandinavica, Karolinska Institutet, S-171 77 Stockholm, Sweden, for material from *Acta Physiologica Scandinavica* used in Figs 10.1, 11.3, 11.11, 15.1, and 15.2; American Association for the Advancement of Science, 1200 New York Avenue, NW, Washington, DC 20005, USA, for material from *Science* used in Fig. 8.12; The American Physiological Society, 9650 Rockville Pike, Bethesda, MD 20814–3991, USA, for material from the *Journal of Neurophysiology* used in Figs 1.5, 1.7, 1.11, 1.12, 1.13, 2.1, 2.2, 2.3, 2.4, 5.1, 6.5, 7.2, 7.4, 8.9, 8.10, 8.11, 8.12,

10.6, 10.8, 11.1, 11.2, 11.4, 11.7, 11.9, 14.1, 14.2, and 15.5; Blackwell Science Ltd., Osney Mead, Oxford OX2 OEL, UK, for material from *European Journal of Neuroscience* used in Fig. 15.3; Cell Press, 1050 Massachusetts Avenue, Cambridge, Massachusetts 02138, USA, for material from *Neuron* used in Fig. 8.6; The Company of Biologists Ltd., Bidder Building, 140 Cowley Road, Cambridge CB4 4DL, UK, for material from the *Journal of Experimental Biology* used in Figs 1.2, 1.3, 1.5, 1.6, 1.11, 1.12, 2.5, 3.4, 4.2, 4.4, 5.2, 5.3, 5.4, 6.1, 6.2, 6.3, 7.5, 7.6, 8.2, 8.13, and 8.14; Elsevier Science, PO Box 800, Oxford OX5 1DX, UK, for material from *Brain Research* used in Figs 2.4, 8.12, 11.1, 11.6, 11.8, 11.9, 11.10, 11.11, 11.12, 13.2, 13.3, 13.4, 13.5, 13.6, 13.7, 13.8, 13.9, and 13.10, for material from *Brain Research Bulletin* used in Fig. 2.4, and also for material from *Neuroscience Letters* used in Fig. 4.3; Elsevier Science, The Boulevard, Langford Lane, Kidlington, Oxford, OX5 1GB, UK, for material from *Posture and gait: development, adaptation and modulation* used in Figs 10.1 and 10.7; Elsevier Trends Journals, 68 Hills Road, Cambridge CB2 1LA, UK, for material from *Trends in Neuroscience* used in Figs 4.4, 8.7, and 9.1; Japan Scientific Societies Press, 2-10, Hongo 6-chome, Bunkyo-ku, Tokyo 113, Japan, for material from *Neurobiological basis of human locomotion* used in Figs 10.5 and 14.2; John Wiley & Sons, Inc., 605 Third Avenue, New York, NY 10158–0012, USA, for material from the *Journal of Comparative Neurology* used in Fig. 7.2, for material from *Journal of Neurobiology* used in Fig. 6.5, and also for material from *Neural control of rhythmic movements in vertebrates* used in Fig. 11.5; Lippincott Williams & Wilkins, 227 East Washington Square, Philadelphia, PA 19106, USA, for material from *Neurology* used in Fig. 15.4; Macmillan Magazines Limited, Porters South, Crinan Street, London, N1 9XW, UK, for material from *Nature* used in Figs 1.7, 1.10, and 2.2; Macmillan Press Ltd., Houndmills, Basingstoke, Hampshire RG21 6XS, UK, for material from *Neurobiology of vertebrate locomotion* used in Figs 9.1 and 11.6; Marcel Dekker, Inc., 270 Madison Avenue, New York, NY 10016, USA, for material from *Neuronal and cellular oscillators* used in Figs 3.1, 3.2, and 3.5; MIT Press Journals, 5 Cambridge Center, Cambridge, MA 021–142, UK, for material from *Neural computation* used in Fig. 11.4; National Academy of Sciences of Ukraine, Bogomolets Institute of Physiology, Bogomolets St. 4, 252601 MSP, Kyiv 24, Ukraine, for material from *Neirofiziologiya* used in Fig. 13.10; Nauka Publishers 90, Profsoyuznaya ul., Moscow 117864, Russia, for material from *Cerebellum and rhythmical movements* used in Figs 13.1 and 13.2, and also for material from *Biophysics* used in Figs 10.3, 10.4, 11.9, 12.2, 13.2, 13.3, 13.6, 13.7, 13.8, and 13.9; Oxford University Press, Great Clarendon Street, Oxford OX2 6DP, UK, for material from *The neurobiology of an insect brain* used in Fig. 6.2, for materials from *Presynaptic inhibition and neuronal control* used in Fig. 8.8; Parey Buchverlag im Blackwell Wissenschafts-Verlag GmbH Kurfürstendamm 57, D-10707 Berlin, Germany, for material from *Insect locomotion* used in Figs. 7.4 and 8.8; The Physiological Society, Shaftesbury Road, Cambridge CB2 2BS, UK, for material from the *Journal of Physiology* used in Figs. 8.2, 9.1, 11.9, and 14.1; Plenum Publishing Corporation, 233 Spring Street, New York, NY 10013–1578, USA, for material from *Stance and motion: facts and concepts* used in Fig. 14.3; Progress in Neurobiology, Department of Physiology and Biochemistry, University of Southampton, UK, for material from *Progress in Neurobiology* used in Fig. 12.3; The Society for Neuroscience, 11 Dupont Circle, NW Suite, Washington, DC 20036, USA, for material from the *Journal of Neuroscience* used in Figs 4.1 and 4.3; Springer-Verlag GmbH & Co. KG, Tiergartenstrabe 17, 69121 Heidelberg, Germany, for material from the *Journal of Comparative Physiology A* used in Figs 3.1, 3.4, 4.3, 5.1, 5.4, 6.5, 6.6, 7.1, 7.3, and 7.4, for material from *Biological Cybernetics* used in Figs 4.1 and 4.2, and also for material from *Experimental Brain Research* used in Figs 1.1, 1.2, 1.4, 1.6, 8.14, 11.2, 11.8, and 13.5; Waverly Press, 351 West Camden Street, Baltimore, Maryland 21201, USA, for material from *Handbook of physiology, the nervous system* used in Fig. 10.3.

The following have been applied to for permission to reproduce copyright material: Academic Press, 525 B street, Suite 1900, San Diego, CA 92101–4495, USA, for material from *Neurobiology of Learning & Memory* used in Figs 2.1 and 3.5; Birkhäuser Verlag, PO Box 133, CH-4010, Basel, Switzerland, for material from *Experientia* used in Fig. 3.1; The Physiological Society, Shaftesbury Road, Cambridge CB2 2BS, UK, for material from the *Journal of Physiology* used in Fig. 14.1; Plenum Publishing Corporation, 233 Spring Street, New York, NY 10013–1578, USA, for material from *Neural control of locomotion* used in Fig. 11.11.

Although every effort has been made to trace and contact copyright holders, in a few instances this has not been possible. If notified, the publishers will be pleased to rectify any omissions in future editions.

Contents

Part I
Locomotion in invertebrates

For the last two to three decades, a few species of invertebrates belonging to different phyla such as Mollusca, Crustacea, etc., have been subjected to a detailed investigation of their neuronal mechanisms of locomotor control. The main reason was that in these animals rather complex forms of behaviour, including locomotion, are controlled by relatively small groups of neurons. In some cases, single neurons are unique individuals, the activity of which is essential for the generation of behaviour. This strongly contrasts with vertebrates, in which the control of the same behaviour requires participation of a large number of neurons. Thus in invertebrates, and especially in molluscs, a description of the system in terms of the activity of individual neurons and their interactions appears to be an adequate language for the analysis of neuronal mechanisms controlling behaviour. In Chapters 1–7 we will present examples of the application of such an analysis to the locomotor control system of a number of invertebrate animals exhibiting very different forms of locomotion—swimming, crawling, walking, and flying.

1

Swimming in the mollusc Clione limacina *based on wing flapping*

1.1 MOTOR PATTERN

The sea angel *Clione limacina* (Mollusca, Gastropoda, Pteropoda), a marine mollusc, has provided excellent opportunities for examining all components of the locomotor control system at the network and cellular level. These studies have been reviewed by Arshavsky *et al.* (1991, 1993*c*, 1998) and Satterlie (1989).

An adult *Clione* (Fig. 1.1A) is 3–5 cm long. It is normally oriented vertically, with its head up, hovering or slowly swimming upward in the water column due to rhythmic movements of its two wings (parapodia). Since *Clione* is slightly negatively buoyant, only these continuous wing oscillations prevent it from sinking. The frequency of wing flapping during hovering or slow swimming is 1–2 Hz, but it can increase up to 3–5 Hz in some other forms of behaviour. The flapping cycle consists of two symmetrical parts (Fig. 1.1B), the dorsal flexion (D-phase) and the ventral flexion (V-phase). Due to the specific configuration of the wing profile, with the posterior edge remaining behind the anterior one (Fig. 1.1B), propulsive force is generated in both phases of the swim cycle (Arshavsky *et al.* 1985*a*; Satterlie *et al.* 1985).

The central nervous system (CNS) of *Clione* has a ganglionic structure which is typical of invertebrates in general. In each ganglion, cell bodies form a layer around the central neuropil area (the site of synaptic interactions). There are five pairs of central ganglia in *Clione* (Fig. 1.1C) with a specific distribution of functions which is characteristic of other gastropod molluscs as well. The pedal ganglia (PedG) contain an essential part of the locomotor pattern generating mechanism. The pedal nerves innervate the wings and the tail, which is used as an effector organ for postural control. The cerebral ganglia (CerG) contain the higher level locomotor control mechanisms, that is the command and behavioural choice systems. In these ganglia, sensory inputs of different modalities are processed and integrated. One of these, the most important one for postural control during locomotion, is input from the statocysts (St), the gravity sensing organs. One pair of statocysts is located on the dorsal aspect of the pedal ganglia and projects to the cerebral ganglia. The remaining ganglia are much less involved in the control of locomotion.

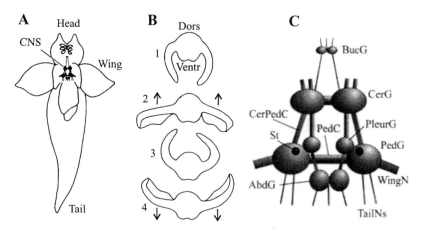

Fig. 1.1 The swimming of *Clione* and the structure of its CNS. A,B: Swimming. A: *Clione* is normally oriented vertically, with its head up. B: One cycle of wing oscillations consists of a dorsal and a ventral flexion of the wing (view from above). C: Structure of the CNS. There are five pairs of ganglia: the cerebral (CerG), pedal (PedG), pleural (PleurG), abdominal (AbdG), and buccal (BucG) ganglia. The two ganglia in a pair are connected by a commissure (the pedal commissure, PedC, is indicated). Connections between ganglia in different pairs are formed by connectives (the cerebro-pedal connective, CerPedC, is indicated). The locomotor organs (wings and tail) are innervated by the wing nerves (WingN) and tail nerves (TailNs) originating in the pedal ganglia. Two statocycts (St) supply the CNS with information about the orientation of *Clione* in the gravity field. Based on Arshavsky *et al.* (1985*a*).

The estimated total number of neurons in the CNS of *Clione* is 5000, of which only a few hundred neurons directly participate in the control of locomotion.

About 40 motor neurons, located in the pedal ganglia, send their axons into the wing nerves. They can be divided into two populations, which innervate muscles on the dorsal or ventral aspects of the wing, and are responsible for dorsal and ventral wing flexions, respectively. The two populations contain about 20 small cells each (Fig. 1.2A$_1$). In addition to the small neurons, two large cells, 1A and 2A, are easily identified in each ganglion (Fig. 1.2A$_2$). Whereas small motor neurons innervate rather limited zones of the wing musculature (Fig. 1.2B$_1$), the large motor neurons innervate the whole extent of the wing (Fig. 1.2B$_2$). The neurons 1A and 2A have been termed 'the general excitors' since they evoke strong flexion of the whole wing (Satterlie and Spencer 1985).

The activity of motor neurons 1A and 2A was recorded simultaneously, by two intracellular electrodes, during swimming in a semi-intact preparation (Fig. 1.2D) (Arshavsky *et al.* 1985*a*). The neurons fire periodically and generate one burst of action potentials per swim cycle (Fig. 1.2F). Bursts in motor neurons 1A and 2A alternate, and excitation of a given neuron is accompanied by an inhibitory postsynaptic potential(IPSP) in the antagonistic neuron. Bursts of discharges in the axons of motor neurons 1A and 2A are seen in the wing nerve, and their amplitude considerably exceeds those of the small motor neurons. Since motor neurons 1A and 2A discharge in the opposite phases of a swim cycle (D and V), the extracellularly recorded activity in the wing nerve has double the frequency of bursting compared with neuron 1A or 2A (Fig. 1.2G).

1.2   CENTRAL PATTERN GENERATOR

An isolated pair of pedal ganglia (*in vitro* preparation, Fig. 1.2E) and even a single ganglion is capable of generating a rhythmic activity similar to that observed during swimming: the burst frequency is 1–3 Hz, and bursts in motor neurons 1A and 2A alternate (Fig. 1.2G) (Arshavsky *et al.* 1985a). This finding indicates (1) that the basic neuronal mechanisms controlling the wing beating (wing controllers) are located in the pedal ganglia, and (2) that these mechanisms may operate without sensory feedback from the locomotor organs (that is, under open-loop conditions). In this case, the wing controller operates as a *central pattern generator* (CPG) (see the Preface). The rhythmic activity of the central pattern generator, in the absence of real movements of the locomotor organs, is usually termed *fictive locomotion*.

The idea of the generation of a rhythmical efferent motor pattern by a special neuronal network that may operate even in the absence of signals about the execution of the motor programme (that is, in the absence of sensory feedback), was first advanced by Brown for the spinal mechanism controlling stepping limb movements in vertebrates (Brown 1911, 1914). This view strongly contrasted with Sherrington's view that reflexes from a moving limb are a necessary component of the pattern generating mechanism (Sherrington 1906a). The existence of a CPG for locomotion was later demonstrated for most investigated species, both vertebrate and invertebrate.

The nervous mechanisms controlling wing beating in *Clione* have been analysed in detail, at the network and cellular levels (Arshavsky *et al.* 1985a–e, 1986a, 1993c; Satterlie and Spencer 1985; Satterlie *et al.* 1985). Each of the two wings is controlled by its own controller, which contains a CPG located in the ipsilateral pedal ganglion. After transection of the pedal commissure (PedC in Fig. 1.2E), these two wing controllers operate independently, at slightly differing frequencies (Panchin 1984), which indicates that the synchronization of the two wings in the intact animal is achieved by mutual commissural influences between the two wing controllers.

A crucial role in rhythmogenesis in *Clione*'s locomotor CPG is played by two groups of interneurons, 7 and 8, with about 10 cells in each group. The axons of these neurons do not leave the pedal ganglia (Fig. 1.2C). Figure 1.2H shows the activity of the interneurons 7 and 8, recorded simultaneously in the isolated pedal ganglia. Each interneuron generates one broad (about 100 ms) action potential per swim cycle; the two cells are active in antiphase. Interneurons 7 and 8 exert an inhibitory action upon each other, and the excitation of a given group of neurons is accompanied by an IPSP in their antagonists (Fig. 1.2H). The IPSP evoked in interneurons 7 by interneurons 8 can be blocked by atropine, suggesting that the transmitter in this synapse is acetylcholine.

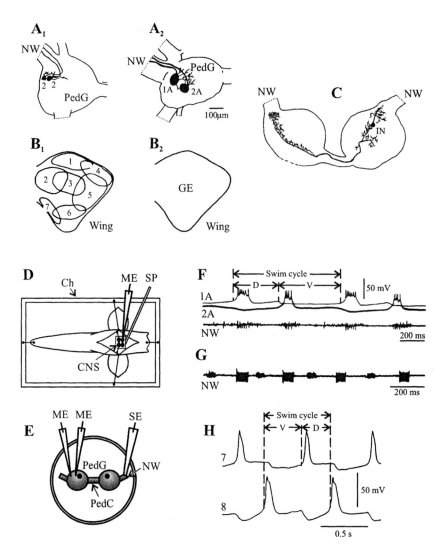

Fig. 1.2 Neural control of wing beating in *Clione*. A–C: Structure of swim motor neurons and interneurons. A_1: Structure of two small swim motor neurons of the group 2. The neurons have a cell body in the lateral area of the pedal ganglion, and the axon that enters the wing nerve. A_2: Structure of the large swim motor neurons 1A and 2A (general excitors). Neuron 1A has a cell body in the lateral area of the pedal ganglion, whereas 2A is located more medially. B_1, B_2: Zones of the wing musculature innervated by different motor neurons. In B_1 the zones innervated by seven small motor neurons are shown. The general excitor innervates the whole extent of the wing (B_2). C: Structure of a swim interneuron. The axon of the neuron has numerous branches both in the ipsilateral and in the contralateral pedal ganglion. D, E: Arrangement for recording the locomotion-related activity of the swim motor neurons and interneurons. D shows the arrangement for *in vivo* recording (semi-intact preparation). The body of *Clione* is secured in the recording chamber (Ch) filled with the sea water while the wings are left free. The CNS is exposed and mounted on

Experiments with simultaneous recording from the locomotor interneurons of groups 7 and 8, and from different groups of motor neurons (Arshavsky *et al.* 1985*b–d*) have shown that the interneurons of group 7 are active in the D-phase of a swim cycle, whereas the interneurons of group 8 are active in the V-phase (Fig. 1.2H). These experiments have also revealed the temporal patterns of activity of different groups of neurons, their relative timing in a swim cycle, and mutual influences between different cell groups. It was also found that there are two principal modes of operation of the locomotor CPG of *Clione*—'slow' swimming (observed during hovering) and 'fast' swimming (observed during hunting behaviour and escape reactions). The two modes differ both in the configuration of the CPG network, and in the pattern of activity of individual neurons. In particular, at slow swimming only some of the group 8 neurons are active (subgroup 8e). Figure 1.3A shows a wiring diagram of the CPG for slow swimming, and Fig. 1.3B shows the activity in the different neuronal groups. Post-synaptic potentials, both excitatory and inhibitory, in all types of neurons are produced by the interneurons of groups 7 and 8. Most of the connections shown in Fig. 1.3A seem to be monosynaptic.

The first goal when studying the organization and operation of any CPG is to identify the neurons that are responsible for rhythm generation. A common method for such a study is polarization of individual neurons by current injection through an intracellular microelectrode (see for example Friesen 1989*a*; Getting *et al.* 1980; Arshavsky *et al.* 1988*a,c*). The 'influential' neurons, i.e. those affecting the frequency or the phase of the ongoing rhythm, may be considered as part of the rhythm generating mechanism. In the locomotor CPG of *Clione*, however, there are numerous electrical connections between different cells (Fig. 1.3A) which do not allow polarization of individual cells without affecting the others. Correspondingly, it was found that most cells in the CPG, both motor neurons and interneurons, are influential (Arshavsky *et al.* 1985*c*).

A different, more successful, approach was photoinactivation of motor neurons (Arshavsky *et al.* 1985*e*) (for the method see Selverston and Miller (1980)). With

---

the supporting platform (SP). The activity of the motor neurons is recorded intracellularly with the microelectrode (ME) and extracellularly from their axons in the wing nerve with a suction electrode. E shows the arrangement for *in vitro* recording (fictive locomotion). The isolated pedal ganglia (PedG) connected by the pedal commissure (PedC) are positioned in a Petri dish filled with sea water. The activity of motor neurons and interneurons is recorded intracellularly by microelectrodes (ME). Activity of motor neurons is also recorded extracellularly (from their axons in the wing nerve, NW) with a suction electrode (SE). F, G: Activity of general excitors during real (F) and fictive (G) locomotion. In F activity was recorded both intracellularly (1A and 2A) and extracellularly, from the wing nerve. In G it was recorded only from the wing nerve. The motor neuron 1A is active in the D-phase of a swim cycle, while 2A is active in the V-phase. H: Activity of two swim interneurons (from groups 7 and 8) during fictive swimming. Interneuron 7 generates a single spike in the D-phase, while interneuron 8 is active in the V-phase. Excitation of a neuron of one group is accompanied by the appearance of the IPSP in a neuron of the antagonistic group. A_1, D, F, and G are from Arshavsky *et al.* (1985*b*). A_2 and H are from Arshavsky *et al.* (1985*a*). B_1 and B_2 are from Satterlie (1993). C is from Satterlie and Spencer (1985).

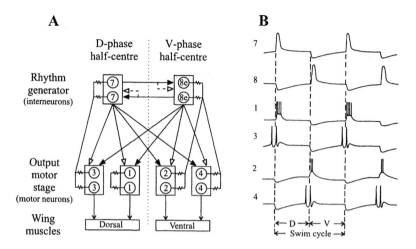

Fig. 1.3 The locomotor CPG of *Clione*. A: The wiring diagram of the CPG in the configuration for slow swimming. Resistor symbols indicate electrical connections between cells, white and black arrows indicate excitatory and inhibitory chemical synapses respectively. The CPG consists of two main parts—the rhythm generator (interneurons of groups 7 and 8e) and the output motor stage (different groups of motor neurons). Interneurons of the two groups exert an inhibitory action on each other, as well as a delayed excitatory action (broken lines). The CPG can also be devided into two 'half-centres'. One of them is driven by interneurons of group 7 and is active in the D-phase of a swim cycle. The other one is driven by interneurons of group 8e and is active in the V-phase. B: Timing diagram of the activity of interneurons and motor neurons comprising the locomotor CPG of *Clione*. Interneurons of groups 7 and 8e have reciprocal inhibitory connections. They also drive motor neurons by producing EPSPs in simultaneously active motor neurons and IPSPs in the motor neurons that are active in the opposite phase. From Arshavsky *et al.* 1985*c*.

this method, all motor neurons of the isolated pedal ganglion were retrogradely filled, through the wing nerve, with a special dye (Lucifer yellow), and the ganglion was then subjected to intense blue light illumination. This resulted in permanent inactivation of the motor neurons. Even when all the motor neurons had been inactivated, the interneurons of groups 7 and 8 continued to generate the normal locomotory rhythm, with a pattern similar to that shown in Fig. 1.2H.

The locomotor CPG of *Clione* can thus be divided into two functional parts (Fig. 1.3A): the *rhythm generator* (interneurons of groups 7 and 8e), and the *output motor stage* (motor neurons of different groups). The latter is not involved in rhythmogenesis, and its function is to transform input from the rhythm generator into more complicated efferent output. A similar structure is characteristic for the locomotor CPGs in different species, both vertebrate and invertebrate.

The rhythm generator in the locomotor CPG of *Clione* consists of two groups of neurons with mutual inhibitory influences. In such a system, both *properties of the neuronal membrane* and *network properties* may contribute to rhythmogenesis (Friesen 1994; Selverston 1985). To assess the contribution of these two factors, experiments with isolation of individual neurons 7 and 8 were performed (Arshavsky *et al.* 1986). The cells were extracted from the ganglia by means of an intracellular microelectrode, while the CPG was generating fictive swimming (Fig. 1.4A$_1$, A$_2$). Figure 1.4B$_1$ shows the activity of the interneuron 7 before extraction. The neuron periodically generates broad action potentials; the mid-cycle IPSPs evoked by the antagonistic (group 8) neurons are also seen (arrowheads). The activity of the same neuron just after extraction from the ganglia is shown in Fig. 1.4B$_2$. The rhythmic activity of the isolated cell persisted, while the mid-cycle IPSPs disappeared. By varying the value of current injected into the isolated cell, one can cover a wide range of locomotor frequencies, from 0.5 to 3 Hz (Fig. 1.4C$_1$). Similarly, spontaneous rhythmic activity was found in the isolated interneurons of group 8.

In some cases, isolated cells exhibited no spontaneous activity. A rhythmical firing could then be evoked by continuous depolarization (Fig. 1.4C$_2$) or by application of serotonin (Panchin *et al.* 1996). A single action potential could be evoked *on rebound* after a pulse of hyperpolarizing current (Fig. 1.4C$_3$). Neurons of different command systems (see Fig. 0.1) exert their action upon the rhythm generator through depolarization or hyperpolarization of interneurons 7 and 8, and thus they can switch the generator on and off and regulate the locomotor frequency (see below).

The two phenomena revealed in the cell isolation experiments, that is the endogenous rhythmic ('pacemaker') activity of individual interneurons and the postinhibitory rebound, contribute to the origin of the periodic oscillations in the rhythm generatory circuit shown in Fig. 1.3A. Due to the mutual inhibitory influences, the two groups of pacemakers (7 and 8) cannot fire simultaneously but only in succession. This network property determines alternation of the D and V phases of a swim cycle (Fig. 1.3B). Under some conditions, however, the postinhibitory rebound becomes of primary importance for rhythm generation. Figure 1.4D shows an experiment where initially the rhythmic activity in the pedal ganglia was absent, most likely because the membrane potential in group 7 and 8 interneurons was below the threshold for endogenous rhythmic activity. Rhythm generation was then triggered by injecting a pulse of the hyperpolarizing current into one of the group 7 interneurons. This cell (and other cells of group 7, electrically connected to it) fired on rebound after termination of current. The group 7 neurons evoked IPSPs in the antagonistic, V-phase neurons (both in the group 8 interneurons and in the motor neurons, Fig. 1.3). In Fig. 1.4D these inhibitory influences are monitored by recording from motor neuron 2A (the IPSPs evoked by interneurons 7 in the motor neuron are marked by white arrows). The group 8 interneurons, when excited, in turn evoked IPSPs in the antagonistic neurons. These IPSPs in interneuron 7 are marked by black arrows in Fig. 1.4D. Thus, due to the postinhibitory rebound, the excitation 'transits' sequentially from the group 7 neurons to the group 8 neurons, and backward. In this mode, the rhythm generator operates in the lower part of the range of locomotor frequencies. Thus, groups 7 and 8 exert not only an inhibitory action upon each other, but also a delayed excitatory action (due to the postinhibitory rebound). These delayed excitatory effects are shown in the scheme of CPG (Fig. 1.3A) by broken lines.

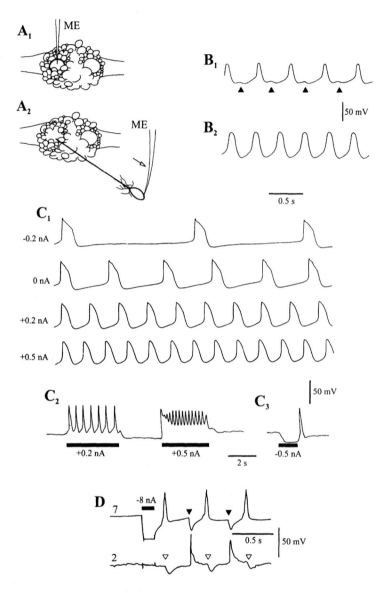

Fig. 1.4 Pacemaker activity and postinhibitory rebound in interneurons 7 and 8 contribute to generation of the locomotory rhythm. A_1–B_2: Experiment with isolation of individual neurons. A neuron is extracted from the pedal ganglion by means of the recording microelectrode (ME) (A_1, A_2). The locomotory rhythm in neuron 7 before isolation is shown in B_1 (arrowheads indicate IPSPs produced by the antagonistic interneurons 8). After extraction, the neuron retained its rhythmic activity (B_2). C_1–C_3: Effects of current injection in the isolated interneuron 7. In C_1 the discharge frequency can be changed in a wide range by hyperpolarizing or depolarizing the neuron. C_2, and C_3 show activation of the silent neuron. A rhythmic firing can be induced by injection of continuous depolarizing current (C_2). A single action potential can be evoked on rebound after injection of a pulse of depolarizing

With a sufficiently strong tonic excitatory synaptic inflow to the generatory neurons (for example from the command systems, Fig. 0.1), they will depolarize and reach a threshold for endogenous rhythmic activity. This inflow can be mimicked *in vitro* by an injection of depolarizing current into the generatory neurons (Fig. 1.4C$_2$). This pacemaker activity of groups 7 and 8 is essential for the generation of locomotory rhythm in the upper part of the range of locomotor frequencies.

1.3 HALF-CENTRE MODEL OF THE CENTRAL PATTERN GENERATOR

A network consisting of two groups of neurons with mutual inhibitory connections (two 'half-centres') was first considered by Brown in an attempt to explain the operation of the nervous mechanism controlling stepping limb movements in the vertebrates (Brown 1911, 1914). Later, this model was extensively discussed in relation to the general problem of generation of rhythmic oscillations in the nervous system (see for example Wilson and Waldron 1968; Friesen and Stent 1977; Lundberg 1980; Grillner 1981; Miller and Selverston 1982). The operation of such a model strongly depends on the properties of each half-centre. Theoretically, the model can produce oscillations even when the half-centres themselves (i.e. when isolated) have no spontaneous rhythmic activity in the range of locomotor frequencies. In this case, the period of oscillations generated by the model is determined by the time that is required for the decay of activity in each half-centre. The reasons for this decay may be different: 'fatigue' (spike frequency adoption), termination of postinhibitory rebound, etc. (Friesen 1994). If inhibitory interaction between the half-centres is supplemented with delayed excitation, the property of 'fatigue' is not necessary for generation of oscillations. In this case, the period of oscillations is determined by the duration of synaptic influences of one half-centre upon another (Getting 1981; 1983a,b). In all these versions of the half-centre model, interaction between the half-centres is necessary for the generation of rhythmic oscillations both in the whole system and in each half-centre. This is the model proposed by Brown. Theoretical and computer modelling studies have shown that the half-centre model can indeed produce stable periodic oscillations (Harmon 1964; Harmon and Lewis 1966; Wilson and Waldron 1968; Perkel and Mulloney 1974; Friesen and Wyman 1979; Grillner *et al.* 1988, 1991; Roberts and Tunstall 1990; Lansner *et al.* 1991; Hellgren *et al.* 1992). Experimental evidence of the possibility of rhythmic oscillations in a system of two real neurons has been obtained by

---

current (C$_3$). D: Contribution of the rebound property of swim interneurons to rhythm generation. In the absence of existing rhythmic activity in the pedal ganglia, the CPG can be triggered by a single pulse of hyperpolarizing current injected into interneuron 7. The black and white arrows show the appearance of IPSPs in interneuron 7 and in the swim motor neuron 2 (activity of this neuron represents the activity of the V-phase half-centre). Due to the rebound, each IPSP gives rise to one half-cycle of the locomotory rhythm. A–C are from Arshavsky *et al.* (1986*a*). D is from Arshavsky *et al.* (1985*c*).

Miller and Selverston (1982). Using photoinactivation they isolated, in the lobster stomatogastric ganglion, a pair of neurons with mutual inhibitory connections and demonstrated that these neurons could generate alternating bursts of spikes.

The operation of the half-centre model changes if each of the half-centres has the ability to produce slow rhythms (Selverston 1985). In this case, interaction between them is necessary not for the rhythmic generation but only for phasing the half-centres. Some theoretical aspects of the operation of such a model have been considered by Kawato and Suzuki (1980), Kahn and Roberts (1982), and Ekeberg *et al.* (1995).

The locomotor rhythm generator of *Clione* belongs to this second class of half-centre models since each of the two antagonistic groups of interneurons (7 and 8) have a capacity for periodic rhythmic discharges with a cyclic duration like that in normal swimming. However, due to the delayed excitatory interactions between these groups of interneurons, the system can also operate like the first version of the half-centre model, i.e. without endogenous rhythmicity in type 7 and 8 interneurons. The two mechanisms (endogenous rhythmicity and postinhibitory rebound) can supplement each other in the process of generation of the loco-motor rhythm. This suggests a considerable redundancy of the rhythm generating mechanisms in *Clione*. The redundancy was directly demonstrated by blocking the inhibitory synapse of interneurons 8 onto interneurons 7 (Panchin *et al.* 1995*c*): after elimination of this connection, the CPG was still able to generate the swim rhythm. A considerable redundancy has also been found in some other CPGs (see for example Harris-Warrick and Marder 1991; Selverston and Moulins 1987; Grillner *et al.* 1993). Redundancy presumably ensures a reliable operation of the CPGs and contributes to their flexibility.

1.4   OUTPUT MOTOR STAGE. SENSORY FEEDBACK

The temporal pattern produced by the locomotor rhythm generator of *Clione* is rather simple: it consists of alternating action potentials in the interneurons of groups 7 and 8. The output motor stage of the CPG (Fig. 1.3A) processes the input from the rhythm generator. Both the network properties, that is specific connections between interneurons and motor neurons, and the properties of the motor neuron membrane contribute to transformation of the input pattern into the more complex output (efferent) pattern. As shown in Fig. 1.3, different groups of motor neurons differ in the pattern of convergence of inputs from the D-phase and V-phase interneurons. Motor neurons of groups 1 and 3 fire in the D-phase of a swim cycle due to excitatory input from the group 7 interneurons. In the V-phase, the motor neurons are inhibited by input from the group 8 interneurons. In contrast, motor neurons of groups 2 and 4 receive excitatory input from the group 8 interneurons, and fire in the V-phase. In the D-phase, they are inhib-ited by input from the group 7 interneurons. This type of control of the motor neurons, with opposite signs of inputs from the antagonistic subdivisions of the rhythm generator, is characteristic of the locomotor CPG in different species, both invertebrate and vertebrate.

Thus, a system of connections from the rhythm generator to the output motor stage contributes to the transformation of the initial rhythmical pattern into the output, efferent pattern. Membrane properties of the motor neurons are also important. As seen from Fig. 1.3B, motor neurons of groups 3 and 4 start their firing before they receive excitatory input from corresponding interneurons. This is due to postinhibitory rebound after the IPSPs evoked by the antagonistic interneurons. Also, the burst duration in the motor neurons of groups 1 and 2 may be relatively long (Fig. 1.2G), considerably outlasting the duration of the EPSP produced by input from interneurons. This is due to the bursting property of the membrane of motor neurons which was demonstrated in experiments with cell isolation (Arshavsky *et al.* 1986a).

Under the conditions of a closed feedback loop, the motor pattern generated by the CPG can be modified to adapt it to the environmental conditions (see the Preface). One important source of sensory feedback in all investigated species is mechanoreceptors located in the moving locomotor organs and affecting the controllers for these organs (Fig. 0.1). In *Clione*, only one type of correction of the ongoing motor pattern initiated by wing mechanoreceptors has been reported, that is withdrawal of the wing. Wing withdrawal in response to tactile stimulation is a graded reaction superimposed upon the locomotory wing oscillations, and is controlled by special groups of inter- and motor neurons located in the pedal ganglia (Huang and Satterlie 1990). Another modification of the wing motor pattern is related to postural control (see Section 1.6).

1.5 ACTIVATION OF THE LOCOMOTOR SYSTEM AND CONTROL OF SPEED

1.5.1 Excitatory and inhibitory command neurons

The locomotor system of *Clione* can be turned on and off and can also produce locomotor activity of different 'intensities', that correspond to different speeds of the animal's progression. The command system for general activation or inhibition of the locomotor CPG in *Clione* (and, therefore, of the wing controllers) consists of more than 10 groups of neurons (about 50 cells in total) located mainly in the cerebral ganglia, but also in the pedal and pleural ganglia (Panchin *et al.* 1995a; Satterlie and Norekian 1995; Norekian and Satterlie 1996a,b). These 'command neurons' affect the interneurons in groups 7 and 8, and in this way the rhythm generator can be activated or inactivated, and the frequency of locomotory rhythm can be controlled (for a discussion of the concept of command neurons see Kupfermann and Weiss (1978) and commentaries of Fredman and Jahan-Parwar (1983)). The command neurons also affect the motor neurons constituting the output motor stage, and regulate the intensity of their rhythmical bursting. The excitatory effect of a command system is illustrated in Figs. 1.5B–D for a neuron of the Cr-SA group ('the cerebral serotonergic anterior cells' (Satterlie and Norekian 1995), most likely identical to CPA1 neurons described by Panchin *et al.* (1995a)). These cerebral neurons project to the pedal ganglia and, due to extensive branching (Fig. 1.5A), may contact numerous neurons of the locomotor CPG. Discharge of the Cr-SA

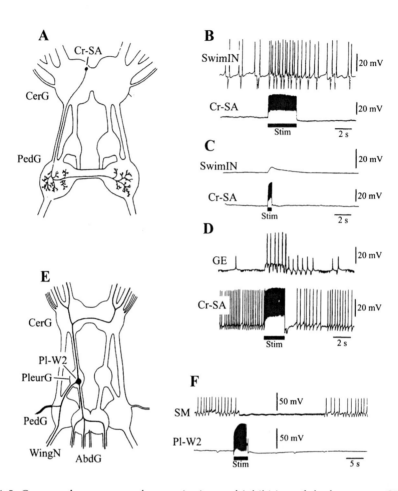

Fig. 1.5 Command neurons produce excitation and inhibition of the locomotor CPG in *Clione*. A–D: The structure and action of a cerebral serotonergic anterior cell (Cr-SA). A: Structure. The cell has its cell body in the cerebral ganglion (CerG), and an axon that descends in the ipsilateral cerebro-pedal connective and branches extensively in both pedal ganglia (PedG). B–D: Cr-SA exerts an excitatory action on swim interneurons and motor neurons. B: Discharge of Cr-SA (induced by current injection) excites the swim interneuron (SwimIN). The EPSP underlying this excitation is seen in C (high Mg^{2+}, high Ca^{2+} sea water). D: Induced activity in Cr-SA evokes excitation of the large swim motor neuron (general excitor, GE). E,F: The structure and action of a pleural withdrawal cell (Pl-W2). E: Structure. The soma of cell is located in the pleural ganglion (PleurG), the cell has numerous axons that transverse the cerebral (CerG), pedal (PedG), and abdominal (AbdG) ganglia and enter several peripheral nerves. F: Induced discharge of Pl-W2 evokes inhibition of locomotor activity. This is reflected in the disappearance of rhythmical PSPs and spikes in a small swim motor neuron (SM). A–D are from Satterlie and Norekian (1995), E and F are from Norekian and Satterlie (1996a).

(evoked by current injection) results in depolarization of the swim interneurons, and in activation of the locomotor CPG (Figs. 1.5B,C). During existing swimming activity, induced firing of Cr-SA accelerated the rhythm. At the level of the output motor stage, the Cr-SA evokes depolarization of motor neurons and their activation (Fig. 1.5D).

An inhibitory effect of the command system is illustrated in Figs. 1.5E,F for a neuron of the group termed 'the pleural withdrawal cells' (Pl-W) (Norekian and Satterlie 1996a). These cells have numerous branches (Fig. 1.5E) and exert a widespread inhibitory effect on different motor systems including inhibition of locomotor activity. As shown in Fig. 1.5F, induced activity in neuron Pl-W2 results in a complete inhibition of the locomotory rhythm. A similar organization of the locomotion-initiating system, with two parallel pathways that have opposite (excitatory and inhibitory) effects on the locomotor CPG, has been demonstrated in some other species, for example in the leech (Brodfuehrer and Burns 1995; see Section 3.5). In Section 1.7 we shall consider the role of different groups of command neurons in the organization of complex forms of behaviour in *Clione*.

1.5.2 Control of speed

In most species, regulation of the locomotory speed is a relatively complicated function of the CNS. *Clione* provides excellent opportunities for elucidating the mechanisms for speed control. In *Clione*, the three primary targets for speed-related modifications are the interneurons of the swim CPG, the swim motor neurons, and the swim musculature.

1.5.2.1 Reconfiguration of locomotor CPG

In Section 1.1 we considered the locomotor CPG for slow swimming (Fig. 1.3A). At fast swimming (which is observed during the escape reaction and hunting behaviour), two additional groups of interneurons (8d and 12) are involved in the operation (Fig. 1.6A). The simple pattern for slow swimming is shown in Fig. 1.6B. The locomotor CPG is driven by two groups of interneurons (7 and 8e) which produce PSPs in motor neurons and mutually in each other. Neurons 8d receive excitatory input from neurons 8e and are triggered later in the V-phase. Due to their activation, an additional component of the EPSP appears in the V-phase motor neurons of type 2, and the burst in these motor neurons becomes prolonged (compare Figs. 1.6B and C). Interneurons 8d also activate interneurons of group 12. The ionic mechanisms generating the membrane potential in interneurons 12 has two stable states: the first one at a potential of about $-50\,mV$ (the 'lower' state) and the second one at $-15\,mV$ (the 'upper' state). In response to depolarizing input, interneurons 12 do not generate ordinary action potentials but they shift to the upper state and generate a long-lasting plateau potential (Arshavsky *et al.* 1985d, 1989b) (Fig. 1.6C). Being in the upper state, interneurons 12 release synaptic transmitter and exert inhibition of the V-phase neurons (both inter- and motor neurons). Due to this negative feedback (by recurrent inhibition), the activity of the V-phase half-centre rapidly terminates. Interneurons 12 also exert an excitatory action upon the antagonistic half-centre (interneurons 7) and promote its activation. Interneurons 12 remain in the 'upper' state until interneurons 7 get

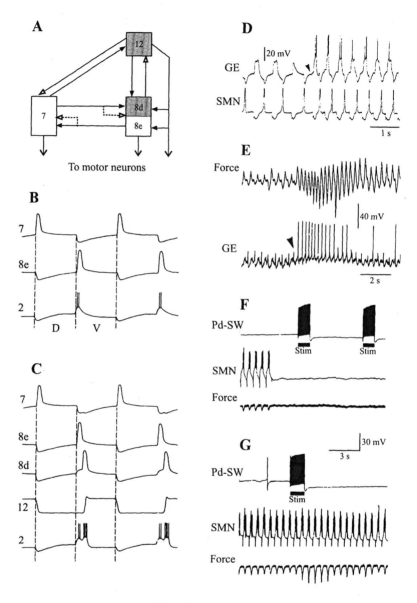

Fig. 1.6 Speed-related modifications of the locomotor activity in *Clione*. A–C. Reconfiguration of the CPG. At slow swimming, the locomotory rhythm is generated by interneurons of groups 7 and 8e (not shaded in A, see also Fig. 1.3A). The corresponding timing diagram of activity of some CPG neurons is shown in B (see also Fig. 1.3B). At fast swimming, two more groups of interneurons (8d and 12, shaded in A) are recruited into operation. The timing diagram for the fast swimming is shown in C. D, E: Recruitment of large swim motor neurons. D: The small swim motor neuron (SMN) is active both during slow fictive

excited. These cells evoke IPSP in interneurons 12 and shift them to the 'lower' state. Thus, the two groups of interneurons, recruited with fast swimming, have the following functions: (1) they promote prolongation of the bursts generated by motor neurons, (2) they promote termination of these bursts, and (3) they contribute to activation of the antagonistic half-centre.

1.5.2.2   Recruitment of large swim motor neurons

Small swim motor neurons, innervating a limited area of the wing (Figs. 1.2A$_1$ and 1.2B$_1$) are active both during slow and fast swimming. In contrast, large swim motor neurons (general excitors 1A and 2A), innervating the whole wing (Figs. 1.2A$_2$ and 1.2B$_2$) are active only during fast swimming (Satterlie 1993). This is illustrated in Fig. 1.6D which shows activity of the large and small motor neurons during fictive swimming generated by the isolated pedal ganglia. At the moment indicated by the arrow, the CPG spontaneously switched to a more intense mode of operation as monitored by an increase in the locomotor frequency. The small motor neuron was active both during slow and fast swimming whereas the large motor neuron only fired during fast swimming. In addition to the small and large motor neurons, a pair of motor neurons has been identified that contributes to wing beating only during the very beginning of the escape reaction—the startle response (Satterlie *et al.* 1997).

1.5.2.3   Recruitment of fast-twitch muscle fibres

Muscles responsible for the wing elevation and lowering contain two types of fibres: (1) slow-twitch, fatigue-resistant fibres innervated by both small and large motor neurons and (2) fast-twitch fatigable fibres innervated only by large motor neurons (Satterlie 1993). Therefore, at the lower speed, when only small wing motor neurons are active, only the slow-twitch fibres are rhythmically contracting. On the contrary, at higher speed, when large motor neurons are recruited, both types of fibres are active. This results in a considerable increase in the force developed by the wing musculature (Fig. 1.6E).

---

swimming (left part of the recording) and during the spontaneously appearing episode of fast swimming (indicated by arrow). In contrast, the large motor neuron (general excitor, GE) becomes active only with onset of fast swimming. E: Discharges of the general excitor in semi-intact *Clione* (which start with the onset of fast swimming, indicated by the arrow) considerably increase the force of contraction of the wing muscles due to activation of fast-twitch muscle fibres innervated by the general excitor. F, G: Enhancement of contractility of the wing muscles by serotonergic modulatory neurons (PD-SW). F: Discharges of a swim motor neuron (induced by periodical current injections) evoke contraction of the wing muscle (left part of the recording). Induced bursts in Pd-SW affect neither the motor neuron nor the wing muscles (right part). Activation of Pd-SW during SMN-evoked rhythmical muscle contractions, however, considerably increases the force of contraction (G). A–C are modified from Arshavsky *et al.* (1985*d*), D and E are from Satterlie (1993), and F and G are from Satterlie (1995).

1.5.2.4 Enhancement of contractility of the wing muscles by serotonergic modulatory neurons

A group of serotonin immunoreactive neurons in the pedal ganglia (Pd-SW) send their axons to the wing muscles. These cells do not directly affect swim interneurons or motor neurons. Neither do they evoke contractions in the swim muscles (Fig. 1.6F). However, discharge of the Pd-SW neurons strongly enhances rhythmic contractions of the wing muscles evoked by the swim motor neurons (Fig. 1.6G) (Satterlie 1995). The Pd-SW neurons and the locomotor CPG have common excitatory and inhibitory inputs from command systems (Norekian and Satterlie 1993). Due to these inputs, enhancement of contractivity of the wing muscles parallels activation of the CPG. The modulatory control of muscles by serotonergic neurons is not a unique feature of the locomotor system of *Clione*. This phenomenon was initially found in the buccal muscles of *Aplysia* (Weiss *et al.* 1978), and has recently been described for the foot muscles of *Aplysia* (McPherson and Blankenship 1992).

1.6 POSTURAL ORIENTATION AND EQUILIBRIUM CONTROL

The most common orientation in the swimming *Clione* is the vertical one, with the head up (Fig. 1.7A_1,B_1). Analysis of the system for postural orientation and equilibrium control has been performed at behavioural and network levels (Panchin *et al.* 1995b; Deliagina *et al.* 1998a,b). The system is driven by the gravity sensing organs, the statocysts, located on the dorsal surface of pedal ganglia (Fig. 1.1C). After bilateral ablation of the statocysts, *Clione* is not able to stabilize any orientation in space, and is continuously looping in different planes (Fig. 1.7C). The two statocysts are functionally equivalent, and removal of one of them does not produce any significant effect on postural orientation.

Two forms of postural correcting response are observed when the orientation of *Clione* has deviated from the vertical (Figs. 1.7A,B). Firstly, the tail is bent upward. This bending occurs approximately in the same plane in which *Clione* has deviated from the vertical: with a lateral deviation (lateral sway, β), the tail bends laterally (Figs. 1.7A_2,A_3); with the deviation in the sagittal plane (sagittal sway, α), the tail bends dorsally or ventrally (Figs. 1.7B_2,B_3). Contractions of the tail muscles are evoked by three groups of tail motor neurons (T1–T3). Secondly, in the case of a lateral deviation from the vertical, the locomotor wing oscillations become asymmetrical, with the amplitude in the 'lower' wing increased and the amplitude in the 'upper' wing decreased (Figs. 1.7A_2,A_3). Four groups of wing motor neurons (W1–W4) are responsible for these reactions. These two forms of gravitational reflexes evoke a turning movement of the animal towards the vertical. Figure 1.8A shows the principal elements of the network for spatial orientation in *Clione*: receptor cells of the statocyst, cerebro-pedal neurons, and motor neurons of the tail and wings.

The statocysts in *Clione* (Fig. 1.8A,B) are spherical organs ($\sim$ 150 μm diameter), with the wall formed by statocyst receptor cells (SRCs) and supporting cells. Each statocyst contains 9–11 SRCs (Tsirulis 1974). In the central cavity of the statocyst, there is a spherical statolith. The statolith exerts a pressure on those SRCs that

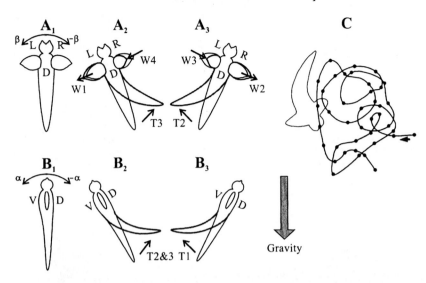

Fig. 1.7 Behavioural characteristics of the postural orientation and equilibrium control in *Clione*. A_1, B_1: The most common orientation in the swimming *Clione* is the vertical one, with the head up (D, V, L, and R denote the dorsal, ventral, left, and right aspects of the body). Deviation from this orientation in the frontal plane (angle β), or in the sagittal plane (angle α), or in any intermediate plane will evoke correcting motor responses. A_2, A_3: Correcting motor responses with deviation from the vertical in the frontal plane (indicated by arrows). B_2, B_3: Correcting motor responses with deviation in the sagittal plane. The groups of motor neurons (W1–W4 and T1–T3) responsible for the motor responses are also indicated. C: After removal of both statocycts, *Clione* is not able to maintain any definite orientation in space. Interval between dots, 400 ms. A and B are based on Deliagina *et al.* (1998*a*), C is from Panchin *et al.* (1995*b*).

are located in the lowermost part of the cavity, and excites them. Gravitational responses in SRCs were recorded intracellularly, in a preparation similar to that shown in Fig. 1.2E. The chamber with the preparation, and the recording micro-electrode were positioned on a movable platform and rotated in space. Figure 1.8B shows that initially the SRC did not contact the statolith and exhibited low activity ($0°$). As the preparation was tilted, the SRC appeared under the statolith, which resulted in its depolarization and firing ($90°$). By gradually tilting the preparation it was shown that the width of spatial zones of sensitivity in individual SRCs range from $90°$ to $135°$. The statolith simultaneously contacts and activates three to four SRCs. Input from SRCs is responsible for postural corrective reflexes as shown in Figs. 1.7A,B. The neuronal mechanisms of these responses are considered below:

1. Tail bending. Tail musculature is innervated by tail motor neurons (TMNs) located mainly in the pedal ganglia (Fig. 1.8A). Some of these motor neurons (about 20 cells) receive input from SRCs and are thus involved in gravitational postural control. Input from SRCs to TMNs is mediated by a special group ($\sim$20 cells) of cerebro-pedal interneurons, CPB3 (Fig. 1.8A) (Panchin *et al.* 1995*a*,*b*).

Due to the input from statocysts, individual TMNs are activated within specific zones of the spatial orientation of *Clione* (Deliagina *et al.* 1998*a*,*b*). All TMNs can

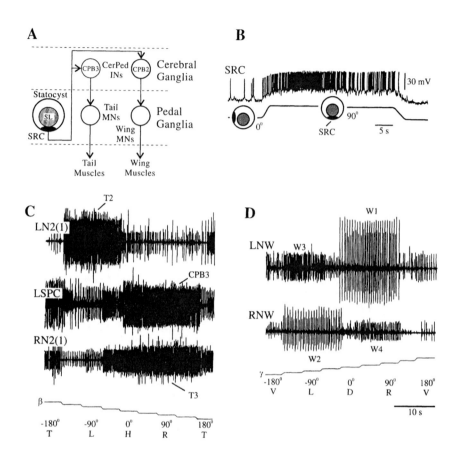

Fig. 1.8 Gravitational reflexes in *Clione*. A: The main groups of neurons involved in gravitational reflexes, and their interconnections. B–D: Responses to gravitational input in different groups of neurons. Recordings were performed in a preparation consisting of the isolated CNS with statocycts. B: Response in the statocyst receptor cell to 90° tilt of the preparation. C: Response in the tail motor neurons of groups T2 and T3 (recording from the left and right tail nerves, LN2(1) and RN2(1)) and response in CPB3 interneurons (recording from the left stump of transected subpedal commissure, LSPC) to changes in the spatial orientation (β is the angle of tilt in the frontal plane). The preparation assumed in succession the orientations corresponding to the tail-up orientation (T), left side up (L), head-up (H), right side up (R), and tail-up (T). D: Responses of the wing motor neurons of groups W1–W4 (recordings from the left and right wing nerves, LNW and RNW) to changes in the spatial orientation (γ is the angle of rotation around the longitudinal axis of the animal, the axis being situated horizontally). The preparation assumed in succession the orientations corresponding to the ventral side up orientation (V), left side up (L), dorsal side up (D), right side up (R), and ventral side up (V). B is from Panchin *et al.* (1995*b*). C and D are from Deliagina, Orlovsky and Arshavsky (unpublished data).

be classified into three groups (T1, T2, and T3) according to the position of their zones of sensitivity in space, as well as according to the motor effect they produce. Figure 1.8C shows gravitational responses of the tail motor neurons belonging to groups T2 and T3. In this experiment, the CNS together with the statocysts was rotated in the plane corresponding to the frontal plane of the animal (lateral sway β in Fig. 1.7A). A deviation of the CNS from the position corresponding to the normal, head-up orientation of *Clione*, evokes activation of a specific group of TMNs: group T2 is excited with the left tilt, and group T3 with the right tilt. Experiments with electrical stimulation and lesion of different tail nerves in semi-intact preparations have shown that T2 motor neurons evoke flexion of the tail to the right, whereas T3 motor neurons, flex the tail to the left. In addition, both T2 and T3 groups evoke dorsal flexion of the tail. Similar experiments have shown that group T1 motor neurons, responsible for the ventral bending of the tail, exhibit the maximal response with inclination of *Clione* in the sagittal plane, when the dorsal side moves down.

Spatial zones of activity in groups T1, T2, and T3 cover the whole range of possible deviations of the animal's longitudinal axis from the vertical (Figs. 1.9A–C). The zones of activity overlap considerably, so that a deviation in a certain direction may activate two groups of TMNs simultaneously. In this case, the direction of the evoked tail flexion will be intermediate to those seen with separate activation of either group. Thus, with any direction of the deviation of *Clione* from the vertical, tail motor neurons will evoke a correcting motor response aimed at restoration of the vertical orientation.

The transformation of input from the statocyst into three-dimensional efferent output (that is, into the activity of groups T1, T2, and T3) is performed by CPB3 neurons which drive the TMNs (Fig. 1.8A). It was found that the gravitational response in CPB3 interneurons is very similar to the response in the corresponding TMNs to which they project, as illustrated in Fig. 1.8C for the TMN of the T2 group (in the nerve RN2(1)) recorded together with the CPB3c interneuron (in the left stump of the transected subpedal commissure, LSPC) sensitive to the lateral inclinations.

2. Asymmetry in locomotor wing oscillations appears with a lateral deviation of *Clione* from the vertical (Figs. 1.7A$_2$,A$_3$). This asymmetry is due to a recruitment into the swimming rhythm of the large swim motor neurons 1A and 2A (general excitors, see Section 1.5.2.2). Figure 1.8D shows activity of wing motor neurons, recorded from the left and right wing nerves, while the preparation was rotated around the longitudinal axis of *Clione*, the axis being situated horizontally. One can see that the general excitors (groups W1 and W2) are recruited into the swim rhythm on the side facing downward, and inhibited on the opposite side. In addition to this inhibition, a motor neuron responsible for wing withdrawal (W3 and W4) is tonically activated on the side facing upward. Thus, both the amplitude of locomotor oscillations and the lateral extent of the wing are reduced on the side facing upward, and increased on the side facing downward. Figure 1.9D shows that the wing motor neurons, eliciting lateral asymmetry in the locomotor wing oscillations, are activated within rather large zones of the deviation of the animal's longitudinal axis from the vertical.

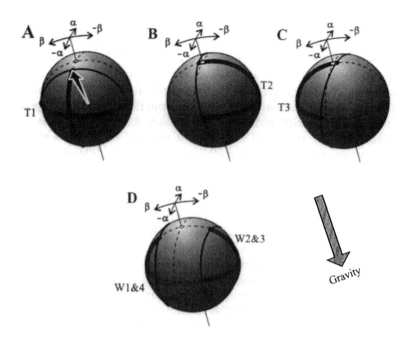

Fig. 1.9 Spatial zones of activity of different groups of motor neurons responsible for the correcting motor responses. A–C. Zones of activity of T1–T3 groups of tail motor neurons. D. Zones of activity of W1–W4 groups of wing motor neurons. Angles α and β characterize the deviation of the *Clione's* axis from the vertical in the sagittal and frontal plane respectively. The radius vector in A represents the orientation of *Clione* in the gravity field. From Deliagina, Orlovsky and Arshavsky (unpublished data).

This type of postural correction (increase or decrease of the amplitude of wing oscillations) occurs without disturbance of the basic locomotory rhythm: due to common input from the rhythm generator, activity in the large motor neurons (general excitors) is always in phase with the activity of the corresponding small motor neurons. In other species, postural corrections are usually incorporated into the ongoing locomotor movements also without disturbance of the basic locomotor pattern (see Sections 11.5, 14.3, and 15.4).

Modification of the pattern of activity in wing motor neurons is produced by a special group of cerebro-pedal interneurons (CPB2) which receive inputs from SRCs and exert an asymmetrical action on the general excitors on the left and right sides (Fig. 1.8A) (Panchin *et al.* 1995*a*). The spatial zones of sensitivity of these neurons have not been characterized yet. In contrast to command neurons, which affect the rhythm generator (for example Cr-SA and Pl-W neurons, Fig. 1.5), the CPB2 neurons affect only the output motor stage of the locomotor CPG.

In most animals and in humans, the postural control system is rather flexible; it can stabilize different postural orientations (see for example Horak and Macpherson 1995; Macpherson *et al.* 1997; Orlovsky 1991*b*). In *Clione*, the system has three distinct modes of operation (Panchin *et al.* 1995*a*; Deliagina *et al.* 1998*a,b*):

(1) Stabilization of the head-up orientation (considered above). This mode is most common, and in the sea or in the aquarium *Clione* is normally found oriented vertically, with its head up. In this mode, deviation from the head-up orientation evokes a tail bending directed upward (Figs. 1.10A$_1$,A$_2$).

(2) Stabilization of the head-down orientation is observed in *Clione* swimming downward from a layer of water with high temperature. This mode is also observed during the hunting behaviour of *Clione*. In this mode, deviation from the stabilized position evokes a tail bending directed downward (Figs. 1.10B$_1$,B$_2$).

(3) In the third mode, *Clione* does not stabilize any specific orientation: the postural control system is inactivated, and postural corrective responses are not generated at any orientation in space. This mode is observed at high water temperature and during defensive reactions.

Switches between the modes with the head-up and head-down orientation are accomplished by reconfiguration of the network for postural orientation. These occur due to changes at the level of the synapses between the SRCs and the cerebropedal interneurons, as illustrated in Figs. 1.10C$_1$–D$_2$. Figure 1.10C$_1$ shows gravitational responses in the tail motor neurons of groups T2 and T3 (from the nerves LN2(1) and RN2(1)), as well as in the interneuron CPB3, at low water temperature (10 °C) when the system stabilizes the head-up orientation. The corresponding connections between the SRC, CPB3, and tail motor neurons are shown in Fig. 1.10D$_1$. With increasing water temperature up to 20 °C, the gravitational response was reversed both in CPB3 and in tail motor neurons (Fig. 1.10C$_2$) which indicates that now CPB3 receives input from the SRCs located on the opposite side of the statocyst (Fig. 1.10D$_2$). It remains unclear, however, if the synapses between SRCs and CPB3 are temperature sensitive themselves, or if they are under the control of special thermoreceptor neurons.

The reconfiguration of the postural control network at different temperatures (Figs. 1.10C$_1$–D$_2$) may explain the reversal of the gravitational tail reflexes in two modes of operation of the postural control system. When the head-up orientation is maintained (Figs. 1.10A$_1$,A$_2$, and D$_1$), the reflex flexion of the tail (caused by deviation from the vertical) occurs contralaterally to the excited SRCs, and upward in relation to the gravity force. When the head-down orientation is maintained (Figs. 1.10B$_1$,B$_2$, and D$_2$), the flexion occurs ipsilaterally to the excited SRCs, and downward in relation to the gravity force.

1.7 INTEGRATION OF LOCOMOTION IN COMPLEX BEHAVIOUR

Any form of complex behaviour results from the coordinated activity of several motor centres. In *Clione*, locomotor activity is a necessary component of almost all forms of behaviour, and this activity is coordinated with activities of other motor

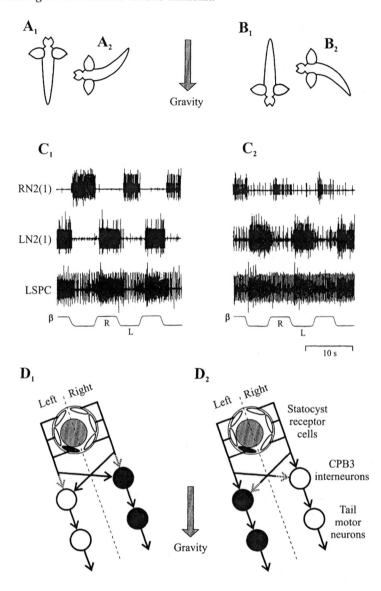

Fig. 1.10 Different modes of operation of the postural control system. A–C: Different forms of gravitational tail reflexes. A_1, A_2: At low temperature, the head-up orientation is maintained. Deflection from this orientation evokes an upward bending of the tail. B_1, B_2: At high temperature, the head-down orientation is maintained. Deflection from this orientation evokes a downward bending of the tail. C_1–D_2: Modifications of gravitational reflexes underlying the head-up and head-down modes. C_1: At 10 °C, tail motor neurons in the left and right tail nerves, LN2(1) and RN2(1), as well as the CPB3 interneuron in the left subpedal commissure, LSPC, are activated with the contralateral roll tilt. C_2: At 20 °C, the same neurons are activated with the ipsilateral roll tilt. D_1,D_2: Wiring diagrams of the postural network in different modes of its activity, corresponding to the recordings of C_1 and C_2. C_1–D_2 are from Deliagina *et al.* (1998*a*).

centres through a complex system of command neurons. Below we shall consider the involvement of locomotor mechanisms in some forms of *Clione*'s behaviour.

1.7.1 Escape reaction

In the normal, non-aroused state, *Clione* slowly swims in the water column. Mechanical stimulation of the tail dramatically increases the locomotor activity, however (Figs. 1.11A$_1$,A$_2$). This escape reaction is mediated by a special group of command neurons (CPB1) located in the cerebral ganglia and projecting to the pedal ganglia, where the locomotor CPG is located (Fig. 1.11B) (Arshavsky *et al.* 1992). Figure 1.11C shows that the CPB1 neuron is excited in response to mechanical stimulation of the tail. In its turn, the CPB1 neuron exerts a strong excitatory action on the locomotor CPG. Figure 1.11D shows that the induced burst of spikes in this neuron results in a considerable acceleration of the locomotory rhythm (monitored by discharges in the type 7 locomotor interneuron).

As shown in behavioural experiments, the locomotor activity and the frequency of heartbeat in *Clione* are strongly correlated: any spontaneous or reflex change of activity of the locomotor CPG is always accompanied by a corresponding change in the heart rhythm (Arshavsky *et al.* 1990). This correlation is partly due to the direct action of the locomotor CPG upon the heart excitatory motor neuron (HE) located in the left pedal ganglion (Fig. 1.11E). One more mechanism linking the locomotory and circulatory systems is a common input from the CPB1 neurons. Figure 1.11D shows that the CPB1 neuron not only activates the locomotor CPG but also excites the heart excitatory motor neuron, HE. Thus, the CPB1 neurons are responsible for different aspects of the avoidance reaction, that is for activation of the locomotor CPG and for acceleration of the heartbeat (Fig. 1.11E).

1.7.2 Passive avoidance reaction

This reaction can be evoked under the normal, non-aroused state of *Clione*, by mechanical stimulation of the head or wings. In response to these stimuli, locomotion is inhibited, and different parts of the body (wings, head tentacles, and tail) are withdrawn (Figs. 1.12A$_1$,A$_2$); then *Clione* passively sinks. A group of command neurons (Pl-W), located in the pleural ganglia (see Fig. 1.5E), is responsible for this reaction. It was shown that mechanical stimulation of the head or wings evoked activation of the Pl-W neurons. The Pl-W neurons in turn affect numerous motor systems. The inhibitory action of Pl-W on the locomotor CPG was considered earlier (see Fig. 1.5F). In addition, Pl-W exert an inhibitory action on the heart excitor HE and an excitatory action on the cerebral motor neurons responsible for retraction of the head tentacles, as well as on the wing retractor neurons (Fig. 1.12B). Thus, the Pl-W neurons evoke all components of the passive avoidance reaction.

1.7.3 Hunting and feeding

This behaviour is the most complex one in *Clione*. *Clione* is a predator; it feeds on a small mollusc, *Limacina helicina*. The hunting and feeding behaviour is triggered

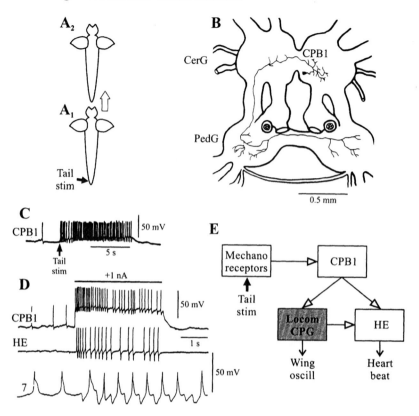

Fig. 1.11 Formation of the synergy for avoidance reaction. A_1, A_2: Mechanical stimulation of the tail evokes fast swimming. B–E: The structure, input, and output of the CPB1 neuron. B: Structure. It has a cell body in the cerebral ganglion (CerG), and an axon that descends in the ipsilateral cerebro-pedal connective and branches in both pedal ganglia (PedG). C: Input from the tail mechanoreceptors. D: Output to a swim interneuron 7 and to the heart excitatory neuron HE, as revealed by activation of CPB1 evoked by current injection. E: Diagram of connections of CPB1. It receives excitatory input from the tail mechanoreceptors, and exerts an excitatory action on the locomotor CPG and on the heart excitor (HE). B is from Panchin *et al.* (1995a). C and D are from Arshavsky *et al.* (1992).

by contact with *Limacina* (due to activation of mechano- and chemoreceptors), and has a number of components (Figs. 1.13A_1,A_2) (Litvinova and Orlovsky 1985; Arshavsky *et al.* 1993a,b; Norekian 1995; Norekian and Satterlie 1993): First, three pairs of tentacles protract forward and capture the prey. At the same moment, the tail bends and the frequency of wing oscillations increases from 1–2 to 3–4 Hz, and *Clione* swims rapidly in circles. When *Limacina* is captured, the feeding apparatus is activated to extract the prey from its shell and to swallow it. The heartbeat accelerates along with the activation of the locomotory system.

A pair of command neurons CPC1 (Fig. 1.13B) plays a crucial role in the control of this complex behaviour (Arshavsky *et al.* 1993b, 1995a; Norekian and Satterlie 1993). They exert widespread effects on different motor systems (Fig. 1.13C):

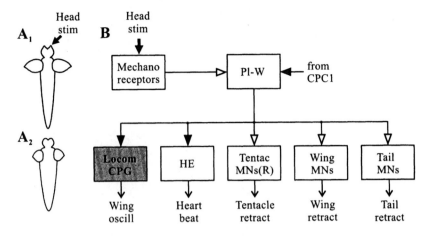

Fig. 1.12 Formation of the synergy for defensive reaction. A_1, A_2: Mechanical stimulation of the head or wing results in termination of locomotion and retraction of the head sensory tentacles, wings, and tail. The command neurons Pl-W (see Figs. 1.5E,F) are responsible for this reaction. B: Diagram of connections of Pl-W. It receives excitatory input from the head mechanoreceptors, and exerts an excitatory action on the tentacular retractor motor neurons (Tentac MNs(R)), wing motor neurons (Wing MNs) and tail motor neurons (Tail MNs), as well as an inhibitory action on the locomotor CPG and heart excitor (HE). Based on Arshavsky *et al.* (1990) and Norekian and Satterlie (1996*a*).

1. They activate the locomotor CPG by exciting both the interneurons of groups 7 and 8, and different groups of motor neurons.
2. The CPC1 neurons excite the efferent pedal neurons (PD-SW), enhancing contractivity of wing muscles.
3. They excite the heart excitatory motor neuron (HE) and thus accelerate the heart rate.
4. They excite a group of cerebral motor neurons (TenMNP) responsible for extrusion of the tentacles and seizing of the prey.
5. They inhibit the cerebral motor neurons (TenMNR) responsible for retraction of tentacles.
6. CPC1 neurons affect the statocyst receptor cells, depolarizing or hyperpolarizing some of them. As a result, the gravitational postural control system is inactivated, *Clione* loses its vertical orientation and, due to the tonic tail bending, swims in circles.

Not all the motor systems involved in hunting and feeding behaviour are activated by the CPC1 neurons. The feeding apparatus (which produces extraction of the prey from the shell, and then its swallowing) is activated by other command neurons, PIN1s (Fig. 1.13C) (Arshavsky *et al.* 1989*a*), which are excited along with the CPC1 neurons, most likely due to a common sensory input (Arshavsky *et al.* 1993*b*). The tentacular motor neurons of the protractor group are under control of both CPC1 and PIN1 interneurons.

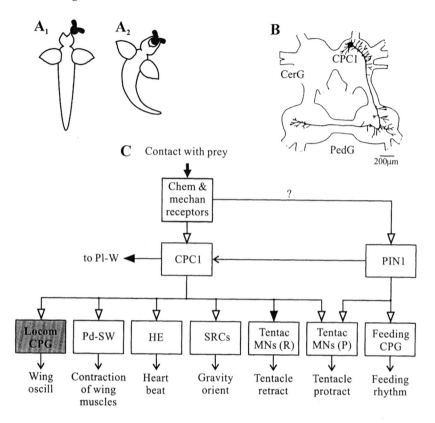

Fig. 1.13 Formation of the synergy for hunting and feeding behaviour. A_1, A_2: Contact with the prey (mollusc *Limacina helicina*) evokes protraction of head tentacles, turning towards the prey, acceleration of wing beating, and (when *Limacina* is captured) feeding movements of buccal apparatus. B, C: Structure, input, and output of the CPC1 neuron. B: Structure. It has a cell body in the cerebral ganglion (CerG) and an axon that descends in the ipsilateral cerebro-pedal connective and extensively branches in the ipsilateral cerebral ganglion and in both pedal ganglia (PedG). C: Diagram of connections of CPC1. The gross synergy for hunting and feeding is primarily formed due to the action of CPC1 upon different motor systems. However, PIN1 neurons also contribute to the formation of this synergy. Targets of CPC1 and PIN1 are: the locomotor CPG, Pd-SW modulatory neurons, heart excitor (HE), statocyst receptor cells (SRCs), tentacular protractor (P) and retractor (R) motor neurons, and feeding CPG. In addition to the effects shown in C, CPC1 may affect different motor systems via the Pl-W command neurons (see Fig. 1.12). B is from Arshavsky *et al.* (1993*b*). C is based on Arshavsky *et al.* (1993*b*) and Norekian and Satterlie (1995).

There is indirect evidence that the two groups of command neurons (CPC1 and PIN1) exert an excitatory effect upon each other, thus promoting formation of a gross hunting and feeding synergy (Arshavsky *et al.* 1993*b*). This synergy is not compatible with the defensive reaction to stimulation of the head (which is controlled by the command neurons Pl-W, see above) and the CPC1 suppress this reaction by inhibiting the Pl-W neurons (Figs. 1.12 and 1.13). Thus, the command system in *Clione* is, to some extent, also responsible for the behavioural choice (Norekian and Satterlie 1993).

From Figs. 1.11 and 1.13 one can conclude that activation of the locomotor CPG may be produced by different command neurons, depending on the behavioural context. The CPB1 neurons activate the CPG during avoidance behaviour, whereas the CPC1 neuron initiates locomotion during hunting and feeding behaviour. In the latter case, inhibition of the Pl-W command neurons by CPC1s results in disinhibition of the CPG, and in this way the Pl-W also contribute to activation of the locomotor CPG.

The role of other groups of command neurons, affecting the locomotor CPG (groups CPA1, CPA2, and CPC2–5 (Panchin *et al.* 1995*a*)) is less clear. They may contribute to activation and inhibition of the locomotor system in forms of behaviour other than feeding and avoidance, for example in reproductive behaviour (Wagner 1885) which has not been investigated electrophysiologically in *Clione*.

Activation of a specific group of command neurons represents the final step in the complex process of behavioural choice. The system responsible for the behavioural choice operates on the basis of multimodal sensory information about the environment and about the internal state of the animal (Fig. 0.1). The problem of behavioural choice is out of the scope of this book. For recent reviews on the problem of selection of motor behaviour, see Grillner *et al.* (1997).

1.8 CONCLUSIONS

1. Swimming in *Clione* is based on rhythmical flapping of two wings. All components of the locomotor control system in *Clione* have been extensively examined at the behavioural, network and cellular levels, and their organization and function have been understood to a considerable extent.
2. Each wing is driven by a separate wing controller. The two controllers interact, which results in their synchronization.
3. Sensory feedback from the moving wings does not play any significant role for the control of locomotion in *Clione*. Thus, generation of the swim motor pattern is performed almost exclusively by the CPG. The CPG consists of the rhythm generator and the output motor stage. The rhythm generator produces a biphasic output pattern. The generator comprises two principal elements—the swim interneurons of groups 7 and 8—possessing pacemaker activity and inhibiting each other. The postinhibitory rebound also contributes to the rhythm generation by promoting transition of activity from one group of interneurons to another. There is, therefore, a considerable redundancy in the rhythm generating mechanism, which ensures reliable operation of the swim CPG. In the output motor stage—wing motor neurons of different groups— the simple input pattern, originating from the rhythm generator, is subjected to transformation in more complicated patterns due to synaptic interactions, as well as due to specific membrane properties of the motor neurons. Anatomical separation of the rhythm generator and the output motor stage may allow for the involvement of a single set of wing motor neurons in multiple behaviours,

for example in wing oscillations, in postural corrections, in defensive wing withdrawal, etc.

4. Activation of the locomotor system and control of speed is performed by the command neurons of different groups. These neurons may affect both the swim interneurons and the motor neurons, and depolarize or hyperpolarize them. In addition to an accelerated locomotory rhythm, faster swimming is characterized by a reconfiguration of the locomotor generator through recruitment of new groups of interneurons, by recruitment of new groups of motor neurons in the output motor stage, and by activation of the fast-twitch fibres in the wing muscles.

5. Postural orientation and equilibrium control is governed by input from the statocysts (gravity sensing organs). There are two actively stabilized postural orientations—head up and head down. Deviation from the stabilized orientation evokes bending of the tail and asymmetry in the locomotor wing oscillations. These postural correcting reflexes are aimed at restoration of the normal orientation. The reflex chains include the statocyst receptor cells (SRCs), the interneurons of CPB2 and CPB3 groups and the motor neurons of the tail or wings. With a switch from the head-up to the head-down orientation, the postural orientation network is reconfigured: inputs to interneurons from the SRCs located on one side of the statocyst are blocked, while inputs from the SRCs located on the opposite side, are activated.

6. Integration of locomotion in different forms of behaviour is achieved by means of a complex system of command neurons. Different groups of command neurons differ in their projections upon the motor systems. Due to this diversity, the locomotor CPG can be activated in combination with different motor systems, the combination being determined by the active group(s) of command neurons. The command neurons may have common inputs from the sensory systems. They may also interact with each other to form gross functional synergies for different forms of behaviour.

2

Other forms of locomotion in molluscs

2.1 SWIMMING IN *TRITONIA* BASED ON WHOLE BODY FLEXIONS

2.1.1 Motor pattern and distribution of locomotor functions in the CNS

In most species of gastropod molluscs, crawling is the main form of locomotion (Miller 1974; Trueman 1983). However, in addition to crawling, certain species can swim. The escape swimming response of the marine mollusc *Tritonia diomedea* can be initiated by a number of noxious stimuli. Under natural conditions, the response is usually initiated by transient epithelial contact with the tube feet of predatory sea stars. The response consists of an initial reflexive withdrawal immediately followed by a series of 2–20 alternating dorsal and ventral flexions (Fig. 2.1A). A swim always starts with a powerful ventral flexion which lifts the animal above the bottom, and terminates on a weak dorsal flexion (Fig. 2.1B).

The CNS of *Tritonia* has the same basic structure as the CNS of *Clione* (Fig. 2.1E). Body flexions are controlled by motor neurons located in the pedal ganglia. Two groups of pedal efferent neurons, presumably motor neurons, display rhythmical bursting activity during swimming. One of the groups (dorsal flexion neurons, DFN) is active when the body is flexing dorsally, and the other one (ventral flexion neurons, VFN) during ventral flexion (Getting *et al.* 1980; Hume *et al.* 1982). This efferent pattern, with alternating bursting activity in DFN and VFN neurons, persists in the isolated CNS, thus indicating that the pattern is, to a large extent, of a central origin. In contrast to *Clione*, where both principal parts of the swim CPG (the rhythm generator and the output motor stage, Fig. 1.3A) reside in the pedal ganglia, the swim CPG of *Tritonia* is distributed between the pedal and cerebral ganglia, with the rhythm generator residing in the cerebral ganglia, and the output motor stage mainly in the pedal ganglia.

2.1.2 Generator of the swim rhythm

A detailed analysis of the swim network in *Tritonia* was carried out by Getting and his colleagues. They identified interneurons and motor neurons involved in the generation of the swim motor pattern and characterized membrane properties

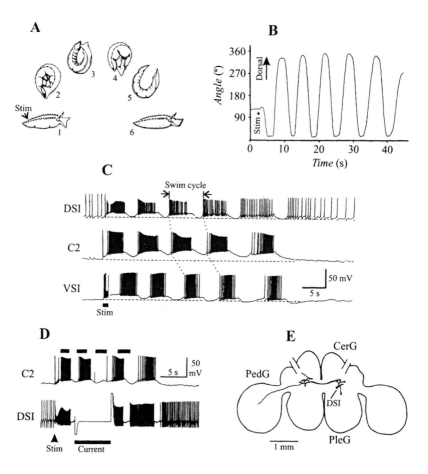

Fig. 2.1 Escape swimming in *Tritonia*. A: A noxious stimulus applied to the tail triggers a stereotyped escape response consisting of a series (2–20) of alternating ventral and dorsal body flexions; successive body configurations (1–6) in two full cycles are illustrated. B: Plot of body angle versus time during a typical swim. Increase in the body angle indicates dorsal flexion. C–E: Three groups of interneurons generate the locomotory rhythm. C: Electrical stimulation (Stim) of a peripheral nerve in the isolated CNS preparation activates the locomotor CPG and evokes fictive locomotion. Simultaneous intracellular recording from the cerebral interneurons DSI, C2, and VSI. Dashed lines indicate the resting potential. D: Phase shift of the swim pattern induced by DSI. Swim sequence was initiated by electrical stimulation (Stim) of the peripheral nerve. Hyperpolarizing current (Current) was passed into three DSIs. The black bars above C2 traces mark the timing of bursts of an unperturbed control swim sequence. E: The structure of the DSI neuron. It has a cell body in the cerebral ganglion (CerG), and an axon that descends in the cerebro-pedal connective and terminates in the contralateral pedal ganglion (PedG). A is from Frost *et al.* (1996), B is from Hume *et al.* (1982), C is from Getting (1983*d*), and D and E are based on Getting *et al.* (1980).

of individual neurons and their synaptic interactions. This allowed them to formulate a model of the locomotor CPG which was subsequently tested in computer simulation experiments.

The swim CPG is formed by three groups of cerebral neurons—DSI, C2, and VSI (Getting *et al.* 1980; Getting 1981). Several morphological features are shared by these neurons. Their somata reside in the cerebral ganglion, and the axon descends to the contralateral pedal ganglion, as illustrated in Fig. 2.1E for a DSI neuron. The DSI group consists of at least three pairs of neurons, three cells in each cerebral ganglion (DSI-A, DSI-B, and DSI-C) slightly differing in their connections with each other and with other cells of the CPG. The VSI group consists of at least two pairs (VSI-A and VSI-B) also slightly differing in their firing pattern and connections. Finally, the C2 group consists of only two neurons located symmetrically in the cerebral ganglia.

Figure 2.1C shows simultaneous recording from one member of each of these interneuron classes during a swim sequence initiated in the isolated CNS by repetitive electrical stimulation of one of the cerebral nerves. During the nerve stimulation, neurons in all the three cerebral neuron classes are excited. This interneuron activity is the neuronal correlate of the reflexive withdrawal that precedes a swim. When the nerve stimulation stops, a rhythmical motor pattern, with a period of 5 to 7 s, is generated; this pattern corresponds to the swimming phase of the behavioural response (Fig. 2.1B).

The initiation and maintenance of swimming in *Tritonia* depends on the establishment of a long-lasting ramp depolarization in both premotor rhythm-generating interneurons, and in the motor neurons. Bursts of activity of the neurons are superimposed on the depolarization, which can be seen in Fig. 2.1C as a displacement of the membrane potential above the dotted base lines.

Bursting activity in the three cell groups during the swim sequence appears and disappears in a strict order in each swim cycle. A sharp activation of the DSI is an easily recognizable event and can be considered as the beginning of the swim cycle (Fig. 2.1C). With some delay, activity in the C2 appears. In each burst, the C2 discharge starts at a low frequency, but the frequency gradually increases to reach 15–20 Hz by the end of the burst. The burst of the C2 terminates later than of DSI. The burst of activity of the VSI occurs in the second half of the swim cycle. Thus, the three cell groups start and stop their firing in the following succession: DSI→C2→VSI (marked by dotted lines in Fig. 2.1C).

One way to verify the participation of a neuron in the production of a rhythmic pattern is to perform phase-shift experiments in which the normal timing of bursts is perturbed by intracellular current injection. If a neuron is involved directly in the generation of the motor pattern, then an imposed change in its normal burst time should influence the burst timing in the whole CPG. In the *Tritonia* swim CPG, resetting of the swim rhythm can be evoked provided both C2 neurons are simultaneously stimulated, or three (out of six) DSI neurons (Fig. 2.1D). Thus, it was directly demonstrated that the C2 and DSI are 'influential' neurons and, therefore, they are involved in the rhythm generation. For the VSI group, resetting of the rhythm was not shown, most likely because only one of the VSIs was stimulated which might be insufficient to drive the whole VSI group. However, strong synaptic interactions of the VSIs with other CPG neurons indicate that this group also belongs to the rhythm generator network.

By using the pairwise recording technique, synaptic connections between the interneurons constituting the rhythm generator, as well as connections between these interneurons and the motor neurons constituting the output motor stage, have been revealed (Fig. 2.2A). In these experiments, none of the identified interneurons (DSI, C2, or VSI) when depolarized with constant current, displayed any endogenous membrane properties which would indicate that they are capable of generating bursts in isolation from network interactions. This led Getting *et al.* (1980) to the suggestion that the bursting pattern produced by these interneurons emerges exclusively from the synaptic interactions among them. This contrasts with the swim CPG of *Clione* for which endogenous rhythmic activity of individual interneurons has been demonstrated (see Section 1.2). The diagram of synaptic connections (Fig. 2.2A) can explain qualitatively the sequential activation of the DSI, C2, and VSI groups in the course of the swim cycle, as well as alternating the activity of the swim motor neurons, DSN and VSN. As shown in the timing

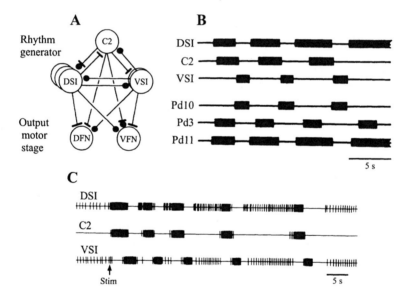

Fig. 2.2 Locomotor CPG of *Tritonia*. A: The wiring diagram of the CPG. Excitatory connections are denoted by bars, inhibitory by circles, and multicomponent synapses by a combination of the two. The CPG consists of two principal parts—the rhythm generator (interneurons of groups DSI, C2, and VSI) and the output motor stage (DFN and VFN motor neurons). B: Timing diagram of activity of the interneurons and motor neurons comprising the locomotor CPG of *Tritonia* during a swim sequence triggered by stimulation of a peripheral nerve. C: Simulated swim pattern. An extrinsic synaptic input to the DSI was stimulated at 10 Hz for 1 s at the arrow to produce a prolonged ramp depolarization of the DSI. Each vertical bar represents the time of firing for each of the three interneuron types. A is from Katz *et al.* (1994), B is from Hume and Getting (1982a), and C is from Getting (1983a).

diagram (Fig. 2.2B), a cycle begins with the onset of DSI firing in response to a tonic ramp depolarization. Firing in DSI has two consequences—DSI inhibits VSI and also excites C2. After some delay, C2 starts firing and, also with some delay, evokes excitation of VSI. When excited, VSI inhibits both DSI and C2, and their bursts terminate. Therefore, VSI eliminates its own source of excitation, and its burst terminates. This results in disinhibition of DSI, and a new cycle begins. Neurons within the same group are bursting simultaneously due to common synaptic inputs, as well as due to mutual electrotonic couplings. The circuit shown in Fig. 2.2A has its symmetrical counterpart in the contralateral ganglia. Synchronization of the two generators is achieved due to electrotonic coupling between bilaterally homologous cells.

An important feature of the swim CPG in *Tritonia* is a considerable delay (1–3 s) in activation of C2 interneurons after the onset of DSI activity. According to Getting *et al.* (1980) this delay is caused by synaptic summation in a slow synapse between DSI and C2. There is also a considerable delay (up to 3 s) in activation of VSI interneurons after the onset of C2 activity. Getting (1983*b*) described two mechanisms for producing this delayed excitation: (1) the integrative properties of dual-component, excitatory–inhibitory synapse from C2 to DSI, and (2) the specific membrane properties of VSI interneurons—these cells exhibit a long delay in the spike response to a constant current depolarization.

A computer 'reconstruction' of the rhythm generator, consisting of interneurons DSI, C2 and VSI, was performed (Getting 1983*a*). In the model, the active and passive membrane properties of the three cells, as well as the time course and strength of monosynaptic connections were matched to physiological data. The reconstructed network appeared able to generate the three-phasic pattern in response to a ramp depolarization (Fig. 2.2C). However, the frequency profile of the bursts generated by DSI and C2 was different from that in the real pattern. In particular, the real C2 exhibits a remarkable increase of the discharge rate towards the end of the burst (Fig. 2.1D) while the simulated C2 does not. The most likely explanation of this discrepancy is that no endogenous bursting properties were attributed to the reconstructed cells, since these properties were not observed in physiological experiments when a cell was depolarized by constant current in quiescent preparation (Getting *et al.* 1980). One cannot exclude, however, that the sensory stimulus, which elicits a swim episode, produces not only the ramp depolarization of the CPG neurons but also modifies their membrane, thus transforming the cells into bursters ('conditional oscillators'). Such a transformation occurs for example in the lamprey spinal neurons under the effect of certain neurotransmitters (excitatory amino acids) (Grillner *et al.* 1995; Wallén *et al.* 1985; see also Section 8.3).

Rhythm generator models of the type shown in Figs. 2.2A,B, with rising activity in one neuron population and cessation of this activity as a consequence of the excitation of another population of inhibitory neurons, have been suggested to explain the work of a number of rhythmic motor systems in other species, specifically, of the medulla oblongata respiratory centre (the model with a 'switch-off mechanism') (Bradley *et al.* 1975; Cohen and Feldman 1977; Euler 1977, 1983, 1986; Wyman 1977; Cohen 1979), and of the spinal centre controlling scratching movements (Berkinblit *et al.* 1978*a,b*). The putative cause of the rising activity in the first neuronal population in the spinal centre has been attributed to a 'chain reaction', i.e. mutual excitation between the individual cells; this was also suggested by Getting *et al.* (1980) for the *Tritonia* swim CPG. In molluscs, the model with a switch-off mechanism satisfactory explains the generation of the feeding rhythm in the snails *Planorbis corneus* (Arshavsky *et al.* 1988*a–c*) and *Lymnaea stagnalis* (Rose and Benjamin 1981; Benjamin 1983; Elliot and Benjamin 1985). In *Planorbis*, experiments with isolation of individual identified cells constituting the CPG have shown that the rising depolarization in the first neuronal population is caused not by mutual excitation but is rather generated in individual cells of this group as a consequence of the properties of their membrane (Arshavsky *et al.* 1988*b*).

2.1.3   Output motor stage

The cells in the rhythm generating network of *Tritonia* (DSI, C2, and VSI) exert rather complex synaptic actions on the motor neurons constituting the output motor stage (Fig. 2.2A) (Hume and Getting 1982*a,b*). The dorsal flexion neurons (DFN) receive excitation from the DSI and C2, and inhibition from the VSI. In contrast, the ventral flexion neurons (VFN) receive excitation from the VSI and inhibition from the DSI and C2. These synaptic connections, as well as specific membrane properties of the motor neurons (spike frequency adaptation) (Hume and Getting 1982*b*), are responsible for the transformation of the three-phasic pattern, produced by the rhythm generator interneurons, into the biphasic output pattern (Fig. 2.2B). However, not all aspects of the output motor pattern can be explained on the bases of synaptic connections from the DSI, C2, and VSI interneurons, and on the bases of motor neuron cell properties. This led Hume and Getting (1982*a*) to the suggestion that the rhythm generator network contains two additional cell groups (X and Y). Several of the properties of these cells were inferred from the study of the synaptic input to motor neurons. These cells have not been identified yet, however. No modifications of the CPG pattern under the effect of sensory feedback have been reported for *Tritonia* swimming.

2.1.4   Command systems

The primary function of the command systems for swimming in *Tritonia* is activation of the CPG. This is achieved by depolarization of both interneurons and motor neurons (Lennard *et al.* 1980). Voltage clamp technique have been used to measure the membrane current responsible for the ramp depolarization in different cell classes (Getting and Dekin 1985). It was found that there are two sources of the depolarization: (1) extrinsic (synaptic drive from a command system) and (2) intrinsic, that is synaptic drive from other neurons of the CPG. The ramp current in the VSI-B is independent of activity within the CPG, that is this current is induced entirely by input from extrinsic sources. In contrast, the ramp current in the motor neurons and in the C2 interneurons is generated largely by activity within the rhythm generator network. In the DSI interneurons, extrinsic input appears to control the first 10–15 s of the ramp current. After this, the activity within the DSI population itself maintains the ramp current. The source of the extrinsic input eliciting the ramp depolarization in the swim CPG remains unknown. Candidate neurons are the sensory cells of the pleural ganglia which respond to cutaneous stimulation. These cells are sufficient for initiation of swimming (Getting 1976, 1977), and may thus play a double role as both sensory and command neurons.

During swimming, *Tritonia* tends to rotate in a tumbling motion about its longitudinal axis (Hume *et al.* 1982). This observation suggests that the postural orientation and equilibrium control systems do not function in this form of behaviour.

In molluscs, defensive reaction is a complex behaviour, with many systems involved in coordinated activity (see for example Arshavsky *et al.* 1994a–c). The defensive behaviour of *Clione* was considered in Section 1.7.1. In *Tritonia*, escape swimming is subject to considerable modifications (for example habituation and iterative enhancement) (Brown *et al.* 1996). The neuronal mechanisms for integration of locomotion in the complex behaviour such as the escape response and for the different modifications of the swim response remain unknown.

2.2 SWIMMING IN *APLYSIA* BASED ON PARAPODIAL UNDULATIONS

2.2.1 Motor pattern and motor neurons

In addition to the basic form of locomotion, crawling, certain species of *Aplysia* ('sea hare'), such as *A. brasiliana*, are able to swim (Porten *et al.* 1980, 1982). Swimming is accomplished by rhythmic undulating movements of two parapodia that cover the dorsum of the body (Fig. 2.3A). In each cycle, a metachronal wave of parapodial closing, followed by another wave of parapodial opening, starts in the anterior parapodia and moves posteriorly (Figs. 2.3B,C). These waves are responsible for generation of the propulsive force moving the animal through the water. The lifting force seems to be generated due to an upward pitch angle of the whole animal during swimming.

The CNS of *Aplysia* has the same basic structure as the CNS of *Tritonia* (Fig. 2.1E) and *Clione* (Fig. 1.1C). Movements of parapodia are controlled by motor neurons located in the pedal ganglia. Experiments with lesions to interganglionic connectives have shown that the pedal ganglia play a crucial role in the control of parapodial undulations. A separate neuronal oscillator resides in each pedal ganglion, and bilateral coordination is mediated via the pedal commissure. The swimming command pathway is located in the cerebro-pedal connectives. Thus, the distribution of functions between different parts of the CNS for the control of swimming in *Aplysia* is the same as for the control of swimming in *Clione* (see Chapter 1).

Motor commands from the pedal ganglia reach the parapodial muscles via three pairs of nerves supplying the anterior, middle, and posterior parts of the parapodia (Fig. 2.3B). Transection of the anterior nerve almost completely abolishes the parapodial undulations, whereas transection of the middle and posterior nerves has little effect. It has been suggested that the parapodial flapping originates in

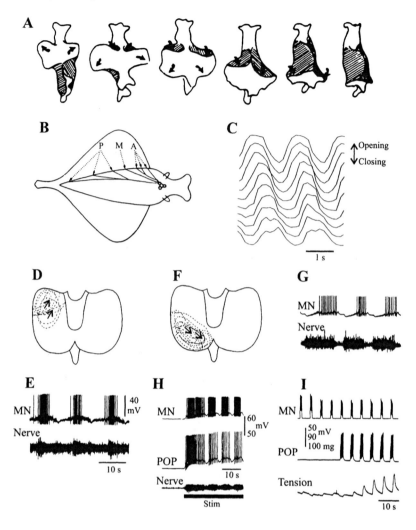

Fig. 2.3 Swimming in *Aplysia*. A: Sequence of parapodial movements during one cycle of swimming (view from above). B: Peripheral distribution of left pedal nerves innervating parapodia (A, anterior; M, middle; P, posterior nerves; parapodia are shown opened). C: Parapodial oscillations recorded as mediolateral displacement of the parapodia border in ten loci along the rostro-caudal extent of the parapodia. D–G: Parapodial motor neurons have different motor fields and fire in different phases of the fictive swim cycle. To define the phase, motor neurons were recorded together with the ENG of the parapodial nerve. D,E: Motor neuron with a rostral motor field (D) fires at the beginning of the cycle (E). F,G: Motor neuron with a caudal motor field (F) fires at the end of the cycle (G). H,I: Rhythmic activity of a motor neuron and a modulatory POP cell that interact peripherally. H: Fictive swimming evoked by continuous stimulation of the cerebro-pedal connective. I: Periodical intracellular stimulation of the motor neuron elicited small muscle contractions (Tension), which increased considerably with simultaneous activation of a POP cell. A and B are from Porten *et al.* (1980). C is from Porten *et al.* (1982), and D–I are based on McPherson and Blankenship (1991*b*,*c*).

the more anterior muscular region, innervated by the anterior nerve, and that the posterior parapodial movement is primarily passive, either through a mechanical linkage (Porten *et al.* 1980, 1982) and/or a peripheral nerve net (Stoll *et al.* 1978). Two additional arguments in favour of these suggestions have been obtained. First, the speed of swimming and the period of parapodial flapping are markedly temperature dependent whereas the timing of the metachronal wave is not (Porten *et al.* 1982). Second, recording of population activity from the anterior and posterior nerves (by implanted electrodes) during swimming has not revealed any phase delay in the posterior nerve in relation to the anterior nerve, suggesting that there is no central command responsible for the temporal offset between undulations of the anterior and posterior parts of the parapodia (Porten *et al.* 1980).

However, experiments with recording from individual parapodial motor neurons during fictive swimming revealed a very specific temporal pattern of firing in the motor neurons projecting to different parts of the parapodia (McPherson and Blankenship 1991*a,b*). The parapodia have eight layers of muscles, differing in the orientation of the muscle fibres. Stimulation of individual motor neurons has shown that they evoke contraction of parapodial muscles in different areas and in different directions, thus suggesting that the motor neurons project to different muscle layers. According to their projections, more than 16 groups of motor neurons can be distinguished. Two of them are shown in Figs. 2.3D,F. To estimate the phase of firing of the motor neurons in the swim cycle, they were recorded during fictive swimming together with one of the parapodial nerves. The activity in this nerve indicated the opening phase of the swim cycle. The phase of bursting activity in different groups of motor neurons occurred distributed over the whole swim cycle. Motor neurons projecting to the anterior part of the parapodium, characteristically fired at the beginning of the swim cycle (Fig. 2.3E), whereas motor neurons projecting to the posterior part, typically fired towards the end of the cycle (Fig. 2.3G). These experiments have clearly shown that the swim CPG in *Aplysia* generates a multiphasic efferent pattern.

A characteristic feature of the locomotor system in gastropod molluscs is a peripheral modulation of the motor effects produced by motor neurons (see Section 1.5.2.4). During swimming in *Aplysia*, two groups of the efferent pedal neurons are activated, the POP cells firing in the opening phase of the swim cycle (Fig. 2.3H), and the PCP cells firing in the closing phase (McPherson and Blankenship 1991*c*; Parsons and Pinsker 1988). These cells cannot alone evoke muscle contractions, but when firing in conjunction with the parapodial motor neurons, they strongly enhance the motor neuron evoked contractions of the parapodial muscles (Fig. 2.3I). Like the corresponding cells in *Clione* (Pd-SW; see Section 1.5.2.4), the modulatory cells in *Aplysia* are also serotonergic (McPherson and Blankenship 1991*c*).

Thus, the rhythm generator of the swim CPG, located in the pedal ganglia, exerts a periodical action on the output motor stage, which includes numerous groups of motor neurons as well as the modulatory POP and PCP neurons. Unfortunately, practically nothing is known about the structure and functioning of the rhythm generator. The most intriguing question is the origin of the temporal offset between different groups of motor neurons.

2.2.2   Command systems

Behavioural studies have shown that swimming in *Aplysia* can start spontaneously or in response to different stimuli. Swimming is goal-directed, involving orientation towards specific environmental cues (Hamilton and Russel 1982). Animals can swim just above the bottom or near the surface when travelling longer distances, but swim less often at intermediate depths (Hamilton and Ambrose 1975). One can thus conclude that the command systems for steering, postural orientation, and equilibrium control in *Aplysia* are well developed. Only a few command neurons, most likely related to the initiation of locomotion, have been identified, however (Gamkrelidze *et al.* 1995). Like the command neurons controlling swimming in *Clione*, they have a cell body in the cerebral ganglia, and send an axon to the pedal ganglia via the cerebro-pedal connective. Three command neuron groups (CN1–CN3) are capable of eliciting the oscillatory, phasic swim motor pattern in the isolated CNS, recorded bilaterally in parapodial nerves. The evoked pattern includes rhythmic bursting in both the swim motor neurons and the modulatory (POP) cells. The CN4 group is less efficient in elicitation of swimming: it causes only a weak activation of the contralateral swim CPG. The command neurons of CN5–CN8 groups, although not capable of inducing the swim motor programme when activated individually, nonetheless have strong synaptic connections with some pedal efferent neurons (POP cells).

An important finding is that different groups of command neurons interact with each other, in some instances monosynaptically. This interaction may be involved in reconfigurations of the command system, necessary for modifications of the swim motor pattern in different behavioural contexts.

2.3   CRAWLING IN *APLYSIA* BASED ON PROPAGATING PEDAL WAVES

2.3.1   Motor pattern and motor neurons

Locomotion in many species of gastropod molluscs, both terrestrial and aquatic, is based on the propagation of waves of muscle contraction along the foot. The configuration of these waves, for example the number of waves simultaneously travelling along the foot, and the direction of their propagation differ between different species (Trueman 1983). In *Aplysia californica*, there are two forms of crawling slightly differing in their motor pattern: escape locomotion and goal-directed locomotion. In both forms, the locomotion is based on the retrograde propagation of a single (monotaxic) wave along the foot (Parker 1917), at the speed from a few to 30 cm min⁻¹. Different speeds are associated with pedal waves which range in frequency from 1 to 12 per minute. Each 'step' (Fig. 2.4A) consists of (1) the extension of the animal's neck over the substrate, (2) planting of the parapodium at maximal extension, and (3) contraction of the caudal segments of the body up to the point of fixation. During the cycle, each part of the body performs in succession: (1) a combined transverse constriction (involving both dorsoventral contraction of the body wall and narrowing of the sole of the foot) and longitudinal extension;

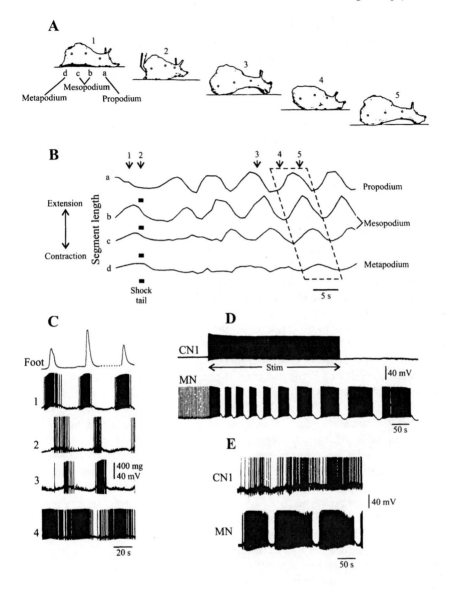

Fig. 2.4 Escape crawling locomotion in *Aplysia*. A: The locomotor sequence (1–5) triggered by shock applied to the tail. A,1 illustrates the division of the animal into equal longitudinal segments by implanted beads. B: Changes in length of the pedal segments during locomotion. Numbers above trace a indicate the points at which the tracings in part A were made. One complete step is demarcated by the dashed parallelogram. C: Pedal motor neurons (1–4) are bursting in different phases of the locomotor cycle defined by the foot muscle contractions. D: Intracellular stimulation (Stim, 5 Hz) of the type 1 command neuron (CN1) activates the locomotor CPG and evokes fictive locomotion in the isolated CNS (monitored by rhythmic activity of a motor neuron, MN). E: The command neuron CN1 is rhythmically modulated by the CPG during spontaneous fictive locomotion. A and B are based on Hening *et al.* (1979), C is based on Fredman and Jahan-Parvar (1980), and D and E are based on Fredman and Jahan-Parvar (1983).

and (2) a combined longitudinal contraction and transversal relaxation (Hening *et al.* 1979). Figure 2.4B shows the length of different body segments as a function of time in a few successive locomotor cycles. Periodical changes of the length in more caudal segments are delayed in relation to more rostral ones; thus a wave of contraction propagates along the body of *Aplysia*. Movements of the foot in *Aplysia* are controlled by motor neurons located in the pedal ganglia. There are two classes of motor neurons: (1) 'longitudinal' motor neurons, eliciting the longitudinal contraction in different areas of the foot, and (2) 'transverse contractor' motor neurons (Hening *et al.* 1979). During locomotion, each pedal motor neuron generates a burst of spikes in a definite phase of the locomotor cycle; phases of activity of different neurons are distributed over the whole cycle (Fig. 2.4C). This pattern strongly differs from the efferent swim pattern in *Clione* and *Tritonia*, with two distinct phases of activity in a cycle corresponding to the dorsal and ventral flexions of the wings in *Clione* (Fig. 1.3B), or the dorsal and ventral flexions of the body in *Tritonia* (Fig. 2.2B). It has been suggested (Hening *et al.* 1979; Fredman and Jahan-Parwar 1980) that the motor neurons, firing in different phases of the locomotor cycle, project to different anterio-posterior regions of the foot. These projections are organized in such a way that different parts of the foot will contract in succession, starting from the anterior part and finishing in the posterior part, which will result in propagation of the wave of muscle contraction along the foot towards the tail. The extreme complexity of the muscular system of the foot, as well as of its nervous control, hampers a direct testing of this hypothesis. An additional complication is the presence of peripheral nerve cells in the foot, which can modify the central commands.

A group of large neurons with the axons projecting to the foot has been discovered in the pedal ganglia. These neurons have no motor effect but, when firing in conjunction with pedal motor neurons, potentiate the force of contractions of the foot muscles. Like motor neurons, they are driven by the locomotor CPG and fire in bursts. These neurons can be stained by 5,7-dihydroxytryptamine (5,7-DHT), suggesting that they are serotonergic (McPherson and Blankenship 1992). They seem to be homologous to Pd-SW modulatory neurons potentiating contraction of wing muscles in *Clione* (see Section 1.2.2.4 and Figs. 1.6F,G), as well as to POP and PCP cells in the swimming system of *Aplysia* (see Section 2.2.1).

The pedal ganglia of *Aplysia*, isolated from the rest of the CNS, are able to evoke the pedal waves but of a reduced amplitude. In the isolated CNS, rhythmical bursting of pedal motor neurons (fictive crawling) can appear spontaneously or in response to stimulation of a peripheral nerve (Hening *et al.* 1979; Fredman and Jahan-Parwar 1980). These findings indicate that the CPG for crawling is located in the pedal ganglia. Very little is known, however, about structure and functioning of this CPG. Most likely, it consists of two major parts, the interneurons (not identified yet) and the motor neurons. Most motor neurons exert an excitatory effect on the foot muscles, but some motor neurons are inhibitory (Fredman and Jahan-Parwar 1980). In both locomotor CPGs of *Aplysia*, for swimming (see Section 2.2.1) and for crawling, there is the temporal offset between the motor neurons projecting to different parts of the locomotor organs. The origin of this offset remains unknown, however. In animals moving due to the propagating metachronal waves (like lamprey, leech, and tadpole), a temporal offset between motor neuron activity in adjacent segments is often viewed as the phase shift between the coupled segmental oscillators (see for example Matsushima and Grillner 1992; Pearce and Friesen 1985*a,b*; Tunstall and Roberts 1991). A chain of coupled oscillators could also be responsible for the generation of motor pattern in *Aplysia*. Another possibility is that the complex, multiphasic pattern is transformed from the initially simpler (mono- or biphasic) pattern due to the complex connections from the rhythm generator to the output motor stage of the CPG (see Section 3.3 for discussion of these two hypotheses).

2.3.2   Command systems

Crawling in *Aplysia* is involved in escape and approach behaviour, is coordinated with orientation movements and defensive withdrawal, and can be modulated by satiation, sensitization, and classical conditioning (Advokat *et al.* 1976; Kupferman 1974; Preston and Lee 1973; Walters *et al.* 1978; Kandel 1979). One can thus expect that a rather complex system of command neurons is responsible for these different behavioural synergies and for their modifications. Only a few command neurons in these systems have been identified (Fredman and Jahan-Parwar 1983). The cell bodies of these neurons are located in the cerebral ganglia, and the axons project to the pedal ganglia through the cerebro-pedal connective. Three types of command neurons have been distinguished, depending on their effect on the locomotor CPG. The type 1 neurons are most efficient—electrical stimulation of a single neuron activates the locomotor CPG (Fig. 2.4D). Type 2 neurons are less efficient. Finally, type 3 neurons do not affect the rhythm generator but produce monosynaptic excitation or inhibition of the pedal motor neurons. The type 1 neurons are excited by sensory inputs eliciting locomotion (nociceptive and food stimuli). One can thus suggest that they participate in the control of escape and approach behaviours.

The type 1 command neurons receive input from the locomotor CPG. Figure 2.4E shows an episode of spontaneous fictive locomotion, with bursting activity in a pedal motor neuron, and with a rhythmical modulation of the discharge rate in the command neuron. A function of this 'internal feedback' in *Aplysia* is not clear. It has been suggested that this feedback is positive, and that it promotes sustained locomotor activity after cessation of the triggering sensory stimulus (Fredman and Jahan-Parwar 1983). A similar internal feedback is characteristic of many other locomotor systems, in both invertebrate and vertebrate animals, and will be discussed further in corresponding sections.

2.4   CRAWLING IN *PLANORBIS* BASED ON CILIARY BEATING

2.4.1   Control of ciliary beating

The ciliated epithelium in various metazoans is an organ for producing a mechanical force. The force can be used for different purposes: for moving mucus, for transporting small particles (for example food), for producing a water stream, etc.

In some species it is used as the propulsive force for moving the animal forward during locomotion (Blake and Sleigh 1974). The nervous control of ciliary locomotion is based on the fact that the frequency of ciliary beating depends on the membrane potential of a ciliated cell. In veligers (larvae of some molluscs) it has been demonstrated that depolarization of a locomotor ciliated cell results in the inhibition of ciliary beating (Arkett 1987; Arkett *et al.* 1987). Thus, the CNS does not participate in generation of the basic motor pattern in the locomotor organs (cilia) but rather activates or inactivates the organs in coordinated fashion.

The ciliated epithelium covering the foot sole is the primary mover in a number of aquatic gastropod molluscs, both freshwater and marine (Miller 1974; Jones 1975; Trueman 1983). The pond snail *Planorbis corneus* (Fig. 2.5A) can crawl, by means of this mover, both on a solid substratum such as the bottom of the pond or river, algae, etc., and below the water surface film at a speed up to $1.5 \, \text{mm s}^{-1}$. Experiments carried out on *Planorbis* (Deliagina and Orlovsky 1990*b*) and on the marine mollusc *Tritonia* (Audesirk 1977, 1978) have shown that the motor activity of the ciliated epithelium is controlled by the CNS in a rather complicated way in relation to different forms of behaviour.

Figures 2.5B,C illustrate the experimental arrangement for studying the nervous control of ciliary beating in *Planorbis* (Deliagina and Orlovsky 1990*b*). Three nerves originating from the pedal ganglia (anterior, middle, and posterior) innervate three separate zones of the ciliated epithelium on the ipsilateral foot sole. Microelectrode mapping of the pedal ganglia (in the pedal ganglia–foot preparation) revealed three symmetrical groups of neurons controlling ciliary beating. Each group comprises a few cells, and is responsible for an activation of ciliary beating in a limited zone on the ipsilateral side of the foot sole (anterior, middle, and posterior, Fig. 2.5C). Figure 2.5D shows the morphology of the excitatory locomotor neuron of the posterior zone, ELN(P), with an axon projecting to this zone through the posterior pedal nerve. With directly driven excitation of the ELN(P), the locomotor activity in the corresponding zone considerably increases (Fig. 2.5E), while the activity in other zones remains unchanged. The transmitter mediating excitatory action of ELNs on the ciliated epithelium has not been identified. However, there is considerable evidence that serotonin (5-hydroxythriptamine, 5-HT) plays an important role in excitation of ciliary beating in gastropods (Audesirk *et al.* 1979; Syed *et al.* 1988; Deliagina and Orlovsky 1990*b*).

2.4.2   Integration of locomotion in different forms of behaviour

Via the ELNs, a differential control of motor activity in various zones of the ciliated epithelium can be exerted, which is necessary for integration of locomotion in different behavioural acts. The simplest mode of coordination between different zones is joint excitation or inhibition. The excitation is observed in some forms of feeding behaviour. Presentation of food evokes a feeding arousal in the snail, one of the components of which is excitation of all the ELNs and activation of ciliary beating in all the zones, as illustrated for the middle zone in Fig. 2.5F. An opposite response—inhibition of the ELNs and of ciliary beating—is observed during the defensive reaction evoked by tactile stimulation of the tentacle (Fig. 2.5G) or dimming of the lights (Fig. 2.5H).

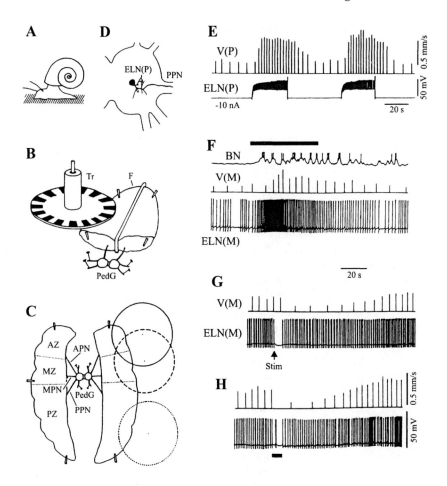

Fig. 2.5 Crawling in *Planorbis* based on cilia beating. A: View of a snail crawling on the solid substratum. B,C: Recording of the summated effect of cilia beating. B: The posterior foot and pedal ganglia preparation. The foot (F) isolated with the pedal ganglion (PedG) is positioned with the ciliated epithelium upwards. Beating of cilia results in rotation of the transducer (Tr), which is recorded by an optoelectronic system. C: The split foot and pedal ganglia preparation. The foot is innervated by the anterior, middle, and posterior pedal nerves. Positions of the transducer to record locomotor activity in the anterior (AZ), middle (MZ), and posterior (PZ) zones are shown. D,E: The structure and locomotor effect of the ELN(P) neuron supplying the posterior zone of the foot sole. D: Structure. It has a cell body in the pedal ganglion and an axon entering the posterior pedal nerve. E: Activation of the ELN(P) neuron (by interruption of the hyperpolarizing current) results in speeding up the rotation of the transducer, V(P). F–H: The ELN(M) neuron mediates various reflex influences on the locomotor speed (semi-intact preparation). F: Touching the lip with a lettuce leaf (bar) evokes the feeding rhythm in a buccal ganglion neuron (BN), activates the ELN(M) neuron projecting to the middle zone, and increases the locomotor speed in this zone, V(M). G: Tactile stimulation of the tentacle (arrow) decreases both the locomotor speed and the neuron activity. H: A brief interruption in illumination of the snail evokes both inhibition of the neuron discharge and decrease of the locomotor speed. From Deliagina and Orlovsky (1990*b*).

A specific inhibition of the motor activity in the middle and posterior zones, while the anterior zone remains active, is observed in the snail when it is located under the water surface and feeds (Deliagina and Orlovsky 1990*a*). This inhibition is mediated by pathways from the cerebral ganglia: transection of the cerebro-pedal connective leads to a selective disinhibition of the ELNs of the middle and posterior zones, and in a considerable increase of motor activity in these zones. An asymmetry in motor activity in the left and right parts of the foot sole is an essential component of a turning behaviour, supplementing the lateral flexion of the foot. Spontaneous switching of the motor activity between the left and right sides was observed in the pedal ganglia—foot preparation, suggesting that there is, in the pedal ganglia, a neuronal mechanism for selective activation of a given side and for reciprocal inhibition of the opposite side (Deliagina and Orlovsky 1990*b*). Thus, selective activation or inhibition of the six zones of the ciliated epithelium (via the ELNs) in different combinations with each other, as well as modifications of the foot shape, is the basis for diverse locomotor patterns exhibited by *Planorbis* in different forms of behaviour.

Central neurons controlling the pedal locomotor cilia were also found in *Tritonia* (Audesirk 1977, 1978). A pair of neurons (Pd21) was identified in the pedal ganglia, the excitation of which initiated ciliary beating. These neurons participated in the control of ciliary beating in various types of behaviour. In many respects these neurons seem to be analogous to the ELNs in *Planorbis*.

Also in *Planorbis*, one can thus expect that a rather complicated system of command neurons coordinates locomotion with the activity of other motor systems. Of these command neurons, a group of neurons (DRN1) eliciting the defensive reaction has been identified in *Planorbis* (Arshavsky *et al.* 1994*b*). The DRN1s are activated by noxious stimuli and some other modalities. In turn, they affect practically all motor systems of the snail. There is direct evidence that the DRN1s evoke body withdrawal into the shell and opening of the pneumostome (the lung). There is also indirect evidence that the DRN1s are responsible for inhibition of ciliary beating, for termination of the feeding rhythm, and for deceleration of the heart rate.

In *Planorbis*, the locomotor system is closely linked with the system for spatial orientation. Behavioural experiments have shown that the direction of crawling of the snail in many cases is completely determined by input from the gravity orientation system (Deliagina and Orlovsky 1990*a*). The corresponding neuronal mechanisms have not yet been identified.

2.5 CONCLUSIONS

1. Swimming of *Tritonia* is based on alternating dorsal and ventral whole body flexions. There are no indications that sensory feedback plays any significant role in swimming. Thus, swimming is controlled by the CPG consisting of the rhythm generator and output motor stage. In contrast to *Clione*, the rhythm generator in *Tritonia* is asymmetrical. It belongs to the class of generators with a switch-off mechanism. A rising activity in one population of the generatory interneurons (DSI and C2) leads to the excitation of the other population (VSI),

which then inhibits the first one and thus terminates the cycle. The rhythm generator produces a three-phasic output pattern, which is transformed into the biphasic motor pattern due to the specific connections from the rhythm generator interneurons to the motor neurons of the output motor stage, as well as due to the specific membrane properties of the motor neurons. The command system for initiation of locomotion transforms a brief triggering sensory stimulus into a long-lasting depolarization of the CPG neurons, which determines the duration of the escape swimming response. No definite body orientation is maintained during swimming.

2. Swimming in *Aplysia* is based on metachronal waves of parapodial undulations. Swimming is controlled by a CPG located in the pedal ganglia. Phases of activity of individual motor neurons, projecting to different parts of the parapodia, are distributed over the swim cycle. Thus, the CPG generates a multiphasic output pattern. The structure and functioning of the CPG are not known. The role of sensory feedback in the coordination of the swim motor pattern is not clear. Some command neurons, responsible for activation of the CPG, have been identified. When swimming, *Aplysia* maintains the dorsal-side-up orientation. The neuronal mechanisms stabilizing this orientation have not been identified.

3. Crawling in *Aplysia* is based on propagating pedal waves. Crawling is controlled by the CPG located in the pedal ganglia. The CPG generates a multiphasic efferent pattern. The structure and function of the CPG are not known, nor the role of sensory feedback. Some command neurons, responsible for activation of the CPG, have been identified. These neurons are excited by sensory inputs (nociceptive and food stimuli) eliciting locomotion.

4. Crawling in *Planorbis* is based on beating of cilia covering the foot sole. In a ciliated cell, the frequency of cilia beating depends on the membrane potential, and thus may be changed under the effect of synaptic input. Accordingly the CNS does not participate in generation of the basic motor pattern but rather activates or inactivates the locomotor organs (cilia) in a coordinated fashion. Six groups of efferent neurons (ELNs) in the pedal ganglia exert an excitatory action on the cilia beating in six zones of the foot sole. The ELNs mediate different central and reflex influences on the locomotor activity of the ciliated epithelium. *Planorbis* has a well developed system for spatial orientation; its locomotion is also integrated in numerous forms of behaviour. The corresponding neuronal mechanisms have not been identified.

Swimming in the leech

3.1 SWIM MOTOR PATTERN

The leech (Annelida, Hirudinea) has presented excellent opportunities for examining all components of the locomotor control system at the network and cellular level. There are two forms of locomotion in the leech—swimming and crawling. The neuronal mechanisms of swimming are better understood (for review see Brodfuehrer *et al.* 1995*a*; Friesen 1989*a*). At rest, the leech has a tubular shape (Fig. 3.1A). At the onset of swimming the body is flattened due to a tonic contraction of dorso-ventral muscles (Fig. 3.1B) and during the locomotion waves of dorsal and ventral flexion start to propagate retrogradely along the body (Figs. 3.1B,C) (Gray 1968; Gray *et al.* 1938; Kristan *et al.* 1974*a*). The swimming undulations are caused by contractions of dorsal and ventral longitudinal muscles. In each of the 21 body segments, these muscles contract in antiphase (Fig. 3.1D). The contractions of dorsal and ventral muscles are phase delayed between successive segments (Fig. 3.1E), so that the locomotor waves propagate along the body. The intersegmental time delay is not constant but varies proportionally to the cycle period. As a result, the phase lag between successive segments is relatively constant (~22°), and about one wave length is expressed along the entire body at any locomotor frequency, from 0.5 to 2 Hz (Fig. 3.1B) (Kristan *et al.* 1974*a*). A similar pattern of intersegmental coordination is observed in the swimming lamprey (see Sections 8.1 and 8.3.7).

Locomotion in the leech is controlled by the ventral nerve cord which includes a chain of 21 midbody ganglia, as well as the 'head' (supra- and sub-oesophageal) ganglia and the tail ganglion (Fig. 3.1F). Each midbody ganglion contains the somata of about 400 neurons (Fig. 3.1G). As in the ganglia of molluscs, these cells form a cortex surrounding the central neuropil. Two large lateral connectives and a small median connective link the ganglia (Muller *et al.* 1981).

Each midbody ganglion gives rise to peripheral nerves supplying the dorsal and ventral longitudinal muscles. For each of the muscles, there are two classes of motor neurons: excitatory and inhibitory (Stuart 1970). The dorsal and ventral excitatory motor neurons in each segment oscillate in approximate antiphase; the inhibitory neurons oscillate in approximately antiphase with excitatory neurons having the same projection (Ort *et al.* 1974).

In the isolated nerve cord, a locomotor-like activity (fictive swimming) can be elicited by stimulation of peripheral nerves (Kristan and Calabrese 1976; Kristan *et al.* 1974*b*). During fictive swimming, the dorsal and ventral excitatory motor neurons are active in antiphase, as in normal swimming. There is also a phase lag between successive segments (Fig. 3.1I). The phase lag during fictive swimming is smaller (6–10°) than the lag seen in intact animals or semi-intact preparation (~22°), however (compare Figs. 3.1H and I), and is not independent of the cycle duration. One can thus conclude that some but not all essential features of the swim motor pattern—specifically the alternating activity of the dorsal and the ventral motor neurons, and the phase lag between adjacent segments—have their neuronal correlates in the swim CPG activity.

3.2 RHYTHM GENERATOR

Analysis of the rhythm generator network in the leech swim CPG appeared a very difficult task because of the great number of neurons involved in rhythmogenesis. It was found that more than ten pairs of neurons in each of the midbody ganglia (and, therefore, more than 400 neurons in the whole ventral nerve cord) met the following three criteria to be considered members of the rhythm generator network ('oscillator neurons'): (1) they exhibit oscillations of the membrane potential phase-locked to the swim rhythm, (2) they have synaptic connections with other members of the oscillator circuit, and (3) experimental manipulations of their membrane potential affects the cycle phase in the whole CPG (Friesen 1989*a*; Friesen *et al.* 1976, 1978). Figure 3.2A illustrates an effect of current injection into one of the oscillator neurons, cell 28. The pulse of current evokes a phase shift both in cell 28 and in a motor neuron (activity of the motor neuron monitors the rhythmic activity of the whole CPG).

Synaptic interactions between different identified oscillator neurons were studied with pairwise recordings. The main attention was given to the connections between cells in one hemiganglion. A typical experiment is illustrated in Fig. 3.2B: cell 28 and cell 115 exert an inhibitory action on each other. The results of such experiments are summarized in Fig. 3.2C which shows connections between oscillator neurons of one hemiganglion (Friesen 1985*a,b*, 1989*b*; Nusbaum *et al.* 1987). Most oscillator neurons are interneurons but two of them are motor neurons (cells 1 and 102). One can see from Fig. 3.2C that most connections between oscillator neurons are inhibitory.

The oscillator interneurons have axons projecting (via the lateral connectives) either rostrally or caudally. The identified interganglionic connections, some of which extend processes for at least five segments (Friesen *et al.* 1978; Poon *et al.* 1978; Friesen 1985*b*) are largely similar to intraganglionic connections (Fig. 3.2E). For example, cell 27 inhibits cell 28 both in its own ganglion (Fig. 3.2C) and in more rostral ganglia (Fig. 3.2E). It was also found that synaptic contacts in distant ganglia are as strong as local ones. Thus, the scheme of Fig. 3.2C may represent not only the intraganglionic connections but, with some reservations, also mutual connections in a large group of ganglia.

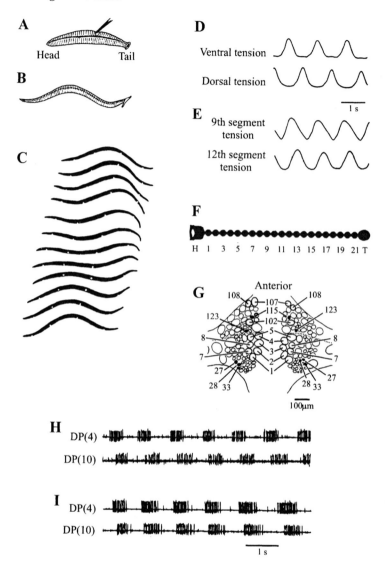

Fig. 3.1 Swimming in the leech. A,B: Mechanical stimulus evokes swimming. C: Body configuration during swimming (lateral view). The images from top to bottom are successive frames of a film taken at 40 ms intervals, of a leech swimming from right to left. One complete cycle is illustrated. D: Contractile rhythm of the ventral and dorsal body wall of a segment during a swimming episode of a partly restrained leech (muscle contraction, up). E: Contractile rhythm of the ventral body wall in the 9th and 12th segments. F: Scheme of the ventral nerve cord, with the head ganglion (H), the tail ganglion (T) and the 21 midbody ganglia. G: A midbody ganglion (dorsal view). The positions of different swim-related interneurons (black circles) and motor neurons (empty circles with numbers) are indicated. H,I: Comparison of motor firing pattern in the semi-intact preparation and in the isolated nerve cord. H: Motor neuron activity recorded from the dorsal posterior (DP) nerves (segments 4 and 10) in a nearly intact, swimming leech. I: Nearly identical activity recorded

In each ganglion, different oscillator neurons are active in different phases of the swim cycle. Figure 3.2D shows phases of maximal depolarization for nine neurons. The phases are distributed unevenly over the swim cycle, and the neurons form three distinct clusters around 20°, 140°, and 260°. Correspondingly, in the diagram of Fig. 3.2C, all oscillator neurons are arranged into three columns active at the beginning, middle, and end of the swim cycle. From Fig. 3.2C one can see that the rule for interactions among oscillator neurons is that the inhibitory interactions occur between neurons in different phase groups but not within the groups. Such a system of interactions is appropriate to prevent co-activation of neurons in different phase groups. To explain generation of oscillations in the leech swim CPG, Friesen and Stent (1977, 1978) and Friesen (1989a, 1994) suggested that excitation 'transits' in succession from one group of oscillator neurons to another one. This hypothesis is, in fact, an extension of Brown's (1911) idea of two half-centres inhibiting each other, which was discussed in relation to *Clione's* locomotor CPG (see Section 1.3). Such a model can generate oscillations with appropriate cycle periods provided the oscillator neurons have suitable 'dynamic' (synaptic and membrane) properties (synaptic fatigue, postinhibitory rebound, adaptation) ensuring a successive transition of excitation from one group of neurons to another (Friesen 1994). Another possibility is that some of the oscillator neurons are endogenous or conditional bursters generating oscillations with a frequency characteristic of swimming (Selverston 1985). In this case, connections within the oscillator circuit (Fig. 3.2C) would serve not for generation of rhythmic oscillations but for mutual phasing of different cell groups (see Section 1.3). However, the physiology of synapses and membranes of oscillator neurons remains insufficiently characterized to assess their role in generating the oscillations (Friesen 1989a).

3.3 INTERSEGMENTAL COORDINATION

From the theory of oscillators it is known that a set of independent oscillators, slightly differing in the cycle period, can be arranged in a chain so that the oscillators will have a common period (Fig. 3.3A) (Cohen *et al.* 1982; Pavlidis 1973; Stein 1976, 1977; Kopell and Ermentrout 1986, 1988). In such a chain, there are phase shifts between the cycles of neighbouring oscillators. These phase shifts depend on two main factors: (1) a difference in the 'intrinsic' cycle periods, and (2) a system of interactions between the oscillators. This model was successfully used to explain generation of the metachronal locomotor waves in different species—lamprey (Matsushima and Grillner 1990, 1992; see Section 8.3.7), frog tadpole (Roberts and Tunstall 1990; see Section 9.2.2), and crayfish (Ikeda and

---

from the same nerve cord following its isolation from the animal. A, H, and I are based on Friesen (1989a), C is from Kristan *et al.* (1988), D,E are from Kristan *et al.* (1974a), and G is based on Friesen (1989b).

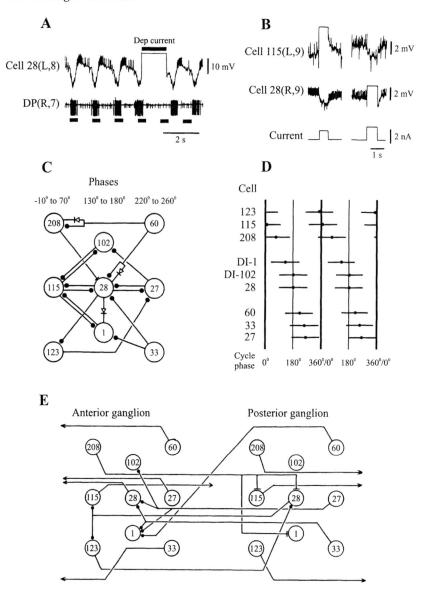

Fig. 3.2 The rhythm generator network of the swim CPG of the leech. A: Identification of the oscillator neuron (cell 28 in the 8th ganglion). Intracellular membrane potential oscillations are phase-locked to impulse bursts of motor neuron DE3, recorded in nerve DP; these bursts are diagnostic of swimming activity in the isolated nerve cord. Injection of a depolarizing current into cell 28 (marked by saturation of the amplifier) results in a shift of the cycle phases. Black bars under DP trace mark the timing of bursts extrapolated from the prestimulus burst sequence. B: Identification of connections between two oscillator interneurons (cells 115 and 28). Excitation of any single neuron in the pair by current injection results in inhibition of the other cell. C: Schematic diagram of intrasegmental interactions between most of the identified oscillator neurons. The cells are arranged into three

Wiersma 1964; Braun and Mulloney 1995; see Section 5.2). Can the leech swimming CPG be also viewed as a chain of coupled oscillators? There are arguments both for and against the application of this model to leech swimming.

An important achievement in the analysis of the leech CPG was the demonstration of the fact that smaller parts of the nerve cord can generate rhythmic oscillations. Even a single ganglion, connected to other ganglia of the nerve cord via the median connective alone, exhibits rhythmical oscillations (Weeks 1981). Through this connective, the 'isolated' ganglion receives very weak phasic input from other ganglia. Nevertheless, the ganglion can generate oscillations with a frequency characteristic of swimming (~ 1 Hz). The efferent pattern generated by a single ganglion, however, differs from that in the intact nerve cord. From this finding one can conclude that the capacity of rhythm generation is distributed over the midbody ganglia. This is a strong argument in favour of the chain-of-coupled-oscillators model. Computer simulations, based on this model, reproduced many aspects of the intersegmental coordination in the leech (Pearce and Friesen 1988).

Against this model, however, speak a number of experimental findings. First, to consider a system as a chain of *independent* coupled oscillators, one has to be sure that each of the oscillators retains some degree of independence (autonomy) when connected to other members of the network. For the leech swim CPG this is not the case, since all oscillator interneurons in each ganglion project to distant ganglia, and their synaptic contacts in distal ganglia are comparable in strength with the local ones. Therefore, each oscillator neuron receives, via the intra-ganglionic connections, only a small proportion of its synaptic input, and the main part of this input comes from other ganglia. Second, the efferent pattern generated by the isolated ganglion strongly differs from that generated by the ganglion with intact connections to adjacent ganglia. Third, the theory of coupled oscillators predicts that, in the chain of oscillators with regular connections, the 'faster' ones (i.e. those which have a shorter cycle period) will lead the 'slower' ones (see for example Matsushima and Grillner 1990, 1992). However, in the leech locomotor CPG, the situation is just the opposite, and the oscillators of the rostral ganglia (having a longer period when isolated) are phase-advanced in relation to the oscillators of the midbody ganglia which have a shorter period when isolated (Pearce and Friesen 1985a,b). These findings indicate that the segmental circuits are very strongly connected with each other over distances comparable with the whole body length and, therefore, they cannot be viewed as independent segmental oscillators. Therefore, a chain of coupled oscillators can hardly

---

columns according to their cycle phases (top). Only one member of bilateral cell pairs is shown. Filled circles indicate inhibitory interconnections, T-bars, excitatory interconnections, and diodes rectifying electrical connections. Most connections are likely to be monosynaptic. D: Cycle phases of the oscillator neurons. Two complete cycles are shown. The reference point ($0°$, cycle onset) is the midpoint of the burst in the motor neuron DE3. E: Schematic diagram of intersegmental interactions between oscillator neurons. Only interactions between neurons in adjacent ganglia are shown. Similar interactions also occur in more widely separated ganglia for some oscillator neurons, however. From Friesen (1989a).

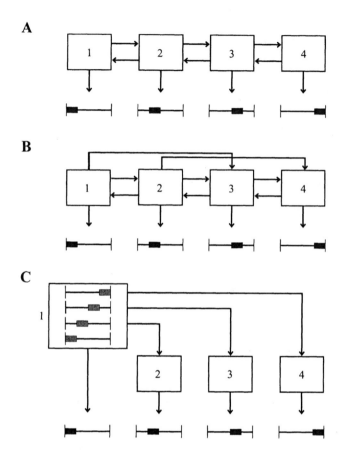

Fig. 3.3 Three different models to explain the origin of the motor pattern in the leech, with the common rhythm and with the phase shifts between segmental outputs. A: A chain of coupled oscillators with only short-distance connections. B: A chain of oscillators with both short-distance and long-distance connections. C: A model containing a single oscillator with numerous phase-shifted outputs.

be regarded as an adequate model for explanation of the coordinated rhythmic activity of the 21 ganglia in the swim CPG of the leech.

As an opposite extreme, one can consider a model containing only one oscillator, the outputs of which are distributed over the swim cycle and addressed to muscles of different segments (Fig. 3.3C). The concept of a single oscillator, formed by merging of segmental oscillators, has been discussed in relation to the spinal CPG for stepping (Grillner 1981) and scratching movements (Deliagina *et al.* 1983) (see Section 11.2). In this model, the distribution of efferent outputs over the locomotor cycle is not caused by the delays between successive oscillators but is centrally programmed in the form of long-distance connections. An intermediate between these two extremes is the model with both short-distance and long-distance connections (Fig. 3.3B) (see also Section 8.3.7). For the leech, this model is supported by the principal experimental finding that the major part of the synaptic drive to the oscillatory segmental neurons comes from other ganglia, including remote ones. No quantitative analysis of the latter two models has been reported, however.

3.4 OUTPUT MOTOR STAGE

The dorsal and ventral longitudinal muscles, the contractions of which evoke body undulations of the swimming leech, are controlled by around 20 motor neurons found in each midbody ganglion (Ort *et al.* 1974). Stuart (1970) has identified two classes of leech motor neurons: excitors and inhibitors, eliciting EPSP and IPSP, respectively, in the muscle fibres. The activity of the inhibitors can counteract the effect of the excitors innervating the same fibres, since in leech muscles, as in crustacea, the tension developed depends on the level of depolarization produced by summation of all inputs. Thus, there are four major groups of motor neurons: excitatory and inhibitory motor neurons of the ventral longitudinal muscles (VE and VI), as well as excitatory and inhibitory motor neurons of the dorsal longitudinal muscles (DE and DI). During swimming, the membrane potential of the motor neurons in these four groups oscillates, and the cells fire bursts of action potentials in a certain phase of the swim cycle (Fig. 3.4A). These are well seen in the peripheral nerves. As shown in Fig. 3.4B, the DE and VI cells are active preferentially, but not exclusively, in the dorsal phase of the swim cycle, whereas VE and DE cells are active in the ventral phase (Ort *et al.* 1974; Friesen 1989*b*,*c*).

Three factors determine the pattern of activity of individual motor neurons— input from the rhythm generator interneurons, mutual interactions between the motor neurons, and specific properties of their membrane. Connections between the oscillatory interneurons and motor neurons in the leech are extremely complex (Poon *et al.* 1978; Granzow and Kristan 1986). Figure 3.4D shows connections from four oscillator interneurons (cells 27, 28, 33, and 123) to the motor neurons. Excitatory connections lead from oscillatory interneurons to both excitatory and inhibitory motor neurons, whereas inhibitory connections lead to only the inhibitory motor neurons. The excitatory motor neurons receive their phasic inhibitory input from the inhibitory motor neurons. This is shown in Fig. 3.4C, which represents a summary of interconnections within the output motor stage. Motor neurons receive inputs both from their own and adjacent ganglia. Thus, the output motor stage of the swim CPG in the leech contributes considerably to the transformation of the rhythm generator output and to formation of the efferent motor pattern.

3.5 COMMAND SYSTEMS

3.5.1 Initiation of swimming

The command system for initiating swimming in the leech has been characterized to a considerable extent. Swimming activity can be elicited in the leech by a wide

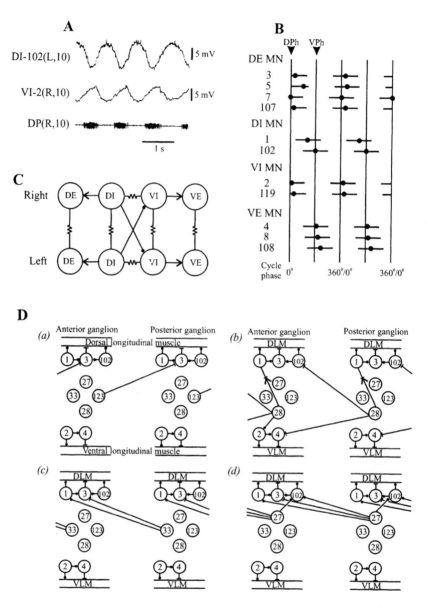

Fig. 3.4 The output motor stage of the swim CPG of the leech. A: Activity of different types of motor neurons from the 10th segment. Intracellular recording of the dorsal inhibitor (DI) and ventral inhibitor (VI), as well as extracellular recording of the dorsal excitor DE3 (in DP nerve). B: Phases of activity of swim motor neurons. The reference point (0°, cycle onset) was obtained from DP records. C: Summary of interactions among swim motor neurons within each midbody ganglion. Symbols (in C and D): resistor, electrical coupling; T-bar, excitatory synapse; filled circle, inhibitory synapse. D: Summary diagram of the direct output of oscillator interneurons (cells 123, 28 33, and 27). A–C are from Friesen (1989b), D is from Poon *et al.* (1978).

variety of natural stimuli, including tactile and noxious stimulation of the skin and water wave vibration (Muller *et al.* 1981; Young *et al.* 1981; Brodfuehrer and Friesen 1984; Debski and Friesen 1987). In the isolated nerve cord, swimming episodes can be evoked by electrical stimulation of a peripheral nerve or by mechanical stimulation of a body wall flap connected by nerves with corresponding ganglia.

Three classes of mechanoreceptors in the leech skin were described by Nicholls and Baylor (1968): the touch (T) cells, the pressure (P) cells, and the nociceptive (N) cells. Each midbody hemiganglion contains three T cells, two P cells, and two N cells. Stimulation of any individual N or P cell, or simultaneous stimulation of two T cells evokes swimming activity in the whole nerve cord (Debski and Friesen 1987).

Initiation of swimming is controlled by two parallel pathways emanating from the head ganglion (see Fig. 3.5F) (Brodfuehrer and Burns 1995). They exert opposite effects on the segmental swim-generating network. A few types of swim-activating ('trigger') neurons were identified in the head ganglion; the most thoroughly investigated of them is the pair of cells Tr1 (Brodfuehrer and Friesen 1986*a–c*). The cell body of these neurons is located in the sub-oesophageal ganglion, and the axon projects to most, if not all, midbody ganglia (Fig. 3.5A). Neurons Tr1 receive excitatory input mainly from N but also from T and P sensory cells located both in the head ganglion and in the midbody ganglia. Figure 3.5B shows that electrical stimulation of a peripheral nerve (which contains axons of sensory cells) results in excitation of Tr1 and in initiation of a swim sequence in the isolated nerve cord. In its turn, excitation of Tr1 (by intracellular current injection) also elicits locomotor activity (Fig. 3.5C). Even a brief burst induced in a trigger neuron is sufficient to evoke a long-lasting episode of swimming. Besides Tr1, there are three other pairs of neurons in the sub-oesophageal ganglion with a trigger function. Cells Tr3 and SE1 can initiate swimming (Brodfuehrer and Friesen 1986*a–c*; Brodfuehrer *et al.* 1995*b*), whereas cells Tr2, when excited, may also terminate an ongoing swim sequence (O'Gara and Friesen 1995).

An essential role in the transformation of a short-lasting activity of the cells Tr1 into the long-lasting excitatory drive to the segmental CPG is played by 'gating' neurons (Cells 204 and 205) (Weeks and Kristan 1978; Weeks 1982*a,c*). These unpaired cells were found in most midbody ganglia. Their axons project for long distances both anteriorly and posteriorly (cell 204) or only anteriorly (cell 205). Cells 204 are more efficient in eliciting swimming. During swim episodes initiated by any means—stimulation of a peripheral nerve or activation of trigger neurons—all 204 cells in the nerve cord are activated (Fig. 3.5C). Activation of any 204 cell by intracellular current injection is in turn sufficient to initiate and maintain the swim motor pattern in the isolated nerve cord, or swimming behaviour in the semi-intact leech (Fig. 3.5D). When excited by input from Tr1, cell 204 remains depolarized and fires throughout the swim episode (Fig. 3.5E).

Pressure ejection of L-glutamate onto a segmental ganglion evokes a long-lasting depolarization of a cell 204, very similar to that evoked by the cell Tr1.

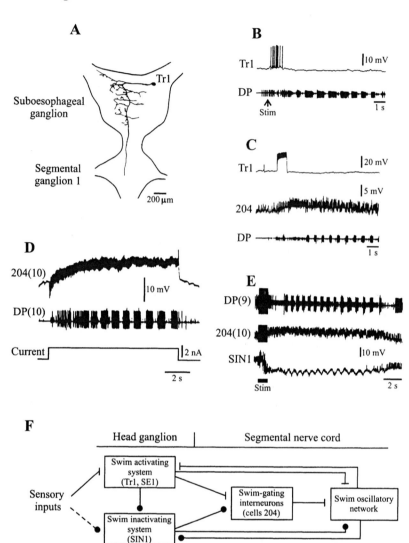

Fig. 3.5 Command system for initiating swimming in the leech. A: Morphology of a trigger cell Tr1. B: Strong mechanical stimulation of a body wall flap (arrow) elicits a burst of spikes in cell Tr1 and swimming activity (monitored by the motor neuron discharges in DP nerve). C: Swimming activity (DP trace) elicited by a brief depolarization of the cell Tr1 with current pulse. The gating neuron (cell 204) is depolarized and intensively firing in response to the Tr1 burst. D: Swim initiation and maintenance by cell 204. The swim sequence was evoked by a long-lasting depolarizing pulse injection into cell 204. E: The gating neuron (cell 204) and the swim inhibitor (SIN1) exhibit different patterns of response to the swim-initiating input (stimulation of DP nerve): cell 204 is depolarized while SIN1 is hyperpolarized throughout the swim episode. F: Summary diagram illustrating interactions between the swim-activating and swim-inactivating systems. A–D are from Friesen (1989a), E,F are from Brodfuehrer and Burns (1995).

This suggested to Brodfuehrer and Cohen (1990), and Brodfuehrer *et al.* (1995*a*) that the transformation of a short-lasting synaptic input from the cell Tr1 into a long-lasting depolarization of the 204 cells occurs due to a specific response of the 204 cell membrane to the release of glutamate by the cell Tr1. The mechanism of this response is currently unknown, however.

The gating neurons (cells 204 and 205) evoke swimming due to their numerous direct excitatory connections with oscillator neurons (cells 28, 115, and 208) in their own and other ganglia (Nusbaum *et al.* 1987; Weeks 1982*a*,*b*). During swimming, the gating neurons exhibit some rhythmical modulation due to the feedback from the swim CPG (Fig. 3.5E). The functional significance of this modulation remains unclear (Kristan and Weeks 1983; Weeks 1981). Besides cells 204 and 205, two pairs of neurons with a command function were identified in midbody ganglia—serotonin-containing cells 21 and 61 (Nusbaum and Kristan 1986). These cells exert a powerful excitatory action on the rhythm generator neurons (Nusbaum 1986).

In the nerve cord consisting of only the isolated segmental ganglia, electrical stimulation of a peripheral nerve or intracellular depolarization of a segmental swim-gating interneuron (cell 204) both elicit swimming with nearly 100 per cent efficacy (Brodfuehrer and Fiesen 1986*d*; Weeks and Kristan 1978). When the head ganglion is connected to the segmental nerve cord, these stimuli become much less efficient, which indicates the existence of inhibitory influences from the head ganglion upon the swim-initiating system. A pair of swim inhibitory neurons (SIN1) with long descending axons was also recently identified in the head ganglion (Brodfuehrer and Burns 1995). When a swim sequence is elicited by stimulation of a peripheral nerve, the SIN1 is hyperpolarized and its spike discharges are inhibited, in contrast to the gating cell 204 which is depolarized and excited (Fig. 3.5E). A directly driven activity in SIN1 results in inhibition of cell 204 and termination of swimming. Thus, SIN1s are the members of a swim-inactivating system (Fig. 3.5F). Whether swimming occurs in response to a particular stimulus depends upon the extent to which the swim-activating system is excited and the swim-inactivating system is inhibited. A similar organization of the locomotor-initiating system, with two parallel pathways that have opposite (excitatory and inhibitory) effects on the locomotor CPG, has been demonstrated in *Clione* (see Section 1.2.1) and the locust (Kien 1990).

The trigger neurons (Tr1, SE1), the gating neurons (204), and the swim inhibitors (SIN1), which constitute the command (swim initiating) system in the leech, are also members of the system making the decision to swim. Moreover, they are components of the more general behavioural choice system. Stimulation of the skin may elicit different behaviours in the leech: body shortening, crawling, and swimming. Experiments of Kristan *et al.* (1988) have shown that the choice between the three possible responses to a given sensory stimulus depends on the value of membrane potential in the cells 204. By driving this value, an experimenter may affect the choice of behavioural response.

3.5.2 Integration of locomotion in feeding behaviour

Behaviours of hungry and satiated leeches are very different (Sawyer 1981). Hungry leeches exhibit alert postures, waving of the body and other exploratory movements including swimming towards the source of the surface water waves. In contrast, satiated leeches are much less active and weakly respond to sensory stimuli. An important role in initiating the feeding behaviour is played by the monoamine serotonin (5-hydroxythryptamine, 5-HT) which can act both as a neurohormone and as an ordinary neurotransmitter in the leech CNS (Nusbaum and Kristan 1986). Four lines of evidence suggest that serotonin is a humoral modulator involved in the integration of locomotion into the feeding behaviour. First, hungry leeches have a higher concentration of serotonin in their blood and nervous system than satiated animals (Lent and Dickinson 1984; Lent *et al.* 1991). Second, the levels of endogenous serotonin in leech blood are positively correlated with the tendency of the animals to swim: with an increase of concentration from 17 to 72 nM, the relative duration of the episodes of spontaneous swimming increases from 1.5 to 42 per cent (Willard 1981). Third, exposure of intact leeches or isolated nerve cords to serotonin increases the frequency with which swimming episodes occur, as well as decreases the latency of swim initiation in response to sensory stimuli (Lent and Dickinson 1984). Fourth, chemically induced serotonin depletion or blockade of serotonin receptors reduces swimming activity (Glover and Kramer 1982; Hashemzadeh-Gargari and Friesen 1989; O'Gara *et al.* 1991).

Serotonin levels strongly affect the probability of swimming, but affect much less the actual performance of this motor programme. The lag between the time of serotonin elevation and the time of occurrence of swimming is also very long—minutes rather than ~1 s that it takes to produce swimming in response to sensory input. This strongly contrasts to the action of neuronal command systems for initiating locomotion in the leech (see Section 3.5.1) or in *Clione* (see Section 1.2.1), which are much faster, and which not only initiate locomotion but can also affect the 'vigour' of the rhythmic motor pattern.

One of the known sources of serotonin in the leech CNS is a pair of Retzius cells (Carretta 1988) located in each segmental ganglion. Intracellular stimulation of a single Retzius cell (for 10 min) results in an increase of the serotonin concentration in the extraganglionic fluid to a level which is sufficient to evoke locomotion (Willard 1981).

There are a number of targets for the serotonin action in the locomotor control system of the leech (Angstadt and Friesen 1993a,b; Mangan *et al.* 1994a,b). In the swim gating neuron (cell 204) serotonin evokes depolarization and spike discharges; besides, serotonin modifies membrane properties of this cell so that shorter depolarization becomes sufficient to evoke swimming. Serotonin also affects the membrane and synaptic properties of several swim-related motor neurons, facilitating oscillatory activity in the swim network.

When swimming, the leech is oriented with its dorsal side up. No organs responsible for gravity sensing have been found in the leech CNS, however. It seems likely that the postural orientation in the leech is not under control of the CNS but is rather passively caused by differences in the shapes of the dorsal and ventral surfaces, and by a shift of the centre of mass towards the ventral side.

3.6 CONCLUSIONS

1. Swimming in the leech is based on metachronal waves of body undulations. Major components of the swim control system in the leech were extensively examined at the behavioural, network, and cellular levels, and their organization and function have been understood to a considerable extent.

2. Generation of a swim motor pattern is performed by the control system distributed over the 21 homologous midbody ganglia. This system produces a multiphasic output pattern, with a phase delay between oscillations in successive ganglia. This phase delay is constant and does not depend on the frequency of undulations. Some essential features of this motor pattern—rhythmicity and phase lag—can be observed in the isolated chains of ganglia. Individual ganglia, when isolated, are able to generate rhythmical oscillations. The generator network in each individual ganglion is constituted by three groups of 'oscillator' neurons, mainly interneurons, with inhibitory interactions between the groups. No endogenous rhythmical bursting activity has been found in the oscillator neurons, and the rhythm generation is supposed to be based on interactions between the oscillatory neurons, that is on the network properties. Connections between oscillator neurons of adjacent and remote ganglia ensure the generation of a common rhythm and the phase lag between the successive ganglia. The output motor stage consists of both excitatory and inhibitory motor neurons controlling the dorsal and ventral longitudinal body muscles. Two major factors determine the efferent motor pattern—input to the motor neurons from oscillatory interneurons in their own and adjacent ganglia, and synaptic interactions between the motor neurons. Sensory feedback seems to contribute to the generation of a proper intersegmental phase lag. In the leech CPG, there is no clear-cut border between the rhythm generator and the output motor stage, since some motor neurons are also the members of the rhythm generating network.

3. Initiation of swimming is controlled by two parallel pathways emanating from the head ganglion. They integrate different sensory inputs and exert opposite, excitatory and inhibitory, effects on the segmental CPG. Swimming occurs in response to a particular stimulus if the evoked activity in the excitatory system is large enough in relation to the activity in the inhibitory system. These command systems are also a part of the behavioural choice system.

4. The nutritional status of the leech strongly affects its locomotor activity, mainly via changes in the serotonin concentration in the blood and nervous system. In hungry animals, the serotonin concentration increases, which results in activation of the command neurons for locomotion, as well as in some modifications in the locomotor CPG, facilitating its oscillatory activity.

4

Walking in the crayfish and lobster

Walking with legs is the main form of locomotion in most species of decapod Crustacea. In addition, some species, like crayfish and lobsters, can swim both forward with the swimmerets and backward with flips of the abdomen. Crustaceans have been extensively examined at the behavioural, network, and cellular levels, and the corresponding neuronal mechanisms have been understood to a considerable extent. In Chapters 4 and 5, we shall consider walking and swimming in the crayfish and lobster.

4.1 MOTOR PATTERN IN A SINGLE LEG

The lobster (Fig. 4.1A) exhibits a walking pattern characteristic of many decapods. It can walk in any direction, using all or only a subset of its ten walking legs. Each of these legs performs periodical stepping movements. The step cycle of a leg consists of two principal parts, the stance phase and the swing phase. In the stance phase, the distal part of the leg is in contact with the ground, the leg is loaded with part of the body weight and produces a force moving the animal forward. During the stance phase of forward walking, the leg gradually moves backward in relation to the body, from the anterior extreme position to the posterior extreme position, which is reflected in a change of the angle between the leg and the body (Figs. 4.1B,C). In the swing phase, the leg does not support the body; it is lifted above the ground and moves forward to be landed at the anterior extreme position. During backward walking, the reverse pattern is displayed: the leg is on the ground when it moves anteriorly, and off the ground when it moves posteriorly (Clarac and Chasserat 1986). Distal joints of a leg also perform periodical flexion—extension movements during walking; these movements are phase-linked to the movements in the proximal joints (Clarac 1977).

More than 20 muscles flex and extend the joints of the leg. The major role in forward and backward walking is played by two pairs of antagonistic muscles flexing and extending the two most proximal joints (thoracocoxal and coxobasal). The remotor muscle moves the whole leg backward whereas the promotor muscle moves it forward. The levator muscle moves the leg upward, whereas the depressor muscle moves it downward. Figure 4.1C shows the reciprocal relationships between the EMGs of muscles responsible for the movement of the leg in the horizontal plane. The EMGs were recorded together with the leg movement during forward walking: the remotor is active in the stance phase, whereas the promotor is active in the swing phase. Similar reciprocal relationships are seen between the levator and depressor muscles responsible for the movement of the leg in the vertical plane. However, phase relationships between the two pairs of muscles are different for forward and backward walking (Chrachri and Clarac 1990). During forward walking, the remotor is active in the stance phase together with the depressor, whereas the promotor is active in the swing phase together with the levator (Fig. 4.1D). When the animal walks backward remotor is active in the swing phase together with the levator, while the promotor is active in the stance phase together with the depressor (Fig. 4.1E).

The most important kinematical variables of a step cycle are the step amplitude, that is the linear or angular distance between the anterior and posterior extreme positions, and the durations of the stance and swing phases. These variables change differently with the speed of locomotion: with an increase of speed, the duration of the stance phase decreases whereas the duration of the swing phase and the amplitude of the step change only slightly (Figs. 4.1F,G). The duration of the stance phase is inversely proportional to the speed of locomotion in a wide range of speeds (Chrachri and Clarac 1990; Clarac and Chasserat 1983*a,b*). Similar relationships between the characteristics of the step cycle and the locomotor speed have been found in insects (Delcomyn 1985; Graham 1985; Pearson 1993; see Section 6.1), cats (see Section 10.1), and humans (see Section 15.1) and reflect similarities in the functional organization of the leg control system (see Section 4.6).

4.2 PHASE SHIFTS BETWEEN LEGS

When a lobster walks forward on a treadmill or on a flat, smooth surface, the two legs in one left–right pair usually move in antiphase at any speed of locomotion (Fig. 4.2A). The phase shift between adjacent ipsilateral legs is around one-quarter of the cycle (Fig. 4.2B) (Clarac and Chasserat 1983*a,b*, 1986). Due to these phase shifts, all ten legs perform stepping in a fixed order, thus forming a specific gait. Figure 4.2C shows the sequential activities of the remotor muscles of the ipsilateral legs 2–5 during forward walking. This order is reversed during backward walking. The phase relationships between the leg movements are not rigidly fixed but can change either spontaneously or due to external influences, as when the animal is walking over the complicated terrain in its natural habitat. Changes in external conditions are reflected in the signals from numerous mechanosensory organs located in the leg (see Section 4.4), and can modify both the stepping movements of individual legs and the interlimb coordination (Clarac and Chasserat 1979; Barnes 1975; Ayers and Davis 1977; Barnes *et al.* 1972). In the cases when walking conditions for different legs differ considerably, their stepping movements become almost independent. Figure 4.2D shows stepping movements of two legs during treadmill locomotion, when the left and right legs were walking over two separate belts of the treadmill which were moved initially with equal speed and subsequently with half the speed for the right belt. With such a complication of the motor task, the stepping movements persisted, but the motor pattern in the 'slower' leg was strongly modified: the amplitude decreased, and the period increased, so

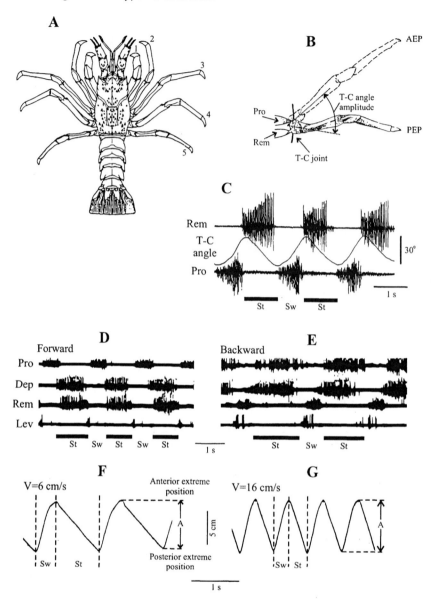

Fig. 4.1 Walking in the lobster: kinematics and EMG pattern of the leg stepping. A: The rock lobster *Jasus lalandii* (dorsal view), with its walking legs numbered (1–5). B: Drawing of the stepping leg 4 in two extreme positions, anterior (AEP) and posterior (PEP). Two antagonistic muscles (promotor, Pro, and remotor, Rem) acting on the thoraco-coxal joint (T-C) are responsible for the movement of the leg in the horizontal plane. C: Stepping movements of the leg 4 during forward walking on the treadmill, recorded together with the EMGs of the remotor and promotor muscles. The two principal parts of the step cycle, the stance phase (St) and the swing phase (Sw) are indicated. D,E: Two different patterns of activity of the leg muscles (promotor, remotor, depressor (Dep), and levator (Lev)) correspond to forward and backward walking. F,G: Leg movement at two different

that the left and right legs were stepping at different frequencies. In some cycles (indicated by arrows) the difference in step periods is so large that the 'faster' leg performs almost two steps during one step of the 'slower' leg. This finding demonstrates that each leg has its own driving mechanism (controller), which generates the rhythmical movements and possesses a relatively high degree of autonomy; the interlimb coordination is based on the interaction between the controllers of individual legs (see Section 4.6). A similar functional organization of the interlimb coordination system is observed in other walking animals, insects (see Section 6.1) and mammals (see Section 10.2).

4.3 CENTRAL PATTERN GENERATOR

The CNS of crustaceans consists of a chain of ganglia. Movements of the walking legs are controlled by the thoracic ganglia. Each of the walking legs receives its innervation from the corresponding hemiganglion, where the leg controller is located. Figure 4.3A shows three of the ganglia and the nerves supplying leg 4 of the crayfish. Each ganglion contains a few hundred neurons of which about 50 are motor neurons (Chrachri and Clarac 1989). An isolated chain of thoracic ganglia, and even a single ganglion, are able to generate a rhythmic pattern. Application of pilocarpine promotes this generation. The generated rhythm is usually slower than the rhythm of walking in intact animals. Nevertheless, the generated pattern has some important features in common with the pattern of walking (Chrachri and Clarac 1987, 1990; Sillar and Skorupski 1986; Sillar *et al.* 1986). First, there is reciprocal, alternating activity in the motor neurons of the 'horizontal' pair (promotor and remotor) and in the motor neurons of the 'vertical' pair (levator and depressor). Second, the horizontal and vertical pairs can be mutually coordinated in two different ways, corresponding to forward walking (Fig. 4.3D) or backward walking (Fig. 4.3B). Third, there is a phase shift, though not very consistent, between the ipsilateral efferent patterns generated by adjacent ganglia. From these experiments one can conclude that the thoracic ganglia contain the CPGs for individual legs which are coordinated due to mutual influences.

The structure and function of the rhythm generator for walking in crustaceans remains unclear. It seems likely that the rhythm of stepping in individual legs is produced by a special group of interneurons, some of which have been identified (Chrachri and Clarac 1989), and that these interneurons supply a rhythmical drive to the motor neurons constituting the output motor stage. A small proportion of the motor neurons, however, seem to be involved in rhythmogenesis since their stimulation may affect the rhythm (Chrachri and Clarac 1990).

---

speeds of treadmill locomotion. An increase of speed results in a considerable decrease of the stance phase duration, while the swing phase and the angle amplitude (A) change only slightly. A–C, F, and G are from Clarac and Chasserat (1986), D,E are from Chrachri and Clarac (1990).

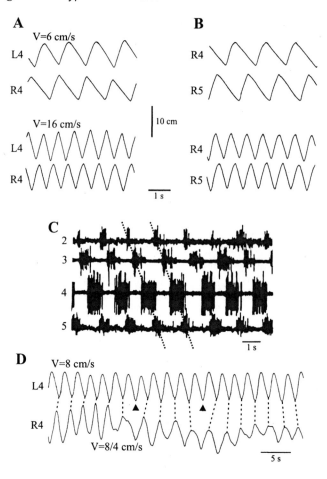

Fig. 4.2 Walking in the lobster: coordination between legs. A: Stepping movements of two symmetrical legs (L4 and R4) are phase-shifted by one half of the cycle both at low and high speeds of walking. B,C: Stepping movements of the adjacent legs (R4 and R5) are phase-shifted by about a fourth of the cycle (B). Due to this phase shift, all the legs on one side of the body are stepping in a coordinated fashion as shown by simultaneous recording from the remotor muscle of ipsilateral legs 2–5 during forward walking (C). D: Walking on the treadmill with split belts. The two symmetrical legs (L4 and R4) are stepping in anti-phase when the speeds of the two belts are equal. After a two-fold reduction of the speed of the right belt, the right leg is stepping with the rhythm differing from the rhythm of the left leg. Arrows indicate the episodes when the left leg performs almost two steps during one step cycle of the right leg. A,B, and D are from Clarac and Chasserat (1986), C is from Clarac and Chasserat (1983*a*).

4.4   SENSORY FEEDBACK

Sensory feedback plays important role in the generation of stepping movements in Crustacea. Mechanosensory information is supplied by a multitude of different

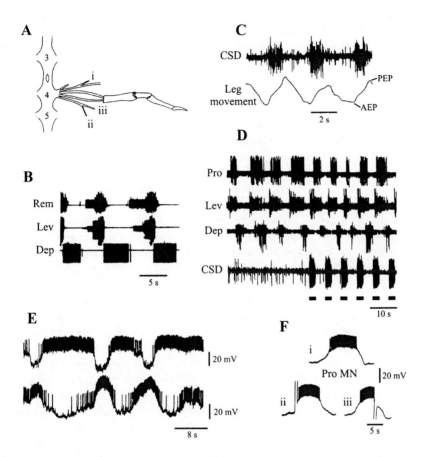

Fig. 4.3 Central and reflex contribution to the generation of stepping. A: An almost completely isolated chain of thoracic ganglia (3–5) of the crayfish that can generate fictive walking. The distal part of the leg 4 is preserved to maintain a tonic activation of the central ganglia. B: Rhythmic activity of the motor neurons in the fourth thoracic ganglion induced by a cholinergic agonist, pilocarpine (10^{-6} M). Recording of the remotor (Rem), levator (Lev), and depressor (Dep) motor neurons from the nerves designated as i–iii in A. The activity pattern corresponds to backward walking. C: Activity of afferents of a proprioceptor sensory organ, the cuticular stress detector (CSD), recorded in an intact crayfish during locomotion together with the stepping movements of the leg. D: Entrainment of the rhythm of fictive locomotion (corresponding to forward walking) by periodical stimulation of the CSD (indicated by bars). E: Anti-phase oscillations of the membrane potential in the two antagonistic motor neurons during fictive locomotion. F: Plateau properties of a leg motor neuron: (i) normal activity of the promotor motor neuron (Pro MN) in the step cycle; (ii) a burst of activity evoked by imposed brief depolarization of the neuron; (iii) termination of the burst by a hyperpolarizing pulse. A,B, and F are from Chrachri and Clarac (1987), C is based on Marchand *et al.* (1995), D is from Leibrock *et al.* (1996), and E is from Chrachri and Clarac (1990).

sense organs. These include proprioceptors such as the chordotonal joint receptors and the muscle receptor organs, and exteroceptors such as the funnel canal organs and the two cuticular stress detectors (Bush 1976; Libersat *et al.* 1987; Marchand *et al.* 1995; Mill 1976).

During walking, different mechanoreceptors are active in particular phases of the step cycle, as illustrated in Fig. 4.3C for a cuticular stress detector. This sense organ is situated in the proximal part of the walking leg, and is maximally active in the stance phase (Clarac 1976; Klärner and Barnes 1986; Marchand *et al.* 1995). Other sense organs, located in the area of the thoracocoxal and coxobasal joints, signal about different aspects of leg movement including position, angular velocity, and muscular forces (Skorupski 1992; Skorupski *et al.* 1992).

Signals delivered by mechanoreceptors affect both components of the leg CPG, that is the rhythm generator and the output motor stage. Influences upon the rhythm generator can be clearly revealed in experiments involving entraining the rhythm of the CPG by means of a periodic sensory input. Even input from a single sensory organ, the cuticular stress detector, which contains only a few afferents, is able to entrain the CPG (Fig. 4.3D) (Leibrock *et al.* 1996; see also Sillar *et al.* 1986).

Sensory influences on the output motor stage give rise to a number of segmental reflexes. Especially important for both the stance and swing phases of the step cycle is the 'resistance reflex', that is the excitation of a muscle when it is stretched (Bush 1962, 1965; Cannone and Bush 1980a,b; Wiens and Gerstein 1976). This reflex is functionally equivalent to the vertebrate stretch reflex (see Section 11.5). Due to the resistance reflex, the depressor muscle, which is active in the stance phase, will contribute to the maintenance of the body at a certain height above the ground (Grote 1981). Without this reflex, the legs would tend to dorsiflex under the weight of the body. In the swing phase of the step cycle, the role of this reflex is different: if the leg hits an obstacle (for example a stone) during its active forward movement, it will develop an additional force aimed at overcoming the resistance. The leg proprioceptors exert their influence not only on the motor neurons of the same joint but also on the motor neurons of other joints of the leg, thus promoting the formation of the functional synergy of the leg muscles (Clarac 1976, 1977; Clarac *et al.* 1978). They may also affect the nervous mechanisms of adjacent legs, thus promoting interlimb coordination (reviewed by Cruse 1990) (see Section 4.6).

The gain in the reflex pathways, that is the strength of response in motor neurons to a given sensory input, is not constant but changes over the step cycle under the effect of periodic synaptic drive from the rhythm generator. There are three sites in the locomotor network for these rhythmic modifications of the reflexes. First, the sensory afferent terminals are subjected to the phase-dependent presynaptic inhibition (Cattaert *et al.* 1990, 1992), with the underlying mechanisms similar to those described for mammals and lower vertebrates (Frank and Fuortes 1957; Kretz *et al.* 1986; Dubuc *et al.* 1988). Second, some sensory afferents affect the motor neurons not directly but through interneurons, which also receive synaptic drive from the rhythm generator. These interneurons represent a gating mechanism in the reflex pathways, and cause a phase-dependent modulation of the reflexes (Skorupski 1992; Leibrock *et al.* 1996). Third, due to a central drive, the motor neurons exhibit depolarization in one phase of the step cycle, and hyper-polarization in the opposite phase (see Fig. 4.3E). Their response to any synaptic input, including sensory input, changes proportionally to the level of depolariza-tion (Skorupski 1992; Leibrock *et al.* 1996; ElManira *et al.* 1991).

The central modulation of sensory transmission is very powerful. It may result not only in a considerable change of the value of reflex responses but, in some cases, even in a phase-dependent reversal of the sign of reflex (DiCaprio and Clarac 1981; Skorupski and Sillar 1986).

4.5   OUTPUT MOTOR STAGE

Each leg muscle is innervated by several motor neurons. Most of these are exci-tatory, but some muscles also receive an input from inhibitory motor neurons. Figure 4.3E shows the activity of two excitatory motor neurons (promotor and depressor) during fictive walking. They are depolarized and fire in one phase of the cycle, and hyperpolarized and silenced in the opposite phase (Chrachri and Clarac 1990). The inhibitory motor neurons are active in antiphase to the excitatory ones innervating the same muscle (Ballantyne and Rathmayer 1981).

The motor neurons innervating the same muscle are electrically coupled, whereas the motor neurons innervating two antagonistic muscles exert an inhibitory action on each other (Chrachri and Clarac 1989). Specific properties of the membrane of motor neurons contribute to the formation of their bursting activity. Figure 4.3F(i) shows a burst in the promotor motor neuron evoked by synaptic input from the locomotor rhythm generator. A similar burst, however, can be evoked by a brief pulse of depolarizing current injected into the neuron (ii). The burst can be terminated immediately by a hyperpolarizing pulse (iii) (Chrachri and Clarac 1987). Thus, interactions between the motor neurons, as well as plateau properties of their membrane, contribute to the transformation of input from the rhythm generator interneurons into the output motor pattern. Sensory feedback influences on the motor neurons (see Section 4.4) will further modify the efferent pattern and adapt it to the environmental conditions.

4.6   INTERACTION OF THE CENTRAL AND REFLEX MECHANISMS. FUNCTIONAL MODEL OF WALKING

4.6.1   Leg controller

Experiments on an isolated chain of thoracic ganglia have shown that the CPG for a single stepping leg produces alternating activation of the antagonistic motor neurons both in the 'horizontal' and in the 'vertical' pairs of muscles (Figs. 4.3B,D,E). This finding indicates that the CPG may perform two basic func-tions necessary for stepping: (1) formation of the muscle synergies for the stance and swing phases of a step cycle, and (2) the periodic switching from one synergy to another one. In real walking, however, leg movements must be coordinated with the movement of the animal in relation to the ground. The task of coordination of the leg CPG activity with the leg movement in relation to the body and to the ground is common for all species with pedal locomotion (Cruse 1990; Pearson 1993). The solution to this task is also similar for different species: the timing of the switch from one muscle synergy to the other one is mainly determined by sensory influences from the mechanoreceptors of the leg rather than by internal processes in the CPG. Experimental results obtained on different species have shown that the most critical point in a step cycle is the transition from the stance phase to the swing phase. This transition terminates the support function of the leg. If the animal is not supported by other legs at the moment of transition, it can fall down.

Figure 4.4 shows a functional model of the leg controller, in which the transition from the stance phase to the swing phase is determined by sensory influences on the CPG. Two parameters may influence the transition—the position of the leg and the load on the leg. Information on these parameters is contained in the afferent signals from leg proprioceptors (sensory input 1, Fig. 4.4A). These peripheral influences ensure that the leg lifts off the ground only provided (1) its position relative to the body is far enough to the rear, and (2) the load under which it stands is small enough, that is the body weight is supported by other legs.

When the leg reaches the posterior extreme position and is unloaded, the leg controller switches to the swing phase, and a new muscle synergy (promotor and levator) is activated (Fig. 4.4A). The leg is lifted above the ground and moves forward to be landed in the anterior extreme position. In this phase, the leg moves in a homogeneous medium without interaction with the ground. Therefore, many fewer sensory corrections of the central programme are needed compared with the stance phase. It remains unclear, however, to what extent the termination of the swing phase requires afference signalling that the anterior extreme position has been reached (sensory input 2, Fig. 4.4A), and to what extent the duration and amplitude of the leg movement in this phase are determined by internal processes in the CPG.

In the stance phase, the speed of backward movement of the leg in relation to the body is determined by the speed of forward movements of the body in relation to the ground. Therefore, the time needed for the leg to move from the anterior extreme position to the posterior extreme position decreases with speed. This gives an explanation of the experimental finding that the duration of the stance phase is inversely proportional to the speed of locomotion (Chrachri and Clarac 1990; Clarac and Chasserat 1983*a*,*b*). The kinematics of the leg movement in the swing phase, on the other hand, is not directly linked with the speed of locomotion.

4.6.2   Coordination between legs

The coordination of the numerous legs in the walking crayfish or lobster is achieved due to the interactions between their controllers. Mutual influences between the leg controllers were revealed in experiments where the movement of one leg was perturbed. One such experiment is illustrated in Fig. 4.4B. The crayfish was walking on the treadmill, and the backward movement of leg 4 was hampered in one of the cycles (indicated by a bar). This resulted in a disturbance of the movements in all legs. By disturbing movements of different legs in different phases of a step cycle, the influences between the legs and their dependence on the phase of the cycle have been characterized (Cruse and Müller 1986; Cruse 1990). It was found that the number of parameters of the step cycle of a single leg depend on the positions of the neighbouring legs. This is true for the timing of the transition from stance phase to swing phase, and vice versa, and for the strengths of the motor outputs in the two phases. Mutual influences between different legs are shown schematically in Figs. 4.4C–E. Between ipsilateral legs, there are both rostrally and caudally directed influences, so that each leg can both exert influences on its neighbours and be influenced by them. The rostrally directed influence (C) is active during the stance phase; it prolongs the swing phase of the anterior leg and can decrease the speed of the leg movement. The caudally directed influence (D) is active at the end of the stance phase and at the beginning of the swing phase; it promotes initiation of the stance phase of the posterior leg. The influences between symmetrical legs occur in the swing phase and in the initial part of the stance phase (E); these influences promote initiation of the stance phase.

The influences shown in Figs. 4.4C–E are aimed at restoration of normal phase relationships between legs after different disturbances of the stepping. It takes about one cycle to restore a normal phasing of ipsilateral legs after a perturbation (Fig. 4.4B). Influences between the contralateral legs are weaker, and it may take a few cycles to restore normal phasing between them. Computer simulations of coordination between the legs has shown that the influences represented schematically in Figs. 4.4C,D are sufficient for maintaining normal gait (Cruse 1983). The existence of other interactions, promoting maintenance of gait, cannot be excluded, however.

The neuronal basis of coordination between the legs is not quite clear. On one hand, the persistence of a common rhythm in all thoracic ganglia during fictive locomotion (Chrachri and Clarac 1990; Sillar and Skorupski 1986; Sillar *et al.* 1986) indicates that the controllers for individual legs have mutual central connections. On the other hand, leg proprioceptors can affect controllers of other legs either through their powerful action on the controller of the same leg or, perhaps, through specific intersegmental paths. It seems likely that both mutual central and reflex influences contribute to interleg coordination.

4.7   COMMAND NEURONS

Experiments with electrical stimulation of axons in the circum-oesophageal connectives in the crayfish revealed at least five command neurons which evoke forward walking, and four command neurons which evoke backward walking (Bowerman and Larimer 1974*a*,*b*). Each of these neurons evokes walking combined with a specific response in other motor systems: cheliped elevation or lowering, abdomen flexion or extension, and swimmeret beating. It has been suggested that different command neurons are responsible for eliciting different forms of behaviour, which involve locomotion as a major component. By combining

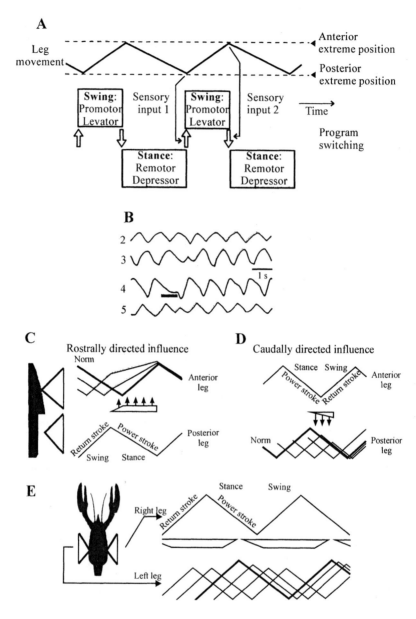

Fig. 4.4 Functional model of coordination within one leg and between legs in the crayfish. A: The single leg controller for forward walking. Sensory inputs (1 and 2) from the leg proprioceptors affect transitions between the stance phase and swing phase motor programs. B: Experiment illustrating the interleg influences. Movements of the ipsilateral legs (2–5) of the crayfish walking on the treadmill are shown (upward deflection means leg protraction). Movement of leg 4 in the stance phase of one of the cycles was hampered, which is shown by a horizontal bar. Due to the corrective movements of all the legs, normal coordination was soon restored. C,D: Two coordinating mechanisms for ipsilateral legs. Each schema is

activation of different command neurons, the animal can produce a wide reper-toire of behaviours (Larimer 1976).

4.8 CONCLUSIONS

1. During stepping in crayfish and lobster, each of the walking legs is controlled by a separate nervous mechanism, or leg controller, located in the corresponding thoracic ganglion. This mechanism generates alternating activity in two groups of leg muscles and thus controls the two principal parts of the step cycle—the swing phase and the stance phase. The muscles in each group (the muscle synergies) are different during forward and backward walking.
2. Both central mechanisms and reflex interactions are important for the gener-ation of stepping. The CPG for stepping determines which muscles should be activated together as groups in the swing and stance phases, whereas the timing of the switches between the different phases of the cycle is largely determined by signals from the leg proprioreceptors. Sensory feedback also affects the output motor stage and thus regulates the level of motor neuron activity. The afferent signals undergo phase-dependent modulation under the effect of input from the rhythm generator. One of the important mechanisms for this modulation is presynaptic inhibition of afferent terminals.
3. Interaction between the controllers for individual legs results in synchroniza-tion of their rhythms and in mutual phasing, and thus determines the gait of the walking animal.
4. The locomotor system can be activated by stimulation of command neurons. These neurons can elicit forward or backward walking in combination with activation of other motor systems, and are thus responsible for the integration of locomotion in a complex behaviour.

---

drawn as if only one of the mechanisms existed. In each case the influencing leg is drawn only once. For the influenced leg several traces are presented to show the effect of the coordinating mechanism. The thicker line shows a normal trace which does not need any corrections. The duration and intensity of the influences are roughly indicated by the length and thickness of the wedges respectively. E: Coordinating mechanism for contralateral legs. Only influences from the right leg on the left are shown. Designations as in C,D. B is from Cruse and Müller (1986); C–E are from Cruse (1990).

5

Swimming in the crayfish and lobster

5.1 SWIM MOTOR PATTERN

The swimmerets of crayfish and lobster are paired segmental limbs located on the ventral side of the abdomen (Fig. 5.1A). They normally beat metachronously when the animal swims forward, walks, or ventilates its burrow. Each cycle consists of a posteriorly directed power stroke that alternates with an anteriorly directed return stroke. The frequency of beating is 1–2 Hz. Swimmerets on each side of the same segment normally beat in phase. Swimmerets on adjacent segments do not beat in synchrony: the oscillations in each segment are delayed in relation to the neighbouring caudal segment by 10–20 per cent of the cycle duration. Due to these delays, a metachronal wave of swimmeret beating propagates anteriorly (Hughes and Wiersma 1960; Davis 1968*a,c*).

Each of the swimmerets is controlled by a separate nervous mechanism (controller) located in the corresponding abdominal hemiganglion (1–5, Fig. 5.1D). Two groups of motor neurons innervate the muscles generating the power stroke and the return stroke of a swimmeret. Each group contains at least six excitatory neurons and one inhibitory neuron (Davis 1968*a*, 1969, 1971). The excitatory neurons in one group burst alternately with the neurons supplying the antagonistic muscles. The phase relations of motor neurons at different segmental levels correspond to the phase relations of the swimmeret movements: Bursts in each segment are delayed in relation to the adjacent caudal segment by 10–20 per cent of the cycle duration.

5.2 CENTRAL PATTERN GENERATOR

An isolated chain of abdominal ganglia can generate a rhythmical efferent pattern either spontaneously, in response to application of some substances (for example neuropeptide proctolin (Mulloney *et al.* 1987)), or in response to stimulation of command neurons (see Section 5.4). The basic characteristics of this pattern are similar to those of the real swim pattern: the frequency of the rhythm is 1–2 Hz, the bursts of activity in the power stroke and the return stroke motor neurons alternate (Fig. 5.1B), the motor neurons on each side of the same segment are active in phase, and the activity in a particular segment is delayed by 150–250 ms in relation to the activity in its caudal neighbour (Fig. 5.1C) (Hughes and Wiersma 1960; Ikeda and Wiersma 1964; Davis 1969; Davis and Kennedy 1972*a*). When the pattern is evoked by stimulation of a command neuron, the basic characteristics of the pattern are established from the very first cycle of the swim sequence (Figs. 5.1B,C). One can thus conclude that the CPG for swimming determines the essential aspects of the motor pattern.

Normally, ganglion 5 leads the rhythm in the whole chain of five ganglia (Fig. 5.1C), which is shown schematically in Fig. 5.1D. This ganglion remains leading even when the excitability of the anterior ganglia (2 and 3) was increased by local application of pilocarpine (Braun and Mulloney 1995). Ikeda and Wiersma (1964) have found, however, that cutting ganglion 5 off from ganglion 4 produces no noticeable influence on the pattern generated by the anterior ganglia (1–4). In this shortened chain, ganglion 4 becomes leading. The completely isolated ganglion 5 retains its capacity to generate the rhythm (Fig. 5.1E). If the cord is transected between ganglia 3 and 4, ganglion 3 becomes leading for the anterior chain (ganglia 1–3) while ganglion 5 leads the posterior chain (ganglia 4 and 5) (Fig. 5.1F). Finally, if the cord is transected between the ganglia 2 and 3, the posterior chain (ganglia 3 and 4) is driven by ganglion 5, while the anterior chain (ganglia 1 and 2) does not generate the rhythm (Fig. 5.1G). On the basis of their experiments, Ikeda and Wiersma (1964) formulated a conceptual model of the swim CPG in the crayfish: 'A single pacemaker cell is considered to be present in each ganglion half, connected with its partner cell in the same ganglion by a side branch as well as with the next anterior ipsilateral pacemaker cell. Within this series, the pacemaker cells show a progressively diminishing excitability, to the extent that the cells of ganglia 1 and 2 fire only when triggered by the posterior pacemaker. Discharge of any of these pacemaker cells is followed almost immediately by discharge of the partner cell and, after a definite latency, by discharge of the next anterior pacemaker.'

The general idea of the functional organization of the swim CPG in the crayfish, with the caudal segments triggering their rostral neighbours, formulated by Ikeda and Wiersma (1964), was later supported by a number of studies (Davis and Kennedy 1972a; Stein 1971, 1974; Murchison *et al.* 1993; Braun and Mulloney 1995; Acevedo *et al.* 1994). These studies have shown, however, that some modification of the initial model is needed. Chrachri *et al.* (1994) have demonstrated that the interganglionic interactions occur not only between the adjacent ganglia. Figure 5.1H shows fictive swimming generated by a chain of five intact ganglia (1–5 in Fig. 5.1D). Then synaptic transmission in ganglion 4 was blocked by low-Ca^{2+} saline applied to this ganglion (Fig. 5.1J). Despite inactivation of ganglion 4, ganglion 5 appeared able to drive those rostral ganglia which remain intact. As shown in Fig. 5.1I, ganglion 2 generates rhythmical output with a delay (in relation to the output of ganglion 5) similar to that in intact chain of ganglia (Fig. 5.1H). Finally, when the cord was divided into two parts (rostral and caudal), and the parts were excited by exposure to the same concentration of charbochol, the rhythm generated by the rostral segments was faster than that from the caudal segments (Mulloney 1997), which contradicts the excitability-gradient hypothesis. Thus, an asymmetric-coupling model, including both local and distant interactions between unitary oscillators (see Section 3.3) offers a more adequate explanation of the generation of swim rhythm in the crayfish.

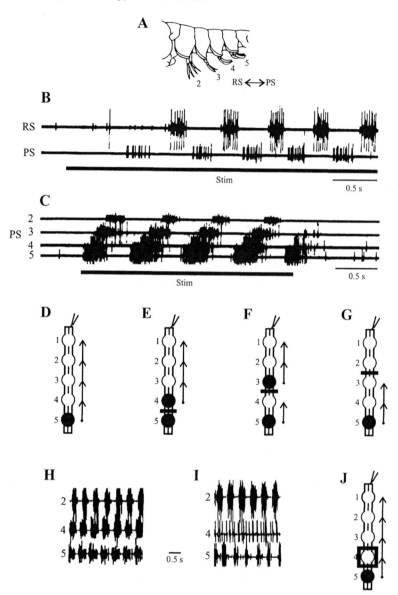

Fig. 5.1 Motor pattern for swimming in lobster and its origin. A: Metachronal wave of beating in swimmerets 5–2 (PS, power stroke; RS, return stroke). B–J: Generation of a fictive swim pattern by an isolated chain of abdominal ganglia in the lobster. B: Rhythmic motor output in the power stroke and return stroke nerves of a swimmeret, caused by stimulation (50 Hz) of a command neuron. C: Rhythmic motor output in the left power stroke nerves of ganglia 2–5, caused by stimulation of a command neuron. D–G: Schematic representation of the experiments with the nerve cord transections at different levels (indicated by bars). The leading ganglion (pacemaker) in each experiment is shown in black. Arrows indicate the sequence of activation of different ganglia in the locomotor cycle. H–J: An experiment demonstrating connections between non-neighbouring ganglia. H: Activity in the power

Extensive studies were carried out to identify the rhythm generator neurons in the abdominal ganglia. A few kinds of neurons resetting the swim rhythm have been described (Paul and Mulloney 1985, 1986; Chrachri *et al.* 1994). The idea that the motor neurons participate in rhythmogenesis (Heitler 1978, 1981) was later found to be unlikely (Sherff and Mulloney 1996). An attempt was also made to separate the rhythm generating neurons from those responsible for interganglionic coordination (Stein 1971, 1974; Paul and Mulloney 1986). Considerable efforts are still needed to characterize interneurons involved in the rhythm generation, their membrane properties, and their mutual interactions, however.

5.3 OUTPUT MOTOR STAGE AND SENSORY FEEDBACK

The power stroke and return stroke motor neurons receive a depolarizing drive from the rhythm generating interneurons in one phase of the swim cycle, and a hyperpolarizing drive in the opposite phase. As a result, the membrane potential of a motor neuron undergoes periodic oscillations with an amplitude up to 20 mV (Murchison *et al.* 1993). Electrical coupling between homonymous motor neurons (Heitler 1985) probably contributes to their in-phase firing.

Numerous proprio- and exteroceptors, located in the swimmerets, give rise to different reflexes. Local reflexes, in the form of sensory influences on swimmeret motor neurons, are much stronger than sensory influences on the rhythm generator (Heitler 1986; Miyan and Neil 1986). Figure 5.2 shows reflex modulation of the power stroke swimmeret motor neurons. Imposed movements of a swimmeret strongly affect the motor neurons, both in the corresponding segment and in the neighbouring caudal segment, but do not affect the swim rhythm. In this respect, the swimmeret system strongly differs from the walking leg system (see Section 4.4), in which afferent input may strongly affect the rhythm generator. The biological expedience of this difference is that walking legs must continuously adapt their movements to irregularities of the substratum, whereas swimmerets oscillate in a homogeneous medium, water.

5.4 COMMAND NEURONS FOR ACTIVATION OF THE SWIMMERET SYSTEM

In the crayfish and the lobster, there are at least five pairs of axons in the connectives between the thoracic and abdominal ganglia. Electrical stimulation of these axons evokes bilateral rhythmic activity in the swimmeret system (Figs. 5.1B,C) (Wiersma and Ikeda 1964; Davis and Kennedy 1972a–c). The axons can be excited by the peripheral stimuli that evoke swimming (Davis and Kennedy 1972a).

stroke nerves of ganglia 5, 4, and 2 in the control condition. I: Activity in the same nerves after blocking synaptic transmission in ganglion 4 (by means of low-Ca^{2+} saline). J: The diagram shows that ganglion 5 can directly drive the rostral ganglia, without involvement of the neuronal network of ganglion 4. B,C are from Davis and Kennedy (1972a), H,I are based on Chrachri *et al.* (1994).

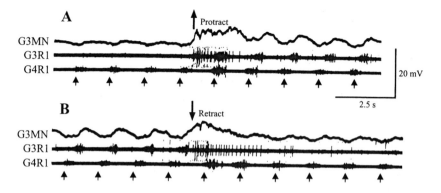

Fig. 5.2 Reflex modulation of power stroke swimmeret motor neurons. The chain of abdominal ganglia was isolated except for a single swimmeret left attached to ganglion 3. Imposed protraction (A) or retraction (B) movement of the swimmeret (marked by arrows) strongly affects the power stroke activity in ganglion 3 but only slightly affects the swim rhythm. G3MN, intracellular recording from the G3 motor neuron; G3 and G4, recordings from the R1 nerves of G3 and G4 ganglia. Small arrows indicate the onset of G4R1 activity in all cycles. From Heitler (1986).

According to these characteristics, the axons can be considered as the axons of command interneurons responsible for initiation of swimmeret swimming.

Detailed study of the command neurons in the lobster (Davis and Kennedy 1972*a–c*) have shown that they are not functionally equivalent but that the swimmeret beating they can elicit differs both in frequency range and in the relative amplitude of the strokes of different swimmerets. Individually, no single command neuron can elicit the full range of normal behaviour. Simultaneous activation of two command neurons can produce the full range of efferent output seen in intact lobsters, however. One can thus suggest that, under normal conditions, not a single but a group of command neurons is activated to elicit swimming.

Swimmeret beating is usually associated with an extended position of the abdomen. A few abdominal interneurons have been identified which simultaneously affect both motor systems and seem to coordinate their activities (Chrachri and Neil 1993).

5.5   CONTROL OF BODY ORIENTATION

In the crayfish and lobster, leg proprioreceptive reflexes, and the resistance reflex in particular (see Section 4.4), contribute to stabilization of body orientation during walking via modifications of the stepping leg movements (see Section 4.6). The leg movements can also be modified under the effect of input from the statocysts (Neil 1985; Murayama and Takahata 1996).

Another group of reflexes, driven by input from the statocysts, include corrective movements of the abdomen and of the tail appendages (uropods), as well as a change of the intensity and direction of swimmeret beating (Davis 1968*b*; Knox and Neil 1991; Neil and Miyan 1986; Yoshino *et al.* 1980; Newland and Neil

1987). These gravistatic reflexes in the lobster are illustrated in Fig. 5.3. During forward walking, the abdomen is partly flexed (Fig. 5.3A). If the animal is held in midwater with its legs out of contact with the substratum, the configuration of the abdomen depends on the inclination of the animal in the pitch plane: head-down tilt evokes extension of the abdomen (Fig. 5.3B) accompanied by closing of the uropods (Fig. 5.3C), whereas head-up tilt evokes flexion of the abdomen (Fig. 5.3B) accompanied by opening of the uropods (Fig. 5.3D). Due to these gravitational reflexes, the animal will rapidly assume the normal, back-up, orientation when released with different body orientations in midwater (Fig. 5.3F).

Roll tilt evokes extension of the abdomen, as well as a number of asymmetrical postural corrective responses. They include opening of the uropod on the side moving downward and closing of the uropod on the opposite side (Fig. 5.3E). In addition, swimmerets on the side moving upward are activated with a considerable lateral component in their power stroke, whereas the swimmerets on the opposite side are inhibited (Figs. 5.3E,G). These motor responses produce a torque around the longitudinal axis of the animal, which results in restoration of the normal, dorsal-side-up, body orientation.

Some of the neuronal mechanisms responsible for postural control in the lobster and crayfish have been investigated. It was found that the superficial extensor and flexor motor neurons, which innervate postural muscles of the decapod tail, can be driven by stimulating specific descending command fibres (Evoy and Kennedy 1967; Kennedy et al. 1966, 1967; Thompson and Page 1982). Some of these fibres control not only the abdominal posture but also the swimmeret activity (Evoy and Kennedy 1967; Williams and Larimer 1981). A strong coupling between these two motor systems of the crayfish abdomen was demonstrated by Chrachri et al. (1994).

In addition to the descending command neurons, a few classes of interneurons have been found in the abdominal ganglia of the lobster ('postural interneurons') the stimulation of which evokes a bilateral flexion response, an extension response, or an inhibitory response (Jones and Page 1986a–c). It remains unclear, however, how these postural interneurons interact with the descending command neurons and how they respond to input from the statocysts.

The gravitational reflexes in the uropods of the crayfish have been analysed in considerable detail by Takahata and his colleagues. The uropod control system is driven by input from two statocysts. Each statocyst consists of a cavity, with about a hundred hair cells aligned in a crescent shape on the statocyst floor (Fig. 5.4A). Under the effect of the statolith, some of the cilia are bent, which results in activation of the corresponding statocyst receptor cells. Axons of these cells form the statocyst nerve. Takahata and Hisada (1979) recorded responses in individual sensory cell axons to deflecting a corresponding statocyst hair in various directions. Figure 5.4A shows the functional polarization, that is the direction of maximal response, for various receptor cells. The response is proportional to the amplitude of the displacement of the hair (Fig. 5.4B). This study suggested that the direction of tilting of the animal is coded in the form of the topographical specification of the excited receptors of the statocyst, that is based on the same principle as coding of information in the statocyst of molluscs (see Section 1.6).

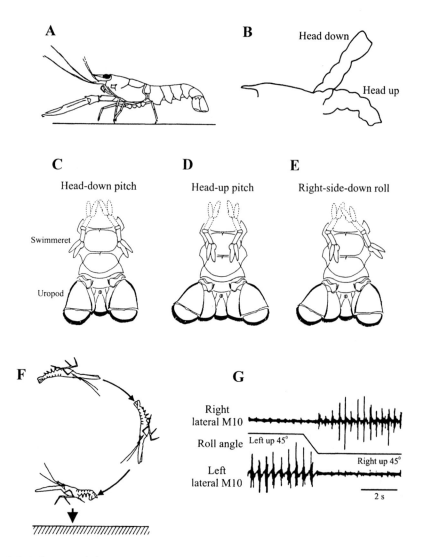

Fig. 5.3 Behavioural characteristics of the postural control in the lobster. A: Posture during forward walking. B: Extension and flexion of the abdomen in relation to thorax in response to head-up (30°) and head down (20°) tilt in the sagittal plane. The animal was suspended in midwater. C–E: Ventral views of the abdomen showing the responses of the swimmerets and uropods to body tilts in different vertical planes: head-down pitch (C), head-up pitch (D), and right-side-down roll (E). F: Schematic representation of the pitch righting response of an animal released from an inverted position in the water column. It turns head-down through a full half-circle before descending to the bottom in an upright position. G: Records of activity from homologous muscles (lateral M10) of the right and left swimmerets during body tilt. Tilting the left side down terminates the beating of the left swimmeret and initiates beating of the right swimmeret. A–E are from Knox and Neil (1991), F is from Newland and Neil (1987), and G is from Neil and Miyan (1986).

Influences from the statocysts on the abdominal postural mechanisms are mediated by four pairs of descending command interneurons ('statocyst interneurons') (Takahata and Hisada 1982a,b): interneuron C_1 responds, both dynamically and statically, to head-up and same-side-down tilting of the body (Figs. 5.4C,D); C_2 responds dynamically to head-up and head-down tilting, as well as same-side-down tilting; I_2 responds both dynamically and statically to head-down and same-side-up tilting; finally, I_1 responds dynamically to tilting in any direction. Collectively, these interneurons supply the abdominal postural mechanisms with specific information about orientation of the animal in space, about transition from one orientation to another, as well as with unspecific signals to initiate movements.

Figures 5.4E–H show the functional connections between the statocyst receptors and the statocyst interneurons deduced from the directional sensitivity of both statocyst receptors and statocyst interneurons, as well as from experiments with partial or total ablation of the statocyst. These connections are polysynaptic.

The statocyst interneurons affect the uropod motor neurons and thus evoke gravitational reflexes. Responses to roll tilt in the uropod motor neurons were analysed by Takahata *et al.* (1985). It was found that the uropod opener motor neurons are activated on the elevated side whereas the antagonistic closer motor neurons are inhibited (Figs. 5.4I,J).

Figure 5.4K shows the functional connections between different type of statocyst interneurons and uropod motor neurons. These connections were deduced from the results of cord hemisection experiments and experiments with unilateral statocyst ablation. The diagram, together with that showing the statocyst-interneuron connections (Figs. 5.4E–H), characterizes interactions of all principal components in the uropod postural system of the crayfish.

The functioning of the uropod postural system in the crayfish is tightly linked with the activity of the abdominal postural mechanisms. Abdomen extension is associated with a subthreshold depolarization of the uropod motor neurons, which is a necessary prerequisite for their response to descending gravitational input (Takahata and Hisada 1986a). This depolarization is caused by a special group of non-spiking interneurons (Takahata and Hisada 1986b). Functioning of the uropod postural system is also linked with the activity of the leg locomotor system: with activation of this system, gravitational responses of the uropods may change and, under some conditions, even reverse (Murayama and Takahata 1996).

5.6 CONCLUSIONS

1. Forward swimming is based on rhythmical oscillations of several pairs of swimmerets, with a metachronal wave propagating rostrally. A controller for each swimmeret periodically activates two antagonistic groups of muscles. The generation of this pattern is performed, to a large extent, by a CPG located in the corresponding abdominal ganglion. The structure and functioning of the CPG remains unclear. Sensory feedback is of minor importance for the rhythm generation but is essential for the control of the amplitude of oscillations.

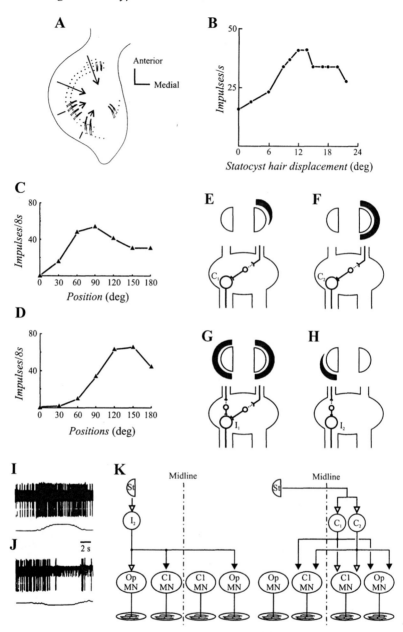

Fig. 5.4 Gravitational reflexes in the crayfish. A: Directions of functional polarization of statocyst receptors located in four representative regions of the crescent. B: Responses (average frequency) of a tonic-type receptor to the stepwise deflection of the specific statocyst hair toward centre of the crescent. C,D: Responses (average frequency) of interneuron C_1 to body tilt in the pitch (C) and roll (D) planes. E–H: Functional connections between the statocyst receptors and four statocyst interneurons (C_1, C_2, I_1, I_2). A pair of semicircles indicates a pair of statocysts. The region of the crescent to which the interneuron connects is indicated in black. I,J: Activity of the uropod closer neurons in response to body rolling with ipsi-side down (I) and contra-side down (J). K: Functional connections between

2. The propagation of the wave of swimmeret beating in the anterior direction is based on the fact that the more posterior segments exert triggering of their anterior neighbours. The most posterior segment thus plays the role of a pacemaker.

3. Activation of the swimmeret system is performed by a few pairs of identified command neurons.

4. Equilibrium control during swimming is governed, to a large extent, by input from the statocysts. Deviation from the dorsal-side-up, horizontal orientation evokes movements of the tail and modulation of the swimmeret beating. The reflex chain includes the statocyst receptor cells, the command neurons with long descending axons (statocyst interneurons), and the abdominal inter- and motor neurons.

a single statocyst and the uropod motor neurons mediated by a set of statocyst interneurons. The ipsilateral pathway is shown on the left and the contralateral one on the right. White and black triangles represent the excitatory and inhibitory connections respectively. A,B are based on Takahata and Hisada (1979), C,D are based on Takahata and Hisada (1982*a*), E–H are from Takahata and Hisada (1982*b*), and I–K are from Takahata *et al.* (1985).

6

Walking in the stick insect and locust

To walk with their six legs is the main form of land locomotion in most insects. Most of the information available on the nervous control of walking in insects has been obtained from three animal models—the stick insect, the locust, and the cockroach. The numerous studies on these models have been reviewed in detail by Graham (1985), Gewecke and Wendler (1985), Bässler (1983), Pearson (1993), and recently by Burrows (1986), Bässler and Büschges (1998). The goal of the present chapter is not to present a detailed review of the field but rather to highlight how the studies of walking in two animal models (the stick insect and locust) have increased our understanding of basic principles of locomotor control.

6.1 MOTOR PATTERN

The insect leg consists of five segments: the coxa, the trochanter, the femor, the tibia, and the tarsus (Figs. 6.1A$_1$,A$_2$). Femor and trochanter are sometimes fused into one segment. Insects can walk both forward and backward. The basic pattern of stepping in insects (Figs. 6.1A$_1$,A$_2$) is similar to that in crustaceans (see Section 4.1). A step cycle consists of two parts—the swing phase and the stance phase. When the animal is walking forward (Fig. 6.1B), the distal part of the leg (tarsus) is on the ground during the stance phase. The leg is loaded by a part of the body weight and develops a force pushing the animal forward. In this phase, the leg gradually moves from the anterior extreme position to the posterior extreme position. During swing, the leg is lifted above the ground and moves forward to be landed at the anterior extreme position.

As in Crustacea, the increase of the locomotor speed in insects is primarily caused by the faster movement of the leg relative the body during the stance phase; an increase of the step amplitude plays a secondary role. As a result, the stance duration and, consequently, the cycle duration decrease as the speed increases. The swing duration is a more constant part of the step cycle (Fig. 6.1C).

About 20 muscles move the leg segments. Movement of the whole leg in relation to the body is due to the contraction of muscles affecting the proximal joints (thoraco-coxal, coxo-trochantal, and trochanto-femoral). According to the net motor effect, these muscles can be divided into two pairs of antagonistic

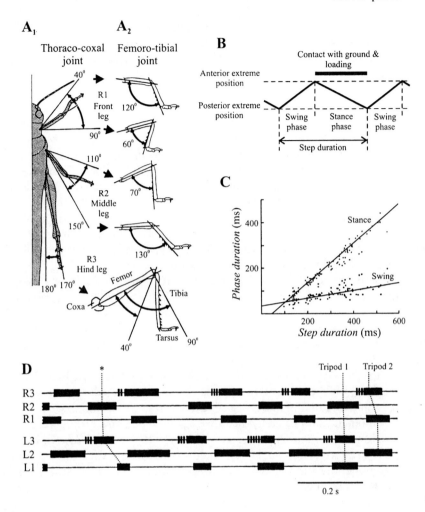

Fig. 6.1 Leg movements of a locust during walking. A_1: Dorsal view of a locust to show the limiting values of the femur–thorax angles. A_2: The limiting tibia–femur angles, corresponding to each of the femur–coxa angles (shown in A_1). B: Main characteristics of the step cycle of an individual leg. C: Duration of the two components of the step cycle (stance and swing) plotted against the step cycle duration. D: Diagram of the tripod gait used when walking. The black bars indicate the time when the leg is off the ground (swing phase); the thin lines show periods of contact with the ground (stance phase), and the broken bars show when the tarsus is dragged on the ground. Spontaneous distortion of the tripod gait is indicated by an asterisk. From Burns (1973).

groups: the protractor and retractor muscles are responsible for excursions of the leg along the rostro-caudal axis; the levator and depressor muscles are responsible for movements along the dorso-ventral axis. A pair of antagonistic muscles affecting the femoro-tibial joint produces flexion and extension of this joint; these movements are phase-linked with movements at the proximal joints (Figs. 6.1A_1,A_2).

The leg controllers are located in the thoracic chain of ganglia. The front legs are controlled by the prothoracic ganglion, the middle legs by the mesathoracic ganglion, and the hind legs by the metathoracic ganglion (Figs. 6.2A,B). Each ganglion contains about 2000 nerve cells, of which about one-tenth of the cells are motor neurons, others are premotor (local) interneurons, intersegmental interneurons, sensory neurons, etc.

Each of the leg muscles is controlled by a small number (up to 10–18) excitatory motor neurons. There are also a few inhibitory motor neurons, each supplying several muscles. The excitatory motor neurons supplying two antagonistic muscles of a joint are typically active in antiphase (Figs. 6.2C,D) in all investigated species (Hoyle 1964; Pearson 1972; Burns and Usherwood 1979; Graham and Wendler 1981; Bässler 1983). Recording from the muscles affecting different joints has shown that the efferent motor pattern of stepping, as a first approximation, can be considered as alternating activities of two groups of muscles, constituting the swing muscle synergy and the stance muscle synergy. These two synergies differ for the forward and backward stepping, as in Crustacea (see Section 4.1). In reality, however, the phase relationships between the antagonistic muscles may slightly differ from the simple alternation; these relationships may vary spontaneously or under the effect of sensory inputs. This is illustrated in Figs. 6.2E,F for two leg muscles (femor protractor and tibia flexor) that were active in antiphase during normal walking (E) but became partly co-active during upside-down walking (F) (Duch and Pflüger 1995).

The most typical gait in insects is the alternating tripod gait in which the front and the hind legs on one side and the middle leg on the other side move together in antiphase with the remaining three legs. During stable tripod walking the body is thus, at any moment, supported by the three legs contacting the ground (Fig. 6.1D) which secures postural stability (Graham 1972, 1985; Burns 1973). Gaits other than tripods are rare (Graham 1978). Interestingly, in the stick insect, the gait changes with age: the tripod gait is observed in younger animals, whereas adult animals use a tetrapod gait (Graham 1972).

None of the investigated insects maintain constant interleg phase relationships even during walking on a smooth terrain. For example, in the grasshopper and locust, spontaneous fluctuations of the interleg phase shifts constitute, on average, 0.1–0.15 of the cycle (Burns 1973). Because of these fluctuations, a tripod support may sometimes alternate with a tetrapod support (Fig. 6.1D). The flexibility of the interleg coordination system allows insects to better adapt to irregularities of the substrate.

6.2   CENTRAL PATTERN GENERATOR

Spontaneous generation of slow rhythms in the isolated or deafferented chain of thoracic ganglia is a rare phenomenon in all investigated species. Rhythmic activity can be elicited in a chain of ganglia or even in a single ganglion, however, by applying the muscarinic cholinergic agonist pilocarpine (Büschges *et al.* 1995;

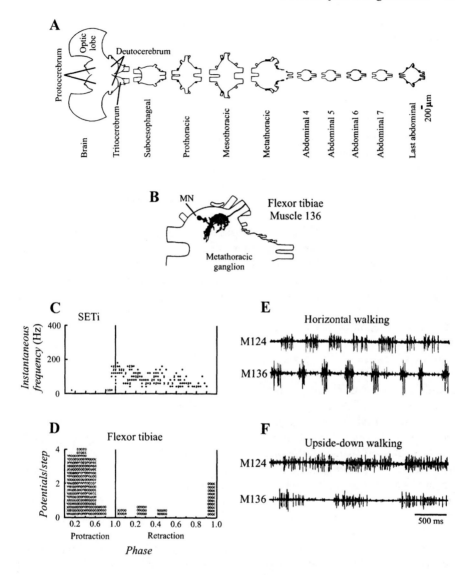

Fig. 6.2 Generation of the efferent motor pattern for stepping. A: General structure of the locust CNS. The legs are controlled by three thoracic ganglia. B: Morphology of the motor neuron in the metathoracic ganglion projecting to muscle 136 (tibiae flexor). C,D: Activity of antagonistic motor neurons controlling the tibia–femur joint of the hind leg as a function of the phase of the step cycle. C: Instantaneous frequency of discharges of the extensor motor neuron (SETi). D: Histogram of discharges of a group of flexor motor neurons. E,F: Activity of motor units in the posterior femur rotator muscle (M124) and in the flexor tibiae muscle (M136) during horizontal walking (E) and during upside-down walking (F). A and B are from Burrows (1996), C and D are from Burns and Usherwood (1979), and E and F are from Duch and Pflüger (1995).

Ryckebusch and Laurent 1993). This has also been shown for crustaceans (see Section 4.3).

6.2.1 Motor output to one leg

The rhythmic activity generated in the absence of sensory feedback has a number of similarities to patterns of neural and muscular activity recorded during walking. First, the bursts in the antagonistic motor neuron pools of a given joint alternate (Fig. 6.3A). Second, the bursts in the swing phase motor neurons usually are shorter and more constant in duration than those in the stance phase motor neurons (Figs. 6.3A,B) (Bässler and Wegner 1983; Büschges *et al.* 1995; Pearson and Illes 1970). Third, in the locust and cockroach, the motor outputs to different joints of an individual leg are coordinated so that the swing motor neuron pools are active in phase with each other; the stance motor neuron pools are also co-active (Pearson 1972; Pearson and Illes 1970; Ryckebusch and Laurent 1993). One can thus conclude that each of the six legs is controlled by its own CPG; the CPG produces alternating activation of the two muscle synergies for the swing and stance phases of the step cycle. In this respect, the function of the CPG for an individual leg in the cockroach and locust is similar to that in crustaceans (see Section 4.3).

In the stick insect (Fig. 6.3E), in contrast to the locust and cockroach, the centrally generated motor outputs to different joints of a leg are poorly coordinated. Usually they have different rhythms (Fig. 6.3C) but in some cycles a tendency of synchronization of the motor outputs can be observed (Fig. 6.3D), with different patterns of mutual phasing that correspond either to forward or backward walking (Büschges *et al.* 1995). This finding strongly suggests that each joint has its own central oscillator, and the oscillators of different joints affect each other. In the absence of sensory feedback, however, these mutual influences between the oscillators are not sufficient for their normal coordination.

Figure 6.4 illustrates two possible principles of the organizations of the intraleg coordination—with a common oscillator for different leg joints (A) and with an individual oscillator for each of the joints (B) (Grillner 1985). It is possible that the leg CPGs in the locust and cockroach are also composed of a set of individual joint oscillators. If the individual oscillators are coupled strongly enough, it is difficult to distinguish experimentally between the two CPG models, with a common oscillator (Fig. 6.4A) and with multiple oscillators (Fig. 6.4B). Autonomous control of individual joints makes the leg controller more flexible and allows, for example, a smooth regulation of the phase shift between different joints (as in the case shown in Figs. 6.2E,F).

The structure and function of the rhythm generator network controlling walking in insects remains unclear. The main difficulty in studying this network is the great number of interneurons, both spiking and non-spiking, involved in the rhythmic activity even in the absence of sensory feedback. Many of them affect the locomotory rhythm when manipulated (Pearson and Fourtner 1975; Büschges 1995). In the stick insect, the rhythm generator network drives the motor neurons

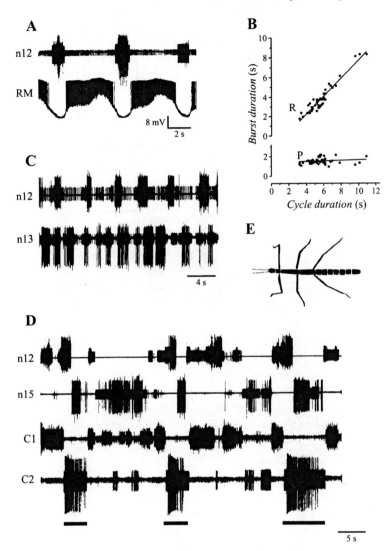

Fig. 6.3 Rhythmic patterns generated by the deafferented thoracic ganglia of the stick insect under the effect of pilocarpine. A: Alternating activity in the excitatory promotor coxae motor neurons (n12, extracellular record) and in the intracellularly recorded retractor coxae motor neuron (RM). B: Dependence of protractor (P) and retractor (R) burst duration on the cycle duration. C: Different rhythms in motor neuron pools controlling different joints. Recordings were performed from the nerves supplying the protractor coxae (n12) and extensor tibiae (n13). D: Simultaneous recording of activity from the nerves controlling two joints, the subcoxal joint (protractor coxae n12 and retractor coxae n15) and the coxa–trochanter joint (levator trochanteris C1 and depressor trochanteris C2). The rhythms in these two groups of nerves are different, but episodes of normal coordination (corresponding to the beginning of the swing phase of forward walking) sometimes appear spontaneously (marked by bars). E: Stick insect (view from above). A–D are from Büschges *et al.* (1995).

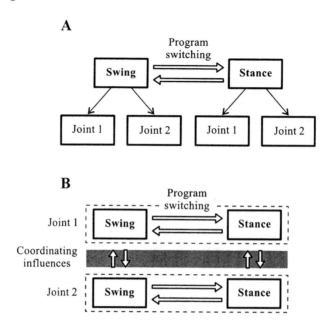

Fig. 6.4 Two possible principles of organization of the leg CPG. A: The rhythm generating mechanism is common for different joints. B: Each joint has its own generator. (See text for details.)

mainly through their phasic inhibition rather than phasic excitation. This phasic inhibition is applied on the background of tonic excitatory drive (Büschges 1998).

6.2.2   Motor output to all legs

When generating rhythmic activity in the absence of sensory feedback, the chain of thoracic ganglia is not able to maintain normal temporal relationships between the efferent outputs to individual legs. Not only may the phase shifts between the efferent outputs be abnormal but even the rhythms of the CPGs for individual legs may differ from each other (Büschges *et al.* 1995; Ryckebusch and Laurent 1993). One can thus conclude that mutual influences between the CPGs for individual legs are not sufficient for their normal coordination.

6.3   FUNCTIONAL ORGANIZATION OF THE LEG CONTROLLER

The functional organization of the leg controller in insects is similar to that in Crustacea (see Section 4.6). The two basic components of the controller are responsible for formation of the swing phase muscle synergy and the stance phase muscle synergy respectively. Switching from one muscle synergy to another one occurs under the effect of signals from several hundred mechanoreceptors of the leg (see Fig. 4.4A). Sensory influences from other legs may also affect the moments of switching and thus contribute to interleg coordination (see Figs. 4.4C,E).

The intensity of the motor output also depends on the sensory feedback. The role of sensory feedback in different phases of the step cycle has been analysed in the stick insect and locust (Weiland and Koch 1987; Cruse 1985, 1990; Bässler 1977, 1983; review in Burrows 1996).

6.3.1   Motor programme for stance

In the stance phase, the movement of an individual leg is not directly caused by the motor commands from the leg controller but is rather determined by the relative movement between animal and ground. Under these conditions, the only regulated value during stance is the force developed by the leg muscles. It was found that hampering the backward leg movement in the stance phase results in an increase of this force. Apparently, numerous mechanoreceptors that signal information about the leg position and movement, as well as about the load applied to the leg, affect the efferent output in this phase (Cruse 1985).

6.3.2   Stance–swing transition

Two sensory inputs are mostly important for timing of the stance–swing transition: (1) input from the sense organs signalling position of the thoraco-coxal joint (Bässler 1977; Cruse 1985), and (2) input from the sense organs (companiform sensilla on the trochanter) measuring the load applied to the leg (Bässler 1977). Due to these inputs, the swing starts only provided the leg is close to the posterior extreme position and is unloaded. The moment of switching from stance to swing is also affected, to some extent, by the stepping movements of the other legs; this mechanism promotes the interleg coordination (Cruse 1990).

6.3.3   Motor programme for swing

The control of swing strongly differs from the control of stance. The leg movement in the swing phase is completely determined by the motor commands coming from the leg controller but not by the relative movement of the body and the ground. The main question regarding swing control is whether this phase is pre-programmed or whether the leg movement can be modified under the effect of sensory feedback. Experiments with application of external forces to the leg during swing have shown that sensory feedback plays an important role, and that the distal point of the leg (tarsus) may reach a close-to-normal anterior extreme position (that is the endpoint of the swing trajectory) despite an external counteraction (Dean 1984). The swing phase programme may thus be termed the 'targeting response' (Cruse 1979; Dean and Wendler 1983). Similar functional organization of the leg controller has also been found in vertebrates; in the dog, hampering the elbow flexion during swing causes an additional activation of the elbow flexors (Orlovsky and Shik 1965) (see Section 11.5.3).

When the leg hits a solid obstacle during its forward movement and is unable to overcome the obstructing force, a new motor programme comes into operation. The leg protraction stops, and the leg is then retracted and lifted. From this new position, the leg moves forward and may thus overstep the obstacle (Cruse 1980;

Bässler 1993). This motor programme is in insects triggered by input from special sensory organs, the campaniform sensilla (Delcomyn 1991; Hofmann and Bässler 1982). A similar adaptive motor pattern, that is overstepping an obstacle, is observed during walking in mammals (see Section 11.5).

The endpoint of the swing trajectory is not fixed but can rather be set by the CNS. This has been clearly demonstrated for the middle and hind legs. In the free-walking stick insect, the distal point of the leg (tarsus) is positioned just behind the tarsus of the anterior neighbouring leg at the end of swing. The biological expedience of this behaviour is evident: where the anterior leg has found a solid foothold, the hind leg will probably also find a foothold just behind (Cruse 1979).

The targeting response requires integration of sensory information about the positions of all joints of the anterior leg. It was found that removal of one or several sense organs in this leg alters the endpoint of the swing trajectory in the neighbouring posterior leg (Cruse et al. 1984). How the sensory information concerning the joint angles is processed and integrated in insects remains unknown. The likely candidates for this function are the intersegmental interneurons identified in different species (Brunn and Dean 1994; Büschges 1998; Laurent 1987).

6.3.4 Premotor interneurons

Leg motor neurons in insects, with almost no exceptions, are output elements of the leg controller, they practically affect neither each other nor other cell groups in the CNS (Burrows et al. 1989). The motor neurons, however, may have active membrane properties like plateau potentials (Hancox and Pitman 1991) and contribute to shaping the drive from the premotor interneurons, as was also shown for the motor neurons in Crustacea (see Fig. 4.3F).

Leg motor neurons receive phasic, step-related inputs from three main sources: (1) sensory neurons that convey exteroceptive and proprioceptive signals (Burrows 1987; Laurent and Hustert 1988; Pearson et al. 1976), (2) local spiking interneurons (Burrows and Siegler 1982), and (3) local non-spiking interneurons that are considered to be the major premotor elements since they integrate not only local inputs (see for example Burrows 1987; Burrows and Laurent 1989; Büschges 1990; Driesang and Büschges 1996) but also signals from the controllers of other legs subserving interleg coordination (Büschges et al. 1994; Laurent and Burrows 1989a,b).

Of the large number of non-spiking interneurons in the stick insect thoracic ganglia, about ten have been individually identified. Most of them have homologues in the locust (Büschges and Wolf 1995). All these interneurons, when stimulated, affect leg motor neurons (Fig. 6.5B). They strongly differ in their pattern of projection upon the motor neuron pools. Some interneurons affect motor neurons of one leg joint only, whereas others may affect two or even three joints (Büschges 1995). The interneurons receive afferent inputs from the leg mechanoreceptors, as illustrated in Fig. 6.5C for the E4 interneuron. The interneurons strongly differ in the pattern of sensory inputs projecting upon them (Büschges and Wolf 1995; Büschges 1990).

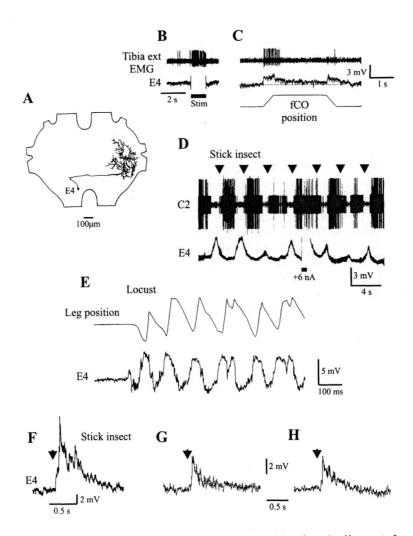

Fig. 6.5 Premotor non-spiking interneurons integrate central and afferent influences. A: Morphology of the E4 interneuron in the mesothoracic ganglion of the locust. B: Stimulation of the interneuron results in activation of a motor neuron projecting to the tibia extensor muscle. C: Passive elongation and relaxation of the femoral chorodontal organ (fCO) induced depolarization of E4 and reflexive activation of the extensor motor neuron. D: Injection of depolarizing current into the E4 interneuron of the stick insect led to a resetting of the rhythm in the depressor trochanteris nerve. The arrowheads mark the occurrence of the bursts during unaffected rhythmicity and the expected occurrence after stimulation. The rhythmic activity in the ganglia was induced by pilocarpine. E: Activity of the E4 interneuron during walking in the semi-intact locust. F–H: Responses of the E4 interneuron from the mesathoracic ganglion of the semi-intact stick insect to tactile stimulation (marked by arrows) of the middle leg (F), front leg (G), and hind leg (H). A–C are from Büschges and Wolf (1995), D is from Büschges (1995), E is from Wolf and Büschges (1995), and F–H are from Büschges *et al.* (1994).

During fictive locomotion elicited by pilocarpine, most interneurons receive phasic input from the rhythm generating network, as illustrated in Fig. 6.5D for the E4 interneuron (Büschges 1995; Büschges *et al.* 1994). Stimulation of an interneuron not only affects the intensity of the activity in the target motor neurons but also resets the rhythm (Fig. 6.5D) or changes its frequency. These findings indicate that the non-spiking interneurons play a double role: they constitute a part of the rhythm generating network and also mediate influences of the sensory feedback upon the stepping leg movements. The contributions of the central and afferent inputs to the activity of the interneurons are of the same order: on average, the oscillations of the membrane potential in these neurons during real locomotion (Fig. 6.5E) are approximately twice as large as during fictive locomotion, when the afferent influences are excluded (Wolf and Büschges 1995).

Some of the non-spiking interneurons integrate not only segmental information but also signals from other segments. Figures 6.5F–H show responses of the E4 interneuron from the mesothoracic ganglion to tactile stimulation of different legs in the standing animal. This neuron is a member of the network controlling the middle leg, but it responds to sensory inputs not only from the middle leg (F) but also from the anterior (G) and posterior (H) legs (Büschges *et al.* 1994). One can suggest that, during locomotion, the E4 interneuron contributes to interleg coordination. Influences of adjacent ganglia on the local interneurons may be mediated by different types of intersegmental interneurons (Laurent and Burrows 1989*a*,*b*; Laurent 1987).

Sensory inputs affecting the non-spiking and spiking interneurons of the leg controller, as well as direct sensory inputs to motor neurons, are subject to step-cycle-dependent presynaptic modulation, like that demonstrated in crustaceans (see Section 4.4). There are three sources for this modulation: (1) interactions between sensory neurons of the same receptor (for example the chorodontal organ) signalling the same movement, (2) signals from different receptors in the same leg and other legs, and (3) outputs of the central neurons of the leg controller (Wolf and Burrows 1995).

6.4 ACTIVATION OF THE LOCOMOTOR SYSTEM

The brain command system for initiation of walking in insects has not been identified yet. From anatomical studies it is known that about 200 pairs of neurons in the brain project to the thoracic ganglia. At least some of them may be involved in initiation of walking (Kien 1990), but the identity and effects of these neurons have yet to be elucidated. The effects of the command system, however, can be estimated indirectly, by observing spontaneous bouts of locomotor activity in semi-intact preparations (Driesang and Büschges 1996).

Different motor behaviours of insects can be divided into two principal categories, associated with locomotion or with a maintenance of a certain configuration of the legs (posture). From this point of view, activation of the locomotor system implies switching the leg controllers from the postural mode of activity into the locomotor mode. In standing animals it was found that the joint control loops, constituting the leg controller, act to reduce an imposed movement and to stabilize the leg posture. In walking animals the same control loops reinforce an ongoing leg movement (Bässler 1976, 1988). Similar results have been obtained for different non-insect species, both vertebrate and invertebrate (DiCaprio and Clarac 1981; Duysens *et al.* 1990; Pearson and Collins 1993; Sillar and Skorupski 1986).

Transformation of the leg controller from a system that prevents movement into a system generating movement is a complex process, only some aspects of which have been discovered. Two kinds of modification of the network controlling movement in an individual joint have been found: changes of the gain in the feedback loop (Bässler 1983; Bässler and Nothof 1994; Büschges and Wolf 1996; Kittmann 1991; Pearson 1993), and a reversal of the sign of motor output evoked by a given sensory input (Bässler 1976).

In the non-locomoting ('inactive') stick insect, passive flexion of the femor–tibia joint elicits activation of the extensor tibia muscles ('resistance reflex'). In contrast, in an animal that is ready to locomote, flexion of the femor–tibia joint elicits a totally different response ('active reaction') (Bässler 1976, 1983). Figure 6.6A shows activity of the same extensor tibia motor neuron during resistance reflex and during active reaction elicited by stretching the femoral chorodontal organ (this receptor signals about movements at the femor–tibia joint). During the resistance reflex, the motor neuron is depolarized and fires action potentials. During the active reaction, the motor neuron receives a strong inhibitory input followed by an excitatory one.

Input from the chorodontal organ to extensor motor neurons is mediated by a group of identified non-spiking interneurons that produce excitation (interneurons E1–E6) or inhibition (interneurons I1, I2) of the motor neurons. The response of these neurons to sensory input was found to strongly differ for the two behavioural states of the animal (Fig. 6.6B). Since the interneurons receive signals from the chorodontal organ via different parallel pathways (excitatory and inhibitory) (Driesang and Büschges 1993; Sauer *et al.* 1995), it seems most likely that a change of the response is caused by a change in the relative strength of these two inputs. One of the possible ways of changing the signal transmission in the afferent pathways is through presynaptic inhibition (Sauer *et al.* 1997) exerted by the system responsible for the initiation of locomotion (Fig. 6.6C). When modified by descending commands, the joint controller does not resist the leg movement any more but instead promotes the transition from the stance to the swing phase of the step cycle (Bässler 1986, 1987).

6.5 GRAVITY AND LIGHT ORIENTATION

When walking in their natural habitat, insects may be oriented in all possible ways in relation to the gravity force or to the sunlight, though in some cases these cues may affect the body orientation. One can thus conclude that usually the leg and body postures are primarily determined by the orientation and shape of the substrate.

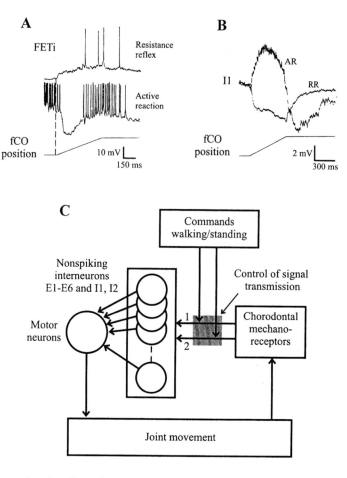

Fig. 6.6 Reversal of the effect of sensory feedback with spontaneous activation of the locomotor system in the semi-intact stick insect. A: Response of the fast extensor tibia motor neuron (FETi) to stretching of the femoral chorodontal organ (fCO). In the passive animal, stimulation results in excitatory response in the motor neuron (resistance reflex). In the active animal the same stimulus results in generation of a complex pattern (active reaction). B: Reversal of the response to stretching of the femoral chorodontal organ in the I1 interneuron (AR, active reaction; RR, resistance reflex). C: A diagram showing modification of the sensory feedback with transition from standing to walking. The extensor tibia motor neuron is driven by a group of excitatory (E1–E6) and inhibitory (I1, I2) non-spiking interneurons. The interneurons receive two inputs from the femoral chorodontal organ—excitatory (1) and inhibitory (2). The relative weights of these inputs are changed by the command system. A and B are from Driesang and Büschges (1996).

Gravity and light, however, may indirectly affect the postural orientation in some cases, primarily by changing the locomotor trajectories (geotaxis and phototaxis). For example, when climbing on a vertical surface, the stick insect assumes a certain body orientation relative to the gravity force and the light incidence (Yagi 1928; Bässler 1983). Sensory hairs on the subcoxial joint and the femoral chorodontal organs participate in the perception of the direction of gravity; input from antennae mechanoreceptors also contributes to this perception (Bässler 1983). Neuronal mechanisms responsible for the sensory-motor transformation underlying gravity and light orientation in walking insects remain unknown.

6.6 CONCLUSIONS

1. The main design of the walking control system in insects is similar to that in Crustacea. Each of the six legs is controlled by a semiautonomous nervous mechanism—the leg controller. Interaction between the leg controllers results in the synchronization of their rhythms and in mutual phasing, that is in the formation of the gait.
2. For the stick insect it was demonstrated that the leg controller, in its turn, can be subdivided into semiautonomous joint controlling mechanisms. Interaction between the joint controlling mechanisms results in synchronization of their rhythms and in mutual phasing, that is in the formation of the leg muscle synergies for the stance and swing phases of the step cycle.
3. Sensory feedback plays an important role both in the generation of the rhythmic activity in the individual joint controlling mechanisms and in their synchronization. The feedback is also necessary for interleg coordination. Deprived of sensory feedback, the CPGs for different legs and, in the stick insect, even the control mechanisms for individual joints of a given leg, generate almost independent rhythms.
4. The segmental network of the leg controller is subject to considerable reconfigurations depending on the behavioural state of an animal. In quiescent animals, the joint controlling mechanisms stabilize a definite joint angle. With activation of the animal, the same mechanism generates a joint movement. This change of the function of the mechanism is caused, at least partly, by a change of the relative weights of two parallel feedback pathways, excitatory and inhibitory.

7

Flying in the locust

7.1 MOTOR PATTERN

Locusts fly by rhythmically flapping their two pairs of wings. Locusts can develop high air speeds (up to $15 \, \mathrm{km \, h^{-1}}$) and can cover long distances (100 km or more) (Baker *et al.* 1981).

The four wings are attached to the thorax by wing hinges that allow the wing to rotate in a large range of angles. A cycle of wing oscillations consists of two parts—an upward movement (elevation) and a downward movement (depression), which are repeated at a frequency of about 20 Hz (Figs. 7.1A,B) (Baker and Cooter 1979). The elevation occupies a shorter part of the cycle than the depression. These basic wing movements are accompanied by the rotatory movements of the wing around its longitudinal axis, so that the anterior edge of the wing is leading both during elevation and during depression. The propulsive force is generated in both phases of the cycle, whereas the lifting force is generated during the down-stroke movement (see for example Wolf 1993).

During steady flying, the left and right wings in each pair oscillate synchronously. The hind pair of wings lag behind the front pair with about one-fifth of the cycle duration, however (Fig. 7.1A) (Weis-Fogh 1956).

Each wing is moved by ten muscles acting around the wing hinge. They are arranged in two antagonistic groups—the elevator and the depressor synergies (Möhl and Zarnack 1977). Each individual muscle is driven by a small number (one to six) of excitatory motor neurons. The motor neurons controlling the front wings are located mainly in the mesothoracic ganglion, whereas those controlling the hind wings are located mainly in the metathoracic ganglion (Fig. 7.1C) (Burrows 1973, 1975, 1996; Robertson and Pearson 1982). The motor neurons discharge in bursts, and the bursts in the elevator and depressor motor neuron pools alternate (Fig. 7.1D). The cycle of efferent activity is not symmetrical: the depressor–elevator interval is longer than the elevator–depressor interval, and this asymmetry accounts for the different durations of the elevation and depression phases in the wing movement cycle. The phase shift between the oscillations of the front and hind wings is caused partly by a corresponding time shift in the motor commands to these wings and partly by differences in the aerodynamic properties of the wings (Wilson and Weis-Fogh 1962).

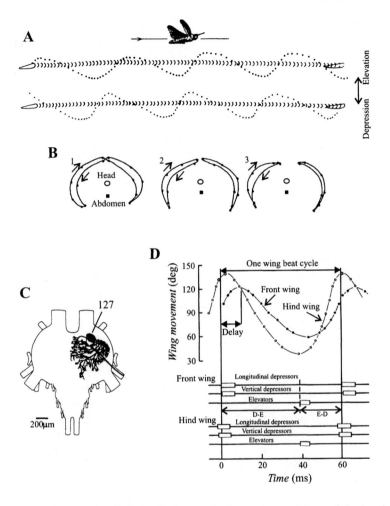

Fig. 7.1 Motor pattern for flight in the locust. A: Successive positions of the head and of the tips of ipsilateral fore wing (upper trace) and hind wing (lower trace) in naturally flying locust (time intervals, 2.5 ms). B: Frontal view of the hind wing tips in three consecutive cycles (1–3). C: Morphology of a motor neuron supplying the depressor muscle 127. D: Main characteristics of the wing beat cycle. A and B are from Baker and Cooter (1979), C is from Hedwig and Pearson (1984), and D is from Burrows (1996).

7.2 GROSS SYNERGY FOR FLYING

Individual locomotor appendages in most investigated animal species are driven by separate, autonomous controllers. This has been shown most clearly in lesion experiments, where individual controllers were anatomically isolated (for the wings of *Clione* see Section 1.1; for the legs in crustacea, insects, and mammals see Sections 4.6, 6.3, and 10.1). Does each wing in the locust have its own controller? It was demonstrated that the locust is able to fly after removal of all ganglia except for the three thoracic ones (Wilson 1961). This finding indicates that the basic part of the wing controlling system is located there. Further reduction of this ganglia chain resulted in distortions of the pattern of flapping of all four wings, however. Especially pronounced distortions were caused by damage to the metathoracic ganglion (Stevenson and Kutsch 1987; Wolf and Pearson 1987). Similarly, a longitudinal split of the thoracic ganglion resulted in discoordination of the flying pattern in the left and in the right pairs of wings (Ronacher *et al.* 1988). Thus, the results of the lesion experiments suggest that the networks controlling individual wings are either distributed over all thoracic ganglia or strongly integrated with each other.

A mass of evidence that strongly suggests that the wing control system in the locust is functionally integrated, and that all the wings are driven by a common rhythm generator has been obtained in physiological experiments (Waldron 1967; Robertson and Pearson 1983):

1. Locust interneurons, particularly in the rhythm generator (for example types 301 and 501, see below), have their neuropilar branches widely distributed throughout the mesa- and metathoracic ganglia, where they form synaptic connections and affect motor and premotor neurons of all four wings (Pearson and Robertson 1987; Robertson and Pearson 1983; see Section 7.3).
2. Different groups of wing afferents project not only to the motor and premotor neurons controlling a given wing, but also to those of other wings, thus promoting formation of the gross flight synergy that includes muscles of all four wings (Tyrer and Altman 1974; Pflüger *et al.* 1981; see Section 7.4).
3. Afferent signals from wing proprioceptors as well as descending signals may affect the phase relationships between different wings (the front wings versus the hind wings, or the right wings versus the left wings) (Wendler 1974; Wilson and Weis-Fogh 1962; Möhl and Zarnack 1977; Zarnack and Möhl 1977; Baker 1979; Simmons 1980). The changes of the motor pattern of individual wings are caused by the descending signals acting on the output motor stage of the wing controlling mechanisms, rather than on the rhythm generating interneurons (Reichert and Rowell 1989) (see Section 7.5).

On the other hand, by applying picrotoxin to the locust CNS, it was possible to partly separate the rhythms of the individual wing oscillators (Ronacher *et al.* 1988; Jarre and Büschges 1995). This makes it likely that each wing in the locust has its own controller, but the individual controllers are linked so strongly with each other that they form a functional unit, similar to the way in which the nervous mechanisms controlling individual joints of the leg form a functional unit—the leg controller—due to their strong interactions with each other (see Section 6.2.1 and Fig. 6.4A).

7.3   CENTRAL PATTERN GENERATOR

In some insects, such as flies, the flight muscles are activated myogenically rather than driven by the CNS. The locust, however, has a very complex nervous mechanism controlling wing beating. That deafferented thoracic ganglia can generate a rhythmic efferent pattern resembling a flying rhythm was first demonstrated by Wilson (1961). This rhythm can be elicited by wind stimuli to the head, or by electrical stimulation of the nerve cord (Wilson and Wyman 1965). The basic features of the motor pattern of flying, that is alternation between bursts of the depressor and elevator motor neurons, synchronous bursting of the homologous motor neurons of the left and right wings, and a phase shift between the motor neurons in the hind and front wings, are observed in the absence of sensory feedback. The frequency generated by the deafferented ganglia is lower than in intact animals, however, but it can be increased by octopamine (Hedwig and Pearson 1984; Stevenson and Kutsch 1987).

In the meso- and metathoracic ganglia, about 40 morphological types of interneurons have been identified that exhibit rhythmic activity during flying, affect the motor pattern when stimulated, and have their neuropilar area of branching overlapping with that of motor neurons or other flight-related interneurons (Pearson and Robertson 1987; Ramirez and Pearson 1988; Robertson and Pearson 1983, 1985a,b; Pearson et al. 1985; Wolf and Pearson 1989). Many of them were also found to be rhythmically modulated during fictive flying, and some of these affected the locomotory rhythm when stimulated (the 'influential interneurons').

Among the influential interneurons, special attention was given to two groups, named 301 (Fig. 7.2A) and 501 (Robertson and Pearson 1983, 1985a). These neurons fire their bursts in succession in the second half of the locomotor cycle; the burst in 501 immediately follows that in 301 (Fig. 7.2B). Stimulation of 301 or 501 resulted in resetting of the flight rhythm (Fig. 7.2D), thus indicating that they are the members of the rhythm generating network.

Experiments with paired recordings from these neurons have shown that 301 excites 501 (Fig. 7.2E) whereas 501 inhibits 301 after a delay caused by the interposed interneuron 511 (Fig. 7.2F). Thus, the two neuron groups form a circuit with a 'switch-off mechanism' (Fig. 7.2G). This type of circuit is capable of rhythmical oscillations and is suggested to be responsible for rhythmogenesis in a number of CPGs: the CPG for the feeding rhythm in the snail (Arshavsky et al. 1988c; Elliot and Benjamin 1985), the locomotor CPG in *Tritonia* (see Section 2.1), the CPG for the scratch rhythm in the cat (see Section 11.3) (Berkinblit et al. 1978b), and the CPG for the respiratory rhythm in mammals (Cohen 1979; Euler 1986). The rhythm generation in the circuit with the switch-off mechanism is based on the fact that the activity in the first neuron group (301) is growing until it reaches the threshold of activation of the second group (502) which inhibits the first one and thus terminates the cycle. The reason for the subsequent activation of the first group can be a post-inhibitory rebound, or spontaneous burst generation if the neurons in this group posess the pacemaker rhythmic activity. This property has not been directly shown for the 301 or 501 cells, but it was demonstrated that some other interneurons of the flight CPG (see below) are conditional bursters: in these neurons, bursting properties are induced during flight (Ramirez and Pearson 1993), probably due to octopamine release (Ramirez and Pearson 1991a,b).

The simple circuit shown in Fig. 7.2G seems to be only a part of the CPG network. Many other neurons receive input from the 301 and 501 cells, and/or

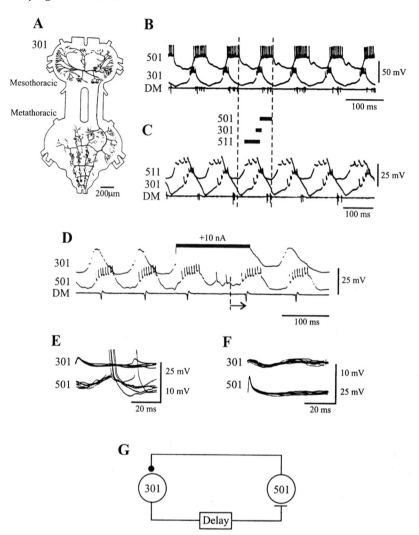

Fig. 7.2 The CPG for flight in the locust. A: Morphology of the 301 interneuron. B,C: Activity of the 301, 501, and 511 interneurons during normal flight sequence evoked by stimulation of the head wind receptors in the deafferented locust. D: Resetting the flight rhythm (shown by arrow) with a short pulse of depolarizing current delivered to the 301 interneuron (in B–D, the DM trace shows activity of the depressor motor neurons). E,F: Pair recordings from the 301 and 501 interneurons to show their excitatory (301→501) and inhibitory (501→301) interactions. G: Diagrammatical representation of connections between the 301 and 501 interneurons. This circuit may be responsible for the rhythm generation in the flight CPG. A–C and E–G are from Robertson and Pearson (1985*a*) and D is from Robertson and Pearson (1983).

exert influences upon them. Activity of one of such neuron (cell 511) is shown in Fig. 7.2C. One of the discovered inputs to 501 is an inhibitory input from 301; in its turn 511 exerts an inhibitory action upon 501. As one can see from Fig. 7.2C, the cell 511 starts firing its burst before 301. The CPG for flight can thus be considered as a three-phasic generator. Computer simulation of this network has reproduced the three-phasic pattern (Grimm and Sauer 1995). It was also shown that, when the basic circuit (cells 301 and 501) was supplemented with the additional cells and connections found in physiological experiments, the robustness of the system against variation of its parameters considerably increased. However, the efferent output of this three-phasic CPG is biphasic, with alternating activity of the elevator and depressor motor neuron pools (Fig. 7.1D).

The wing motor neurons receive inputs from numerous premotor interneurons (Figs. 7.3C,D); the inputs are excitatory in one phase of the cycle and inhibitory in the other phase. Simultaneous recordings from the elevator and depressor motor neurons (Fig. 7.3A) have shown that inputs to these antagonistic motor neurons are not symmetrically timed. This was especially well seen when the duration of the locomotor cycle changed spontaneously: with lengthening of the cycle, the elevator phase changed proportionally, whereas duration of the depressor burst remained relatively constant (Fig. 7.3B). The low variability of the events occurring at the end of cycle is a characteristic feature of a generator with a switch-off mechanism (Wolf and Pearson 1988). This is an additional indication that the circuit shown in Fig. 7.2G plays an important role in rhythmogenesis.

7.4   ROLE OF PROPRIOCEPTION IN FLIGHT CONTROL

Various wing mechanoreceptors are activated during flight (Figs. 7.4A,B). Deafferentation of the wings dramatically affects the activity of the flight control mechanisms: the wing beat frequency decreases from about 20 Hz to 10 Hz, and the temporal patterns of activity of motor neurons change correspondingly (Wilson 1961). Figures 7.4C,D show activity of the elevator and depressor motor neurons during flight before (C) and after deafferentation (D). In the depressor motor neuron, the wave of depolarization remains almost unchanged, whereas in the elevator motor neuron the wave changes considerably. This is especially well seen in Fig. 7.4E, where the two curves are superimposed. In intact locust, the elevator depolarization has steep rising and repolarization slopes, and is of short duration. In the deafferented preparation, the elevator depolarization commences more gradually, and the initial depolarization slope is followed by a fairly steep final depolarization. The repolarization, by contrast, remains almost as steep as in the intact animal. The late wave of depolarization, however, can be observed not only in the deafferented animal but also in the intact locust when it flies with low wingbeat frequency (Fig. 7.4E, the upper trace). From these findings one can conclude that the afferent input has a double function in the elevator phase of the cycle: (1) it initiates the early, steep wave of depolarization, and (2) at higher wingbeat frequency, it eliminates the late wave of depolarization (Wolf and Pearson 1988).

Two classes of wing proprioceptors are mainly responsible for transformation of the CPG pattern into the normal flight pattern—the stretch receptors and the

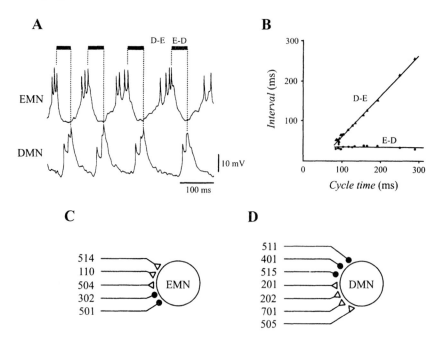

Fig. 7.3 Output motor stage of the wing-controlling mechanism. A: Activity of the elevator (EMN) and depressor (DMN) motor neurons in the deafferented locust during a flight sequence with gradually increasing cycle duration. The bars show the constancy of the interval (E–D) between offsets of the elevator and depressor bursts. B: Graph showing that variations in the cycle duration are caused by variations in the D–E interval but not in the E–D interval. C,D: Convergence of different interneurons on the elevator (C) and depressor (D) motor neurons. A and B are from Hedwig and Pearson (1984) and C and D are based on Robertson and Pearson (1985*b*).

receptors of the tegula. Both sense organs are located close to the hinge of each wing, and are affected by the wing movements. The stretch receptor contains a single afferent neuron that fires its burst at the beginning of the wing beat cycle, around the peak of wing elevation; the number of spikes in the burst is proportional to the value of elevation (Fig. 7.4A) (Möhl 1985). The numerous tegula afferents are active later in the cycle, during the wing depression (Fig. 7.4B).

Input from the wing stretch receptor is responsible for suppression of the late component of depolarization in the elevator motor neurons (Wolf and Pearson 1988). After removal of this input, the initial rapid depolarization was still generated, but it was followed by a large second wave, especially at low wingbeat frequencies. In the deafferented locust, electrical stimulation of the stretch receptor afferent in a proper phase of the wingbeat cycle results in suppression of the late wave of depolarization, and in a corresponding shortening of the cycle (Fig. 7.4F) (Pearson and Ramirez 1990).

Input from the tegula afferents is responsible for the initiation of the early component of depolarization (Wolf and Pearson 1988). Abolition of tegula discharge removes this component. In contrast, electrical stimulation of the tegula afferents in the proper phase of the cycle results in the appearance of the early, steep wave of depolarization, and in a further shortening of the wingbeat cycle (Fig. 7.4F). Thus, the two sensory inputs, from the tegula and from the stretch receptor, are responsible for initiation and termination of the elevator phase of the cycle respectively. In contrast, the timing of depressor activity is much less dependent on proprioceptive input (Figs. 7.4C,D) and is thus essentially controlled by the CPG itself. There is, therefore, some similarity in the organization of the wing and leg control systems. In the stepping leg, duration of the swing phase is, to a large extent, centrally programmed, whereas duration of the stance phase strongly depends on proprioceptive input (see Sections 4.1, 6.3, and 11.5).

In contrast to the timing of the cycle, the level of efferent activity in both phases of the cycle is not much affected by afferent signals. Due to the high wingbeat frequency, the feedback signals from the stretch receptor, generated at the beginning of the elevator phase of the cycle, produce their action only at the end of this phase; that is too late to modify the ongoing motor command (Pearson and Ramirez 1990). This may account for the considerable variability of the wingbeat amplitude during flight (Fig. 7.1B). Afferents of a given wing affect different groups of motor neurons of all four wings (Fig. 7.5) and thus contribute to formation of a gross flight synergy.

7.5 COMMAND SYSTEMS FOR FLIGHT

7.5.1 Equilibrium and steering control

During steady flight, the locust maintains a definite orientation of its body in the external coordinate system (horizontal, dorsal side up) and also maintains a definite direction of flight. Information about orientation of the animal in relation to the horizon (that is in the roll and pitch planes, Fig. 7.6A) comes mainly from two compound eyes, but also from the three luminosity detectors, the ocelli (Rowell and Pearson 1983; Taylor 1981a,b). Information about the orientation in relation to the direction of wind comes from the five groups of hairs on the head (Weis-Fogh 1949; Camhi 1969a,b). These sensory inputs are processed and integrated, and then affect the animal's orientation.

Any deviation of the flying locust from the normal orientation (the roll tilt α, the pitch tilt β, and the yaw angle γ, Fig. 7.6A) elicits a correcting motor response aimed at restoration of the normal orientation (reviewed by Rowell 1988; Möhl 1989; Hensler 1989) (for a review of earlier studies on insect orientation, see Wehner (1981)). This response includes, first of all, shifts in the relative timing of oscillations of different wings (left/right or front/hind) caused by corresponding shifts in timing of action potentials in different wing muscles (Möhl and Zarnack 1977; Zarnack and Möhl 1977; Taylor 1981a,b; Thüring 1986). Each of these shifts alters the flight motor pattern and evokes a torque rotating the animal in a certain plane (roll, pitch, or yaw). For turning in the pitch and yaw planes, the ruddering effects produced by bending the abdomen in the corresponding plane are also used; for the yaw plane, they may be accompanied by the supination of the extended hind legs (Camhi 1970; Arbas 1986).

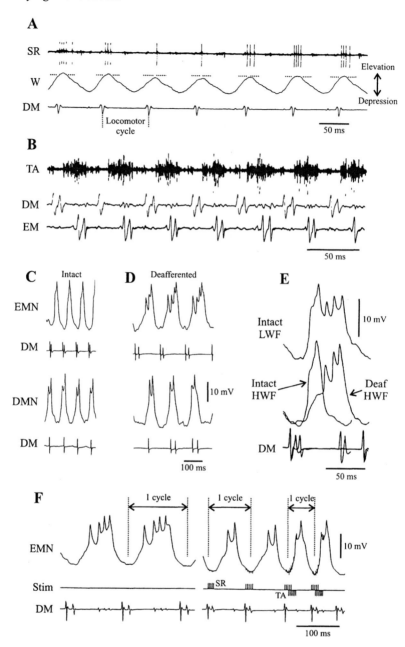

Fig. 7.4 Afferent influences on the flight motor pattern. A,B: Discharges of the stretch receptor afferent (SR in A) and tegulae receptor afferents (TA in B) during flight in the intact, tethered locust. Afferent activity was recorded together with wing movements (W in A) and EMGs of the elevator and depressor muscles (EM and DM in B). C,D: Activity of the elevator (EMN) and depressor (DMN) motor neurons recorded during tethered flight in the intact (C) and deafferented (D) locust (DM, the depressor muscle EMG). E: Recordings from the elevator motor neuron in the intact locust obtained at the low and high wingbeat

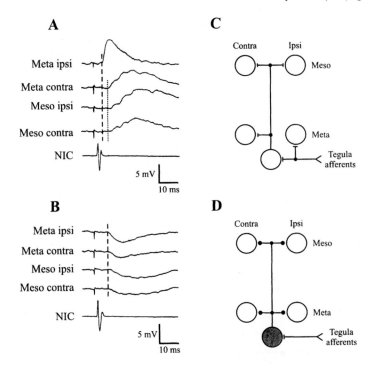

Fig. 7.5 Excitatory and inhibitory connections of the hind wing tegula afferents with the motor neurons of different wings. A,B: Electrical stimulation of the tegula nerve evokes compound EPSPs in the elevator motor neurons (A) and IPSPs in the depressor motor neurons (B); the neurons were recorded from different ganglia and the bottom trace shows the afferent volley (NIC). C,D: Schematic diagrams showing the connections of tegula afferents to the motor neurons in the meso- and metathoracic ganglia. From Pearson and Wolf (1988).

Sensory inputs from eyes, ocelli, and wind detectors are processed and integrated to form the commands addressed to the thoracic and abdominal ganglia where they elicit postural and steering corrections. These signals are transmitted by different groups of command neurons. Figure 7.6B shows the experimental apparatus for studying activity of the command neurons and for recording the correcting motor responses that they elicit during flight in the tethered locust. Figure 7.6C shows rhythmical activity of the left and right depressor muscles during flight. Normally,

---

frequency (LWF and HWF), and a recording from the same neuron after deafferentation of wings. F: Combined stimulation of tegula and stretch receptor afferents in the deafferented preparation results in a pattern of elevator motoneuron depolarization resembling that in intact animals. Upper trace: the elevator motor neuron (EMN); middle trace: stimulation of the stretch receptor (SR) or tegula afferents (TA); lower trace: EMG of the depressor muscle. A is from Möhl (1985), B is from Neuman (1985), and C–F are from Wolf and Pearson (1988).

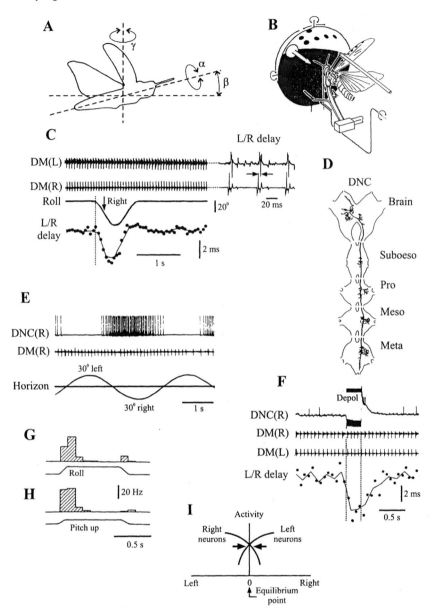

Fig. 7.6 Equilibrium and steering control in the flying locust. A: The spatial orientation of the animal is characterized by three angles—roll (α), pitch (β), and yaw (γ). B: Experimental apparatus for studying motor and neuronal responses in the intact locust to movements of an artificial horizon during tethered flight. C: Postural correcting response to the roll tilt of the horizon. The tilt evokes, in about 10 cycles, a delay in activation of the left depressor muscle, DM(L), in relation to the right one, DM(R). D: Morphology of the DNC command neuron. E: Response of the DNC neuron to the roll tilt of the horizon. F: Intracellular stimulation of the DNC neuron evokes, in about 10 cycles, a delay in activation of the left depressor muscle in relation to the right one. G,H: Roll tilt (28°) or pitch tilt (14°) of the artificial horizon evoke similar responses in the PI(2)5 command

their motor units generate action potentials almost in phase. However, inclination of the artificial horizon to the right, that simulates a roll tilt of the animal to the left, is immediately detected by the eyes and, via the command system, elicits a modification of the motor output. This includes an induction of a time shift between the motor units of the right and left wing depressors, which is the basis for postural corrections in the roll plane.

One of the numerous command neurons, responsible for elicitation of corrective motor responses, is the DNC neuron (Rowell and Reichert 1986; Hensler and Rowell 1990). This neuron is driven mainly by visual input from the compound eyes and from the ocelli, but it also receives signals from the wind detectors. The axon of the DNC projects from the brain to the sub-oesophageal, thoracic and fused abdominal ganglia (Fig. 7.6D). At the normal relative orientation of the animal and the horizon, the neuron has low activity, but it becomes active with inclination of the horizon to the right (Fig. 7.6E). The symmetrical neuron of the DNC pair has an opposite response, that is it is activated with the inclination of the horizon to the left. Activation of the DNC by current injection evokes a time shift between the motor units of the right and left wing depressors (Fig. 7.6F), that is a roll-correcting motor response similar to that evoked by inclination of the horizon (Fig. 7.6C).

The numerous command neurons that elicit corrections of the body orientation differ in their spatial areas of sensitivity, in the pattern of convergence of different sensory inputs, and in their motor effects (reviewed by Rowell 1988; Hensler 1989). For example, the pair of TCG neurons (Bacon and Möhl 1983; Möhl and Bacon 1983; Bacon and Tyrer 1978) receive inputs primarily not from the eyes (as the DNC neurons) but from the head wind detectors. The left and right TCG respond in an opposite way to asymmetrical wind stimuli. These neurons project to the thoracic ganglia and affect wing motor neurons. It is suggested that TCGs participate in the stabilization of the flight direction contrary to the wind. They may also initiate the flight in response to wind stimuli. The corrective commands delivered by different command neurons affect the output motor stage of the wing control system rather than the rhythm generating network, which was demonstrated by recording responses to movement of the artificial horizon in the CPG interneurons and in the motor neurons (Reichert and Rowell 1989).

An essential common feature of different command neurons controlling equilibrium and steering is the large size of their spatial zones of sensitivity, as well as a poor directional specificity. This is illustrated in Figs. 7.6G,H for the PI(2)5 command neuron (Hensler 1988). This neuron responds equally well to roll (G) and pitch tilt (H) of the artificial horizon. By relying only on the activity of this neuron, it is impossible to judge about the real body orientation, and to generate the necessary postural corrections. It is evident that the information required for

neuron, presented as post-stimulus histograms. I: A conceptual model of the roll control by two antagonistic groups of the roll-sensitive command neurons. The arrows indicate the compensatory roll evoked by the corresponding group. The system has an equilibrium point at 0° (the dorsal-side-up orientation). B–F are from Hensler and Rowell (1990) and G and H are from Hensler (1988).

generation of postural corrections is coded in the form of the population activity of command neurons, and is decoded in the wing motor centre on the basis of comparing activities of different command neurons. For example, by comparing activities of the left and right PI(2)5 neurons, one can distinguish between the reaction to roll (when the two responses are highly different) and the reaction to pitch (when they are similar) (Figs. 7.6G,H). A conceptual model for stabilization of the dorsal-side-up orientation, based on the comparison of the activity of command neurons signalling about the left and right roll tilt (Fig. 7.6I), was proposed by Hensler (1988). This model stabilizes the orientation at which the activities of two antagonistic groups of command neurons are equal to each other. Similar models explain the equilibrium control in *Clione* (see Section 1.6) and in the lamprey (see Section 8.5.2).

7.5.2   Initiating flight

The locust often starts to fly by jumping into the air. It is suggested that the movement of the animal relative to the air during the jump stimulates the wind receptors, that give rise to a reflex activation of the locomotor system. A loss of contact with the ground also promotes initiation of flight. Most of the command neurons participating in the equilibrium and steering control, when stimulated in quiescent animals, may activate the flight system (Rowell 1988, 1989; Bicker and Pearson 1983). One cannot exclude, however, the existence of special command neurons for flight initiation (Pearson *et al.* 1985; Ramirez and Pearson 1988). The general behavioural state of the animal strongly influences the flight threshold, probably due to altering concentration of different hormones and neuromodulators associated with each behavioural state.

7.6   CONCLUSIONS

1. Wing beating in the locust is controlled by the nervous mechanism located in the thoracic ganglia. This mechanism contains a rhythm generator that is common for all four wings, and output motor stages that are separate for the individual wings. This design of the control system allows the separate regulation of amplitude and phase in individual wings without affecting the wing beat frequency.
2. The wing control system contains a three-phasic CPG operating as a circuit with a switch-off mechanism. In the presence of sensory feedback, however, the transitions between the elevator and depressor phases of the wingbeat cycle are determined not by the CPG but by signals from the wing proprioceptors.
3. During flight, the locust maintains a definite body orientation in relation to the horizon and a definite direction of flight. The control system for spatial orientation is driven by visual and wind stimuli. The descending commands for postural and steering corrections are represented in the activity of the whole population of command neurons. Decoding of these commands and generation of corrective motor responses take place in the wing motor centre in the thoracic ganglia.

Part II
Swimming locomotion in lower vertebrates

8

Swimming in the lamprey

Swimming by means of undulatory movements of the trunk is the main form of locomotion in most aquatic vertebrate species (fish, frog tadpole, etc.). Most information available on the nervous control of swimming has been obtained from two animal models—the lamprey, which is considered in this chapter, and the toad tadpole, discussed in the next chapter.

The lamprey (cyclostome) originates from a group of animals that diverged from the main evolutionary line of the vertebrates around 450 million years ago when ordinary fish had not yet appeared. The anatomical structure of the lamprey brainstem, spinal cord, sensory organs, and motor apparatus is in many respects similar to that in higher vertebrates (Kappers *et al.* 1936; Rovainen 1979*b*; Nieuwenhuys *et al.* 1998). The functional and cellular organization of the locomotor control mechanisms are also similar. The lamprey presents good opportunities for analytical studies of the neural networks controlling different motor functions. This is because the lamprey has orders of magnitude fewer nerve cells of each type than higher vertebrates; secondly, an *in vitro* preparation of the brainstem and spinal cord has been developed which can remain in good condition for several days; and thirdly the motor pattern underlying locomotion can be elicited in this isolated nervous system (Fig. 8.1). These conditions thus allow an analysis of the motor control mechanisms at the network and cellular levels. The lamprey has been used extensively as an experimentally amenable animal model for studying the basic principles of the locomotor control (for reviews see Grillner *et al.* 1984*b*, 1986, 1988*a*, 1990, 1993, 1995; Grillner and Wallén 1985; Grillner 1997). Below we will discuss the forebrain control of locomotion, followed by a review of the network including a detailed account of the contribution of different types of ion channels, and the importance of presynaptic modulation and synaptic plasticity involving peptidergic modulation of glutamatergic pathways, followed by the control of body orientation and steering.

8.1 MOTOR PATTERN AND ITS ORIGIN

The lamprey swims by producing alternating lateral undulating movements of the body, usually with a frequency range of 1–8 Hz. The alternating contractions of the myotomes along the body takes place with a phase lag from rostral to caudal, resulting in laterally directed flexions, starting from the anterior part a

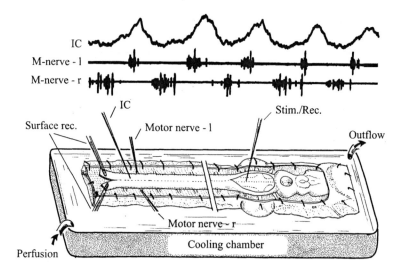

Fig. 8.1 *In vitro* preparation of the lamprey CNS. The brainstem-spinal cord of the lamprey can be maintained alive for several days in isolation, and the motor pattern underlying locomotion can be produced by stimulating the brainstem locomotor centers. The motor activity can be recorded in the ventral roots (motor nerves) that normally activate the musculature on the left (l) and right (r) sides. The activity in single or pairs of cells can be recorded intracellularly with microelectrodes (IC). An intracellular record (IC) of a network neuron with subthreshold membrane potential oscillations is shown above together with the alternating motor activity in the ventral roots on the left and right sides. The experimental chamber is kept cold (4–7°C), and it is continuously perfused with physiological solution.

wave propagated towards the tail (Fig. 8.2A). These caudally directed undulatory waves push the animal forward through the water. The higher the speed of propagation of the locomotor waves, the faster the lamprey will swim.

The mechanical wave of body undulations is caused by a corresponding wave of muscle contraction. The body musculature in the lamprey has a segmental organization. Altogether, there are about 100 muscular segments (myotomes); each segment is innervated by the left and right ventral roots from the corresponding segment of the spinal cord. Each myotome consists of a superficial layer of red (slow) muscle fibres and a deeper layer of white (fast) muscle fibres. Muscle fibres of a few successive segments are mechanically linked together to form a chain that produces a body flexion when the fibres contract (see Rovainen 1979b).

Each myotome is subdivided into dorsal and ventral parts that are innervated by two separate pools of motor neurons. When excited alone, the two parts elicit dorsolateral and ventrolateral body flexion respectively. During rectilinear swimming, both the dorsal and ventral parts of a myotome contract simultaneously and to an equal extent, which results in pure laterally directed body flexions without dorsal or ventral components (Grillner and Kashin 1976; Alexander 1969; Wallén *et al.* 1985; Williams *et al.* 1989).

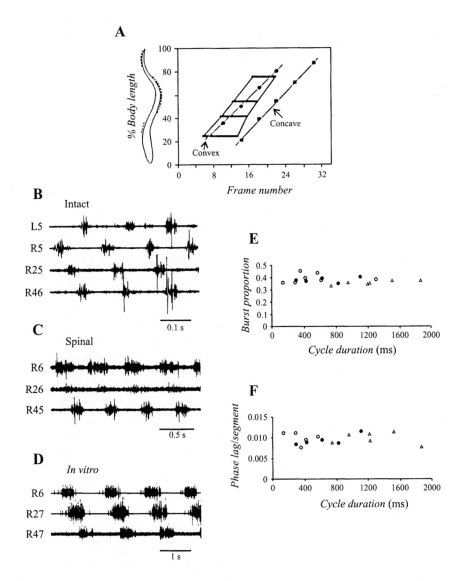

Fig. 8.2 Motor pattern for swimming in the lamprey and its origin. A: Rostrocaudal prop-agation of neural (EMG) and mechanical activity during one swimming cycle. Position of maximal concave/convex curvature (squares and circles) along the body, and the periods of the EMG activity at four electrodes positioned at different rostro-caudal levels (horizon-tal bars) are shown. The body outline is shown for frame 16 (80 frames/s); dashed lines show active muscles. B–D: The EMG activity during active swimming (B,C) compared with the ventral root activity during fictive swimming (D). Segment numbers, counted from the last gill opening are indicated to the left. E,F: The burst proportion (E) and phase lag per segment (F) plotted against the mean cycle duration for the three preparations shown in B–D: intact (triangles), spinal (empty circles), and *in vitro* (filled circles). A is from Williams (1989) and B–F are from Wallén and Williams (1984).

By recording EMGs from the myotomes (Wallén and Williams 1984), and by comparing the EMG pattern with the mechanical pattern (Williams *et al.* 1989) it was found that:

1. In any myotome, the burst of activity lasts about 40 per cent of the locomotor cycle, and up to 40 per cent of the myotomes on one side of the body are contracting simultaneously.
2. The excitation of the ipsilateral myotomes is accompanied by the relaxation of their contralateral counterparts.
3. The wave of myotomal excitation ('electrical wave') propagates in the caudal direction.
4. The electrical wave propagates slightly faster than the mechanical wave.
5. The speed of propagation of the electrical (or mechanical) wave and the frequency of undulations change approximately in direct proportion to each other. This remarkable feature is characteristic not only of the lamprey but also of a number of investigated species of fish (Grillner and Kashin 1976; Williams *et al.* 1989).

The tight linkage between the frequency and the speed of the wave has one major consequence. The wavelength of the mechanical (or electrical) wave remains constant and does not depend on the locomotor frequency. In the lamprey, the mechanical wave is about 0.8 of a body length, and the electrical wave is about one full body length during forward swimming at constant rate. In other words, the phase lag between oscillations of two different points along the body axis is constant and does not depend on the frequency. For the electrical wave, the phase lag per segment at any frequency is around 1 per cent of the locomotor cycle. By contrast, the time lag changes in inverse proportion to the frequency. These findings impose constraints on the possible models for explaining the generation of locomotor pattern in the lamprey.

There is convincing evidence that the motor pattern for swimming is generated by the spinal cord, and that the basic features of this pattern persist after elimination of sensory feedback. Wallén and Williams (1984) compared the patterns of muscle activity during swimming in the intact lamprey (Fig. 8.2B) and in the lamprey after high spinal transection (Fig. 8.2C). Then these patterns were compared with the patterns of activity in the ventral roots of the isolated spinal cord, in which rhythmic activity was induced by bath application of excitatory amino acid (D-glutamate) (Fig. 8.2D). In all preparations, the activity in a given segment alternated between the left and right sides (as in B) with the burst duration constituting about 40 per cent of the cycle duration at any frequency (Fig. 8.2E). In all preparations, activity propagated in the caudal direction (see 8.2B,C, and D), and the time delay per segment was proportional to the cycle duration. The proportionality constant, or the phase lag per segment, did not significantly differ between the different preparations (Fig. 8.2F) but, in fictive swimming, its value may vary considerably between different experiments (Matsushima and Grillner 1992). These findings, nevertheless, clearly indicate that the spinal cord of the lamprey contains the CPG which, when activated, determines basic features of the motor pattern of swimming, although when providing additional excitatory drive the phase lag may change to some degree (Tegnér *et al.* 1997).

A small piece of the lamprey spinal cord (a few segments in length) dissected from any region of the cord (rostral, medial, or caudal), and activated by the bath application of NMDA or other excitatory amino acids, is able to generate the rhythmic efferent pattern with alternating bursts of activity of motor neurons on the left and right sides (Cohen and Wallén 1980; Poon 1980). The frequency of the generated rhythm is directly correlated with the amino acid concentration (Grillner *et al.* 1981). NMDA receptor activation will elicit swimming in a low frequency range and AMPA kainate in a higher range.

8.2   FOREBRAIN CONTROL OF LOCOMOTION

Locomotion can be initiated from a diencephalic (ventral thalamus—zona incerta) and mesopontine area (Figs. 8.3 and 8.4), both of which project to glutamatergic reticulospinal neurons, which in turn activate the spinal network underlying locomotion (McClellan and Grillner 1984; El Manira *et al.* 1997; Viana di Prisco *et al.* 1997). These different structures are presumably involved in the control of

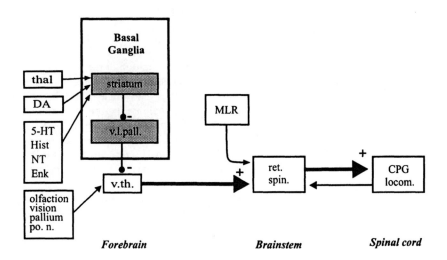

Fig. 8.3 Forebrain and brainstem structures important for initiation of locomotion in lamprey. The striatum of the basal ganglia receives dopaminergic (DA), serotonergic (5-HT), histaminergic (Hist), and peptidergic (NT, Enk) inputs, as well as input from the thalamus (thal) and telencephalon. GABAergic striatal neurons project to the ventrolateral pallium (v.l. pal.), which in turn sends GABAergic projections to the ventral thalamus (v. th). This nucleus also receives olfactory and visual input, and projects to the brainstem where reticulospinal neurons are excited. In addition to this diencephalic locomotor control, the mesencephalic locomotor region (MLR) area also may initiate locomotion by exciting reticulospinal (ret. spin) neurons. The brainstem reticulospinal neurons will then in turn activate the locomotor central pattern generator (CPG locus) in the spinal cord.

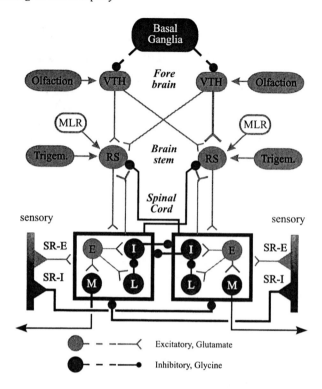

Fig. 8.4 Lamprey locomotor network. A schematic representation of the forebrain, brain-stem, and spinal components of the neural network that generate locomotor burst activity. All neuron symbols denote populations of neurons rather than single cells. The reticulo-spinal (RS) glutamatergic neurons excite all classes of spinal interneurons and motor neu-rons. The excitatory interneurons (E) excite all types of spinal neurons, that is, the inhibitory glycinergic interneurons (I) that cross the midline and inhibit all classes of neurons on the contralateral side, the lateral interneurons (L), which inhibit I interneurons and motoneu-rons (M). The stretch receptor neurons are of an excitatory type (SR-E) that excites neurons on the ipsilateral side and an inhibitory type (SR-I) that inhibits all neurons on the contralat-eral side. RS neurons receive excitatory synaptic inputs from cutaneous afferents (Trigem.), the mesencephalic locomotor region (MLR), and from the ventral thalamus (VTH), which in turn receives inputs from the basal ganglia.

goal-directed locomotion in different behavioural contexts (Grillner *et al.* 1997). The diencephalic locomotor area in turn receives fibre projections from the olfac-tory bulb and the ophthalmic nerve—two sensory inputs which are known to activate goal-directed locomotor behaviour (Kleerekoper 1963; Ullén *et al.* 1997).

The lamprey basal ganglia have a neural organization that histochemically appears closely related to that of mammals and primates (Pombal *et al.* 1997a,b). The striatum contains neurons with extensive dendritic trees with spines dis-tributed in the neuropil. Striatal neurons consist of GABAergic neurons and cells with substance P and ACh-esterase immunoreactivity. The input to striatum (Fig. 8.3) includes a dense dopaminergic, 5-HT-ergic, and histaminergic inputs, as well as peptidergic (galanin, enkephalin, neurotensin) inputs and presumed glutamatergic input from thalamus and telencephalon. GABAergic projections from the striatum extend to the ventrolateral pallium, which contains GABAergic neurons that in turn project to the ventral thalamus. The latter nucleus gives rise to the diencephalic locomotor control. Stimulation of the ventral thalamus elicits locomotor activity which can be recorded in the ventral roots of the isolated brainstem–spinal cord. The basal ganglia may thus exert a gate control of goal-directed locomotion elicited by olfactory and visual stimuli. Since olfactory and visual stimuli are both potent activators of locomotion, it is likely that these effects are exerted over the ventral thalamus. This would mean that goal-directed locomotion can be elicited via an oligosynaptic pathway which involves only two relays (ventral thalamus, reticulospinal nuclei) from sensory structures to the spinal cord.

8.3 BRAINSTEM–SPINAL CORD NETWORK CIRCUITRY, MEMBRANE PROPERTIES, AND ION CHANNELS

The cellular components of the brainstem–spinal cord network underlying locomotion are shown in Fig. 8.4. It consists of glutamatergic excitatory and glycinergic inhibitory neurons (see Grillner *et al.* 1995). These provide dynamic interactions on the millisecond time scale. In addition there are a number of G-protein mediated modulatory effects exerted by monaminergic and peptidergic systems.

The brainstem reticulospinal (RS) neurons are responsible for initiating and maintaining the excitatory drive to the locomotor pattern generators. They exert their effects through both NMDA and AMPA kainate receptors onto all neurons in the spinal network (Ohta and Grillner 1989). The main components of the spinal network that are responsible for the actual pattern generation are the ipsilateral excitatory interneurons (EIN, or E), which provide a phasic excitatory drive to motor neurons during each locomotor cycle (Buchanan and Grillner 1987), and also to glycinergic interneurons with crossed axons (CCIN, or J) that inhibit all contralateral network neurons, including motor neurons (MN, or M), at the segmental level (Buchanan 1982; Grillner 1985). The inhibitory interneurons provide phasic inhibition during contralateral activity. In addition there are in the rostral part of the spinal cord other types of inhibitory interneurons called lateral interneurons (LIN, or L) which receive phasic depolarization and hyperpolarization during locomotor activity. They do not appear to play any major role in pattern generation (Fagerstedt *et al.* 1995). The motor neurons on the left and right side show alternating activity. All motor neurons undergo one half-cycle with excitatory drive and another half-cycle with inhibitory drive (Russell and Wallén 1983; Wallén *et al.* 1985). During slow activity many motor neurons generate subthreshold oscillations while at higher burst rates the motor neurons are recruited progressively.

The total number of neurons in a hemisegment is estimated to 500 (Rovainen 1979*b*). There are about 100 motorneurons, five to nine inhibitory commissural interneurons with caudally projecting axons (CCIN), and at least 20 excitatory interneurons (Buchanan 1982; Buchanan and Cohen 1982; Dale 1986; Dale and Grillner 1986; Buchanan *et al.* 1989; Ohta *et al.* 1991). In addition there are a limited number of large lateral interneurons in the rostral part of the spinal cord (Rovainen 1974, Buchanan 1982).

Dynamic interactions between network interneurons are responsible for the pattern generation. The more tonic excitatory drive the interneurons are provided with (from the brainstem or by administering glutamate agonists (Grillner *et al.* 1981*b*) in the bath) the faster the network will oscillate (range 0.2–10 Hz). The reciprocal inhibition is of prime importance for generating the alternating pattern (Grillner and Wallén 1980; Hellgren *et al.* 1992). During activity on one side, both excitatory and inhibitory interneurons will be active. The net result will be that ipsilateral motor neurons are excited, while contralateral interneurons and motor neurons become inhibited. This inhibition is strong enough to overcome the excitatory drive from the brainstem. One crucial factor in a network like this is the control of the locomotor burst termination. In the isolated spinal cord, the membrane properties of the inhibitory interneurons play an important role. In particular, these include the calcium-dependent potassium channels (K_{Ca}) which are of two types, activated by (1) the calcium entry through high-voltage-activated calcium channels of N and P/Q type (El Manira *et al.* 1994; Tegnér 1997; Wikström *et al.* 1997; see Fig. 8.5A), and (2) a separate set of K_{Ca} channels that are activated by calcium entry through NMDA channels (Tegnér 1997). Frequency adaptation in the interneurons through summation of the after-hyperpolarization due to K_{Ca} is one major factor for controlling burst termination. Plateau-like depolarizations elicited by activation of NMDA channels (Fig. 8.5B) may also contribute, as well as low-voltage-activated calcium channels (Wallén and Grillner 1987; Grillner *et al.* 1995; Tegnér *et al.* 1997).

The network can thus operate at different burst rates. To prove that the K_{Ca} channels have a critical role, experiments with channel-specific toxins have been carried out. Apamin blocks the K_{Ca} channels activated by the calcium entry through N and P/Q channels occurring during the action potential (Wikström and El Manira 1998). If apamin is administered during continuous burst activity, interneurons will fire at a higher rate and the burst duration will increase, and consequently the burst frequency decrease. At lower frequencies the burst pattern will break down altogether (El Manira *et al.* 1994). Endogenous modulators like 5-HT, that also act on K_{Ca} channels, cause more intense bursts with much longer burst durations (Harris-Warrick and Cohen 1985; Wallén *et al.* 1989; Zhang *et al.* 1996).

Low voltage-activated (LVA) calcium channels are also present in network neurons (Matsushima *et al.* 1993; El Manira and Bussières 1997). These are activated when the cells are depolarized from a comparatively hyperpolarized level, and open below the threshold for the action potential. The LVA Ca^{2+} channels can thus boost the membrane depolarization enabling it to reach the threshold for an action potential. The calcium entry through LVA Ca^{2+} channels thus provides a post-inhibitory rebound. This can contribute to the stability of network activity (Tegnér *et al.* 1997), since during rhythmic burst activity, a blockade of LVA Ca^{2+} channels in modelling experiments may cause a change from a strict reciprocal pattern to more or less irregular activity. Thus, both LVA Ca^{2+} channels and voltage-dependent NMDA channels may contribute to burst stability.

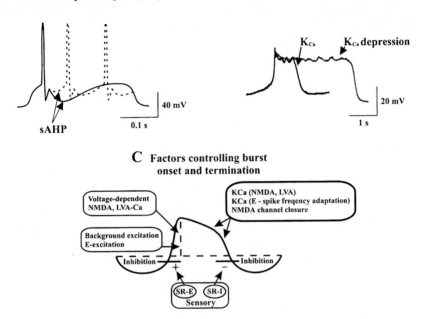

A **sAHP and spike frequency regulation**

40 mV

0.1 s

sAHP

B **K$_{Ca}$ and NMDA-plateau potentials**

K$_{Ca}$ K$_{Ca}$ depression

20 mV

1 s

C **Factors controlling burst onset and termination**

Voltage-dependent NMDA, LVA-Ca

KCa (NMDA, LVA)
KCa (E - spike freqency adaptation)
NMDA channel closure

Background excitation E-excitation

Inhibition   Inhibition

SR-E   SR-I
Sensory

Fig. 8.5 Spike frequency regulation, NMDA-plateau potentials, and control of burst termination. A: The amplitude of the slow afterhyperpolarization (sAHP) will determine whether one or several action potentials will occur during the phase of synaptic excitation in locomotor cycle. A large and long-lasting sAHP will make locomotor bursts shorter. B: Ca^{2+}-dependent K$^+$ channels (K$_{Ca}$) not only cause the sAHP but will also promote the termination of NMDA-receptor induced plateau potentials. The control plateau (solid trace) is markedly prolonged in the presence of the K$_{Ca}$-channel blocker apamine (dotted trace). C: Several different factors contribute to the initiation of the depolarizing phase, its maintenance, and its termination. In addition to conventional synaptic excitation, voltage-dependent NMDA receptors and low-voltage activated Ca^{2+} channels (LVA-Ca) are activated. Ca^{2+} will enter the cell through these channels, cause activation of K$_{Ca}$, and thereby a progressive hyperpolarization leading to closure of the NMDA channels. The initiation of the depolarizing phase is facilitated by activation of ipsilateral excitatory stretch receptor neurons (SR-E), while the termination of the depolarized phase is partially a result of activation of contralateral inhibitory stretch receptor neurons (SR-I). E indicates an excitatory interneuron.

Figure 8.5C summarizes several different factors which are important for determining burst onset and termination. Each neuron undergoes a phasic inhibition followed by excitation. The background excitation contributes to the depolarization and in addition the excitation from E-interneurons. There are in addition two factors that boost the membrane depolarization, the post-inhibitory rebound which activates low-voltage-activated calcium channels, and secondly the voltage-dependent NMDA channels which play an important role. During normal swimming there is in addition excitation from stretch receptor neurons (SR-E; see below). During the plateau depolarization there will be a progressively increasing activation of K_{Ca} channels due to the Ca^{2+} entry during three different sources, that is NMDA, LVA Ca^{2+}, and N-channels, activated during the action potential. The burst termination will occur due to a decreasing level of depolarization, which in turn will lead to NMDA channel closure and a more rapid repolarization. In addition during active swimming there will be a stretch receptor evoked inhibition (SR-I).

8.3.1   Calcium imaging in lamprey neurons

Calcium imaging experiments with high temporal and spatial resolution in the spinal cord of the lamprey (Bacskai *et al.* 1995), show that in both soma and dendrites of the network there is an entry of Ca^{2+} ions during activation. During an action potential, Ca^{2+} entry occurs in both soma and dendrites (Fig. 8.6A) and during synaptic activation (subthreshold EPSPs) there are local increases of calcium in the dendrites at the synaptic region (Fig. 8.6B). The Ca^{2+} entry during the glutamatergic EPSPs was due to both NMDA channels (50 per cent) and to

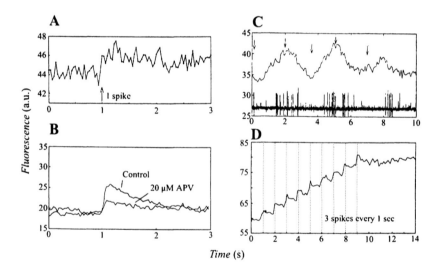

Fig. 8.6 Calcium dynamics in lamprey neurons. A: Fluorescence increase (Fluo-3; arbitrary units) in a portion of a proximal dendrite of a motoneuron, in response to a single action potential, evoked by intracellular stimulation. B: Calcium transients recorded in a small portion of a distal dendrite of a motoneuron, elicited by synaptic activation (resulting in subthreshold EPSPs) via stimulation of reticulospinal axons. The NMDA-receptor blocker 2-APV did not completely block the calcium transient. C: Phasic fluctuations of the calcium level in a motoneuron dendrite during ongoing fictive locomotion. Lower trace is the corresponding ventral root recording. The peak of the calcium trace occurs in phase with the burst, corresponding to the depolarizing phase of the locomotor cycle. D: A train of three action potentials was evoked by intracellular stimulation every 1 s. Calcium increases in a stepwise fashion with each spike train. Modified from Bacskai *et al.* (1995).

LVA Ca^{2+} channels, or possibly AMPA channels. During locomotor activity there is a phasic Ca^{2+} entry occurring in the dendrites in neurons, even in the absence of action potentials. This synaptically driven Ca^{2+} entry peaks during the ipsilateral burst and reaches a minimum during the trough (Fig. 8.6C). To what extent these changes in Ca^{2+} levels during the locomotor cycle affect the activation of K_{Ca} channels is thus far unknown.

8.3.2 Role of sensory feedback

The segmental network can thus operate in its physiological frequency range with a surprisingly simple drive signal from the brainstem or by changing the level of excitatory drive in the bath, that is the level of excitatory amino acid (Cohen and Wallén 1980; Grillner *et al.* 1981*b*). Under normal conditions, however, the undulatory movements of the body provide phasic sensory feedback from stretch receptors located at the lateral margin of the spinal cord (edge cells) (Grillner *et al.* 1982, 1984*a*). The stretch receptor neurons are of two kinds (see Fig. 8.4), one that provides excitation to ipsilateral interneurons and motor neurons, and a second that provides inhibition contralaterally (Viana Di Prisco *et al.* 1990). The sensory input is powerful enough to entrain the central network activity. Sensory feedback thus provides an overlay that can adapt the motor activity to different types of perturbations that may occur during locomotion under natural conditions, for instance by changing water currents. It is easy to realize that the connectivity discussed above can produce entrainment of the central network. Essentially, if the muscles on one side contract, the curvature of the other half of the segment will be affected and the stretch receptors on this side activated. This will result in an inhibition of the ongoing activity on the contracting side and ipsilateral excitation. This coupling will thus make the activity of the central pattern generator become entrained by peripheral movements within a certain range above or below the rest rate of the spinal network.

8.3.3 Mathematical modelling of the locomotor network

Even with a fair knowledge of the properties of each type of neuron, the types of synaptic interaction, and the neuronal activity that occurs, it is very difficult to intuitively understand how the network operates (cf. Fig. 8.4). This is due to the fact that an immense number of events occur in parallel in each cell, as well as in the interaction between a number of cells. In order to rigorously test if different plausible interpretations could apply, mathematical modelling is a very useful tool. Therefore, biophysical models of each type of neuron in the network have been developed (Ekeberg *et al.* 1991). These neurons are simulated with five different compartments, each of which may have Na^+, K^+, Ca^{2+}, K_{Ca} conductances, as well as synaptic conductances for EPSPs and IPSPs and voltage-dependent NMDA receptors. These neurons are thus assigned a certain input resistance and respond to simulated current injection in a similar way to their natural counterparts (Fig. 8.7A). The neurons thus exhibited an action potential and a fast and slow after-hyperpolarization.

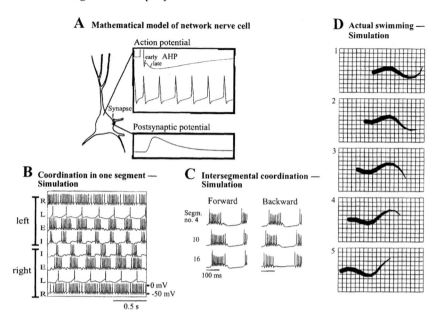

Fig. 8.7 Modelling of the lamprey locomotor network—simulations at neuronal, network, and behavioural levels. A: Neurons of the network were simulated in a realistic fashion, with the different voltage-dependent (Na^+, K^+, Ca^{2+}), Ca^{2+}-dependent K^+ channels, and ligand-gated channels (AMPA/kainate, NMDA, glycine). Action potentials with early and later afterhyperpolarization (AHP), and spike frequency adaptation, can be simulated, together with postsynaptic potentials occurring in different compartments. B: Simulation of the segmental network using a pool of excitatory (E) and inhibitory (I) interneurons and lateral (L) interneurons. The activity is driven by excitatory reticulospinal neurons (R). Activity on the left and right sides alternates. C: Pattern of intersegmental coordination, produced by a simulated network of 60 segments. This circuitry will produce a rostro-caudal phase lag along the simulated spinal cord, and this lag can be reversed if the excitability is increased in the caudal end, which results in backward locomotion. D: Simulation of actual swimming movements using a neuro-mechanical model. Frames show steady-state swimming at 4 Hz, resulting from tonic excitation of the network, with the model lamprey moving forward at a speed of 0.73 m s^{-1}. Time interval between frames is 50 ms. See text for further details. B–D are from Grillner *et al.* (1995).

Populations of excitatory and inhibitory interneurons with properties varying as in the natural population of cells were then connected as in the network described above (Hellgren *et al.* 1992; Tråvén *et al.* 1993). Such a network will respond to excitatory drive with burst activity with the appropriate phasing of the different cell types (Fig. 8.7B). The simulated network can be made to cover the physiological range of burst rates between 0.2 and 10 Hz. This means that the simulated network can mimic the segmental central pattern generator, and consequently that sufficient biological information is available to account for the behaviour. Although this does not mean that all relevant factors have been identified, what we have can itself explain the behaviour.

If in addition, segmental networks along the cord are connected in series, a rostrocaudal pattern of activation with a constant phase lag can be achieved, similar to that occurring in the swimming lamprey. This means that the intersegmental coordination can also be mimicked (Fig. 8.7C) (Wadden *et al.* 1997). Subsequently, this network was used to control a segmental viscoelastic muscle model such that motor activity in the rostral segments control rostral myotomes, which are coupled in series with caudal myotomes, which in turn are controlled from caudal network oscillators. By also simulating the viscous properties of water, it is possible to simulate actual swimming movements. The lamprey's movements are controlled by the neural network which activates the different segments along the body in the appropriate sequence. This results in a mechanical undulatory wave that is propagated from head to tail and which pushes the lamprey model through the simulated water (Fig. 8.7D) (Ekeberg *et al.* 1995). The model was initially made in two-dimensional space but later developed into a three-dimensional model that can 'swim' through the simulated water and turn left, right, upward, downward, and even produce screw-like movements. This is achieved by dividing the myotomes into dorsal and ventral compartments (cf. Wallén *et al.* 1985; Wannier *et al.* 1998) on each side, which in turn is controlled by a dorsal and ventral compartment of the ipsilateral spinal network. The actual motor pattern of this model lamprey is similar to its biological counterpart, not only with regard to the propulsive movements but also with regard to the movement pattern used during turning. At the network level, turning is produced by providing extra excitation via reticulospinal neurons to different combinations of the spinal compartments. For example, providing extra excitation to the dorsal and ventral compartments of the network on one side will produce turning toward this side. Correspondingly, an excitatory bias of the dorsal compartments on the left and right side will produce an upward turning movement.

8.3.4 Presynaptic modulation of sensory, interneuronal, and descending neurons

At the interneuronal level in the pattern generator network, a phasic GABAergic modulation of synaptic transmission occurs from both excitatory and inhibitory interneurons to motor neurons, which results in a gating of the synaptic efficacy in phase with the locomotor burst activity (Alford *et al.* 1991).

A similar GABA$_B$ modulation occurs at the sensory side and there is also a phasic modulation of afferent neuron synaptic transmission (Figs. 8.8A–C) (Christenson and Grillner 1991; El Manira *et al.* 1998). Sensory dorsal cells provide glutamatergic excitation to target interneurons. Small bipolar interneurons which contain both GABA and NPY immunoreactivity (Söderberg 1996; Parker *et al.* 1997*a*) form close appositions onto the axons of the dorsal cells. Both GABA (via GABA$_B$ receptors) and co-stored NPY cause a depression of synaptic transmission by a presynaptic action. The action of GABA is shorter-lasting than that of NPY. NPY is stored in dense core vesicles in the terminals and GABA immunoreactivity occurs over clusters of small vesicles. It would therefore seem likely that GABA is released during low levels of activity in the bipolar interneurons, whereas NPY would be released from the dense core vesicles only when the level of cytoplasmic calcium is

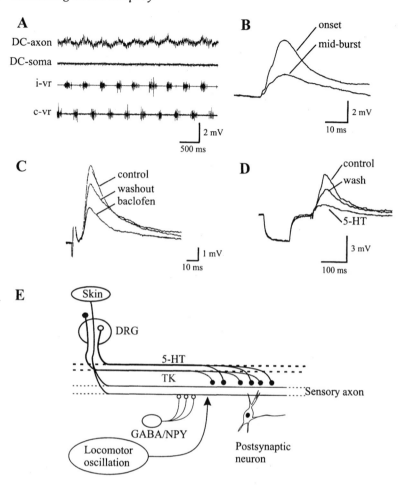

Fig. 8.8 Phasic membrane potential depolarization and modulation of sensory transmission. A: Dual intracellular recordings are made from a dorsal cell soma (DC-soma) and its axon (DC-axon) during fictive locomotion. The DC-axon recording shows phasic membrane depolarizations with the peak amplitude at the midpoint of the ipsilateral ventral root (i-vr) burst, whereas the membrane potential of DC-soma shows no phasic modulation. B: Monosynaptic compound EPSPs elicited in the giant interneuron by stimulation of the dorsal column, which activates axons of dorsal cells as well as other sensory neurons. The EPSP amplitude is smaller when the stimulation is delivered at the midburst, as compared with the burst onset. C: The GABA$_B$ receptor agonist baclofen depresses a sensory-evoked monosynaptic EPSP. D: 5-HT reduces the amplitude of monosynaptic EPSP elicited in a giant interneuron by dorsal column stimulation. E: Presynaptic modulation of sensory transmission. Dorsal root ganglion (DRG) contains small cells with 5-HT immunoreactivity and tachykinin fibres with their cell body in the peripheral dorsal root. 5-HT causes presynaptic inhibition of sensory dorsal cells' synaptic transmission. GABA and NPY, which are co-localized in bipolar interneurons also mediate presynaptic inhibition of sensory transmission. The locomotor oscillator also provides presynaptic modulation of excitatory glutamatergic transmission to postsynaptic neurons. A–D are from El Manira *et al.* (1998).

elevated, as will occur during high activity levels. If so, the presynaptic GABAergic action would be potentiated by co-released NPY only during high levels of activity. The dorsal root monosynaptic sensory transmission is also modulated by 5-HT (Fig. 8.8D) (El Manira *et al.* 1998) which provides presynaptic inhibition and a depression of calcium channel of the N-type, and by tachykinins which instead generate presynaptic facilitation (Parker and Grillner 1996). Both these modulatory inputs, 5-HT and tachykinins, appear to originate from sensory afferents with smaller diameters than glutamatergic dorsal cells which mediate touch and pressure (see scheme in Fig. 8.8E).

Synaptic transmission from the large reticulospinal axons is the target for presynaptic modulation by metabotropic group II and III glutamate receptors (mGluR), which are co-localized on the same reticulospinal axon (Fig. 8.9) (Krieger *et al.* 1996, 1998). This glutamatergic presynaptic inhibition of a glutamatergic synapse will thus presumably serve to provide autoinhibition, perhaps during overflow of glutamate during high levels of activity. In addition to the presynaptic group II and III mGluR, there are also post-synaptic group I mGluRs that increase the excitability of network neurons and increase the frequency of the locomotor rhythm. mGluR receptors can be activated by their specific agonists, and the presynaptic receptors require somewhat higher glutamate concentration than the post-synaptic metabotropic glutamate receptors belonging to the type I category.

The reticulospinal synapses are also subject to presynaptic modulation from 5-HT/DA interneurons in the spinal cord (Fig. 8.9B) (Buchanan and Grillner 1991; Wikström *et al.* 1995) and neuropeptides (Parker, unpublished). This means that segmental interneurons can determine the efficiency of the descending control signals from the brainstem.

8.3.5   Modulatory effects

The prime targets for different monoamine modulators (dopamine, 5-HT), metabotropic GABA and glutamate receptors, and peptides (somatostatin, NPY, tachykinins) are the different types of Ca^{2+} channels, K_{Ca} channels, and K^+ channels in the network neurons. Each of the target ion channels may affect either the somadendritic membrane properties of the interneurons, or synaptic transmission. This will in turn affect the firing properties of the cells and the strength of synaptic transmission. The properties of the cells then determine the activity pattern of the network. Dopamine and $GABA_B$ receptors act on N and P/Q Ca^{2+} channels (Matsushima *et al.* 1993; Schotland *et al.* 1995; El Manira and Bussières 1997; Bussières and El Manira 1997), and reduce Ca^{2+} entry occurring during the action potential, thereby reducing the activation of K_{Ca} channels. This will result in a smaller post-spike after-hyperpolarization and thereby higher frequency of firing, and at the network level, longer bursts. At the presynaptic level, dopamine and $GABA_B$ receptors reduce Ca^{2+} entry and thereby depress synaptic transmission (Christenson and Grillner 1991; Alford and Grillner 1991).

Just below the central canal in the midline of the spinal cord there is a group of cells that are immunoreactive to 5-HT, dopamine, and tachykinins (Schotland *et al.* 1995). They form a dense bilateral plexus at the ventromedial surface of the

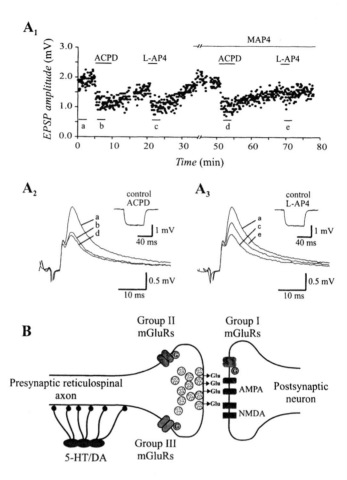

Fig. 8.9 Metabotropic glutamate receptor-mediated presynaptic inhibition of reticulo-spinal synaptic transmission. A_1: The effects of the mGluRs agonists (1S,3R)-ACPD and L-AP4 on the amplitude of the reticulospinal evoked EPSP were tested before and dur-ing application of the group III mGluRs antagonist MAP4. A_2: The decrease in the monosynaptic EPSP amplitude by (1S,3R)-ACPD was not antagonized by MAP4. A_3: The L-AP4-induced decrease of the monosynaptic EPSP was antagonized by MAP4. Neither (1S,3R)-ACPD nor L-AP4 affected the electrical component of the EPSP or the input resist-ance of the postsynaptic target neuron. B: Two types of mGluRs are co-localized on single reticulospinal axons and mediated presynaptic inhibition. These receptors are pharma-cologically similar to group II and III mGluRs. Group I mGluRs are present at the post-synaptic soma-dendritic level where they increase the excitability of neurons and thereby increase the frequency of the locomotor rhythm. Reticulospinal axons are also subject to presynaptic inhibition by 5-HT and dopamine (DA). Both 5-HT and DA are co-localized in neurons located ventral to the central canal and make close apposition with reticulospinal axons. From Krieger *et al.* (1996).

spinal cord. In this plexus the network interneurons and motor neurons distribute their ventromedial dendrites. The varicosities in this plexus do not form point to point synapses, and thus rely on paracrinic release of the transmitters (Christenson *et al.* 1989). The plexus extends throughout the spinal cord and is very dense. The concentration of transmitter/modulator in the ventromedial part of the spinal cord will presumably be substantial. Co-release of 5-HT and dopamine will target K_{Ca} and calcium channels, respectively, on network interneurons, and thereby exert complementary actions (see above). Furthermore, both dopamine and 5-HT elicit presynaptic inhibition on synaptic transmission from reticulospinal axons (Buchanan *et al.* 1989; Wikström *et al.* 1995). The fact that the neurons of the 5-HT/dopamine plexus are distributed along the spinal cord and are activated by sensory as well as descending fibres means that the activity in this plexus can be regulated segmentally (Schotland *et al.* 1996). This in turn suggests that the level of presynaptic inhibition along the reticulospinal axons can be regulated locally. In fact, the segment can presumably control how efficient synaptic transmission from descending supraspinal fibres will be. Consequently the level of descending drive may be varied through segmental presynaptic inhibition in different parts of the spinal cord.

8.3.6 Long-lasting synaptic plasticity induced by tachykinins in the locomotor network

Tachykinins are also distributed in the ventromedial plexus as well as in the dorsal horn and in sensory afferents (van Dongen *et al.* 1985, 1986). If tachykinins are applied to the bath during ongoing fictive locomotion, they cause a concentration-dependent increase in the locomotor rate. At higher, but still physiological, concentrations (1 μM) a short-lasting (10 min) application of tachykinins may cause a doubling of the locomotor burst rate, and this increased burst rate will remain elevated over 24 hours (Parker *et al.* 1998). The initial increase in burst rate is due to a protein kinase-C mediated increase in NMDA mediated synaptic transmission lasting over a period of 1–2 h. This leads to a potentiation of synaptic transmission in glutamatergic synapses, which involves activation of post-synaptic NMDA receptors. The subsequent period (2–24 hours) requires protein synthesis. Synthesis blockers like anisomysin applied prior to or within 1 h of the short-lasting tachykinin application will entirely block the second phase of facilitation of the burst rate, while the first NMDA-dependent component remains unchanged.

8.3.7 Coordination of unitary oscillators along the spinal cord

When the locomotor pattern is generated by the spinal cord, the unitary (segmental) oscillators are coordinated so that a wave of excitation of motor neurons travels along each side of the cord (Fig. 8.2D), and the waves on the left and right sides are in antiphase to each other. Two different views have been formulated to explain this coordination. According to the first view (Kopell and Ermentrout 1986, 1988), all the unitary oscillators in the spinal cord are equivalent to each other, and the direction of propagation of the waves is determined by the asymmetry of connections of each oscillator with its rostral and caudal neighbours. The alternative view (Cohen 1987; Rand *et al.* 1988; Matsushima and Grillner 1990, 1992) suggests that the oscillators are not equivalent to each other and that differences between the oscillators is the primary factor determining the direction of propagation of the waves as well as the speed of propagation.

Arguments that support the idea that excitability differences could play an important role were obtained in the following experiments (Matsushima and Grillner 1990, 1992). A chamber with a piece of the spinal cord was separated into three pools perfused with NMDA solutions of different concentration (Fig. 8.10A). By this method, the activity of oscillators in different regions along the cord (their 'excitability' and 'intrinsic frequency') could be manipulated separately. With equal NMDA concentration in the three pools, the pattern with caudally propagating waves was observed in most experiments (Fig. 8.10B). This may be due to different factors, including some asymmetry in the intersegmental connections formed by excitatory interneurons (EIN), inhibitory interneurons with crossed axons (CCIN), and lateral interneurons (LIN) (see for example Wallén *et al.* 1993). The speed of propagation of the locomotor waves strongly differed between the experiments, however. As shown in Fig. 8.4E, the value of the phase lag per segment in different experiments ranged continuously from +2 per cent to −1 per cent (the negative values correspond to the rostrally propagating waves). Thus, the spinal machinery is able to generate a continuum of the patterns of coordination between the unitary oscillators.

By applying NMDA of different concentration to different regions of the cord, one could change the pattern of coordination in a predictable way. A reduction of concentration in the rostral and middle pools resulted in reversal of the direction of propagation, from rostro-caudal (Fig. 8.10B) to caudo-rostral (Fig. 8.10C). A reduction of concentration in both rostral and caudal pools resulted in the formation of two waves, propagating from the middle region both in the rostral and in the caudal direction (Fig. 8.10D).

These findings may be explained if one suggests that the difference in the NMDA concentration creates a difference in intrinsic frequency of the unitary oscillators in different regions along the cord. These effects may be superimposed upon the effects of coupling rostro-caudal asymmetry. To illustrate this idea (the 'trailing oscillator' hypothesis) (Matsushima and Grillner 1990), let us consider a simple network that contains three unitary oscillators (Fig. 8.10F). Each of the oscillators consists of two parts (half-centres) with mutual inhibitory connections. The half-centres on each side of the oscillator have excitatory connections with their neighbours, thus forming two chains, the left and the right ones.

Activity of the half-centres on one side of the spinal cord (for example on the left side) is shown in Figs. 8.10G and H for different patterns of coordination. In G is shown the case when the cycle duration in the oscillator 1 (T_1) is shorter than the cycle duration in the oscillator 2 (T_2) and in the oscillator 3 (T_3). In each cycle, activation of the half-centre 2 is caused, with some delay (d_{1-2}), by input from the faster oscillator 1 rather than by the intrinsic oscillatory properties of the oscillator 2. The same relates to the oscillator 3 driven by the faster oscillator 2. Thus, the whole chain of unitary oscillators follows the faster ('leading') oscillator

1, and the wave of activation of the ipsilateral half-centres propagates caudally. The same considerations can be applied to the chain of half-centres on the right side of the cord. The antiphase relationships between the waves propagating on the left and right sides are caused by the system of reciprocal inhibition between the contralateral half-centres. This pattern, with caudally propagating waves, corresponds to forward swimming. If the most caudal oscillator 3 has the shortest cycle duration, the waves on the two sides will propagate rostrally, which corresponds to the backward swimming (Fig. 8.10H).

In this model, the control strategy to change the locomotor pattern is very simple. In addition to the uniform activation of all unitary spinal oscillators (which is necessary for eliciting their rhythmic activity), the supraspinal centres have to initiate a local excitation in a small portion of the spinal cord, either rostral (for forward swimming) or caudal (for backward swimming), and thus to create a leading oscillator.

In the model (Fig. 8.10F), the neuronal substrate for interactions between the unitary oscillators may be the excitatory interneurons (EINs) that are also the principal component of the unitary oscillators (Fig. 8.4). Their axons extend for several segments in the rostral or caudal direction (Dale 1986). The CCINs, with their caudally projecting axons (Buchanan 1982) may also contribute to the inter-segmental coupling.

An interesting feature of the model with the chains of interacting half-centres is that it can, in principle, generate not only periodical oscillations but also a single unilateral propagating wave. If one of the half-centres of the oscillator 1 is excited by supraspinal input, it will evoke excitation of the ipsilateral half-centre 2, which will then evoke excitation of the half-centre 3. This mode of operation of the model corresponds to the unilateral propagating wave that can be observed in the lamprey during lateral turns (see Section 8.6).

In the model (Fig. 8.10F), the speed of propagation of the locomotor waves is determined by the latency of the response in a given half-centre to the excitatory drive from the preceding half-centre. This latency depends on many factors, one of which is the level of the population activity of the EINs projecting to the half-centre. In Figs. 8.10J,K, the value of this activity is presented as the amplitude (A) of oscillations. With larger amplitude of the input signal, which is usually associated with faster swimming, it is easier to excite the follower half-centre, and the delay will be shorter. An increased descending excitatory drive, presumably associated with faster swimming, will also contribute to faster excitation of the follower half-centres. This gives one of the possible explanations for the shortening of the time delay between the motor neuron bursts in the successive segments when the locomotor frequency increases. This factor may contribute to the maintenance of the constancy of the intersegmental phase lag at different frequencies of swimming (Fig. 8.2F). The high precision of the maintenance of the phase lag (and, consequently, of the wavelength) in the lamprey and many species of fish suggests a contribution of some other mechanisms, however. One of these may be long intersegmental connections. To stabilize a wavelength of one body length, the crossed excitatory descending influences have to be exerted at the distance of one-half body length or approximately 50 segments (Fig. 8.10K). The lateral

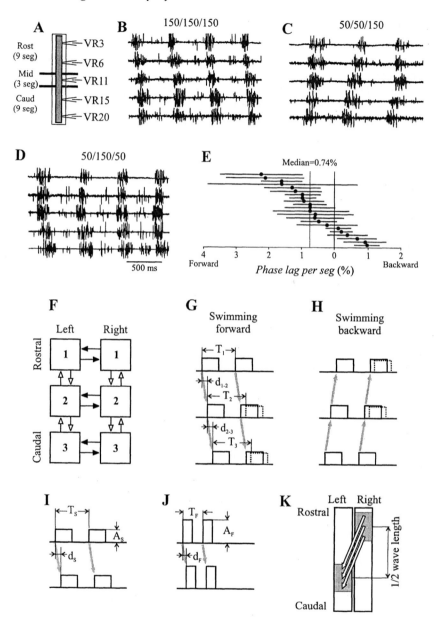

Fig. 8.10 Coordination of unitary oscillators. A: Experimental arrangement for separate manipulation with the excitability of neurons in different parts of the spinal cord. A chamber with a piece of the spinal cord was separated into three pools (rostral, middle, and caudal) perfused with NMDA solutions at different concentration, and the activity of the motor neurons was recorded from five ventral roots. B–D: The motor pattern generated by the spinal cord depends on the NMDA concentration in different pools (indicated in μM for the rostral/middle/caudal pools). B: With equal concentration in all the pools, the wave propagates caudally. C: With higher concentration in the caudal pool, the wave propagates rostrally. D: With higher concentration in the middle pool, there are two waves propagating rostrally

interneurons, that are activated by unitary oscillators (see Section 8.2), are good candidates for this role (Rovainen 1986). Their axons project caudally at distances comparable with the body length; they inhibit the ipsilateral CCINs and may thus disinhibit the contralateral hemisegments (Rovainen 1974).

8.4   COMMAND SYSTEM FOR THE INITIATION OF SWIMMING

8.4.1   Reticulospinal projections

The lamprey has two main behavioural states (Rovainen 1979*b*, 1982), quiescent and active. In the quiescent state the animal is attached to a substratum, for example the bottom of the aquarium, by its sucker mouth, and the trunk musculature is almost completely relaxed. Only a few postural reflexes can be observed in quiescent animals (Deliagina 1997*a*). In the active state, the animal is detached from the substratum and swims. The transition from the quiescent to active state is due to the activation of the reticulospinal (RS) system.

The RS system is present throughout the vertebrate kingdom, even in the phylogenetically oldest groups (Brodal 1958; Kuypers *et al.* 1962; Pompeiano 1973; Peterson 1979; Ten Donkelaar 1982; Cruce and Newman 1984; McClellan 1986). The lamprey has four reticular nuclei (Fig. 8.11A): the mesencephalic reticular nucleus (MRN), as well as the anterior, middle, and posterior rhombencephalic reticular nuclei (ARRN, MRRN, and PRRN) (Nieuwenhuys 1972). All of them give rise to RS pathways. The nuclei include mainly small and mid-sized neurons (4–20 µm) but also a few larger neurons (50–100 µm), the Müller cells (M, I, and B groups), the Mauthner cells, and a group of V cells. The Müller and Mauthner cells, as well as their axons in the spinal cord, can be individually identified (Figs. 8.11A,B) (Rovainen 1967, 1978). The estimated number of RS neurons is 2500, half of which are located in the PRRN (Bussières 1994).

The axons of the RS neurons descend mainly along the ipsilateral side of the spinal cord. About half of them terminate in the rostral and middle areas of the

---

and caudally. E: With equal concentration of NMDA in all pools, the spinal cord preparations ($n = 22$) differed in the value of the phase lag per segment. F–K: Schematic illustration of the idea of trailing oscillators (Matsushima and Grillner 1992). In the chain of three oscillators (F), the oscillator with a shorter cycle period automatically becomes the leading one. If the rostral oscillator (1) has the period (T_1) shorter than the other oscillators (T_2 and T_3), the wave propagates caudally (G); if the caudal oscillator (3) has the shorter period, the wave propagates rostrally (H). The delay between activation of successive oscillators in this model depends, among other factors, on the amplitude of oscillations. At slow swimming (I) with a long period (T_s) and small amplitude (A_s), the delay (d_s) is larger than at fast swimming (J). K: Illustration of the idea (Rovainen 1986) that long propriospinal descending axons, with the excitatory action on the contralateral hemisegments, may contribute to stabilizing the length of the propagating wave. Active areas on the left and right sides of the spinal cord are shaded. Long arrows show excitatory influences of the rostral area on the caudal area. The configuration of two excited areas travels caudally. A–E are from Matsushima and Grillner (1992).

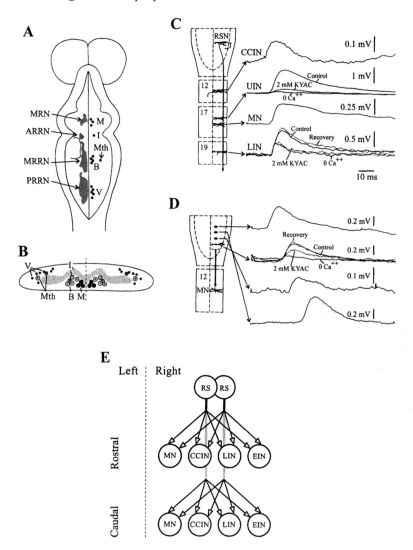

Fig. 8.11 The reticulospinal system. A: The four main reticular nuclei of the brainstem: the mesencephalic (MRN), and the anterior, middle, and posterior rhombencephalic reticular nuclei (ARRN, MRRN, and PRRN), outlined on the left side of the brain. On the right side, the M, I, and B groups of large Müller cells, the Mauthner cell (Mth), and a group of V cells are shown. Position of the spinal axons of these cells on the cross section of the spinal cord are shown in B. C: Divergence of monosynaptic excitatory effects from a single reticulospinal neuron (RSN) from PPRN, to different types of spinal neurons. Intracellular stimulation of the RSN produced EPSPs in four types of spinal neurons (CCIN, MN, LIN, and unidentified interneuron, UIN) tested in different spinal segments (indicated by numbers in the drawing). The EPSPs in UIN and LIN were depressed by the excitatory amino acid blocker kynurenic acid (KYAC). In Ca^{2+} free solution, the transmission was further depressed in UIN and not changed in LIN. D: Convergence of monosynaptic EPSPs from several individual PRRN neurons to a single motor neuron. Four PRRN neurons elicited EPSPs in the motor neuron. The excitatory amino acid transmission was confirmed

spinal cord, but many reach the most caudal part. Thus, the RS system is the main descending system in the lamprey. The vestibulospinal system in the lamprey is formed by much fewer cells, located in the vestibular (octavomotorius) nuclei; their axons project only to the rostral part of the spinal cord (Rovainen 1979*b*; Bussières 1994).

The connectivity between the large and mid-sized RS neurons and their target nerve cells in the spinal cord has been elucidated in paired intracellular record-ing experiments (Rovainen 1974; Buchanan and Cohen 1982; Buchanan *et al.* 1987; Ohta and Grillner 1989). Most of the fast-conducting RS neurons from all reticular nuclei produce monosynaptic EPSPs in the spinal cells by means of dual electrical and chemical transmission. Spinal projections of individual RS neurons were investigated in detail for the PRRN (Ohta and Grillner 1989). Intracellular stimulation of single PRRN neurons produced monosynaptic EPSPs in simultan-eously recorded motor neurons and premotor interneurons of different classes (EINs, CCINs, and LINs, see Fig. 8.4) on the ipsilateral side of the spinal cord. An individual RS neuron can project to different segments along the spinal cord, where it affects spinal neurons of different classes (Fig. 8.11C). Conversely, several RS neurons can converge on individual spinal neurons (Fig. 8.11D). The diver-gence and convergence of the ipsilateral RS projections is schematically shown in Fig. 8.11E.

The EPSPs produced by the PRRN neurons in their target cells contain chemical and electrical components. The electrical EPSPs remained when Ca^{2+} was substi-tuted with Mn^{2+} in the ordinary physiological solution. The chemical component of the EPSPs was depressed when a broad-spectrum excitatory amino acid antag-onist (kynurenic acid) was applied, suggesting that the chemical component was due to excitatory amino acid transmission (Figs. 8.11C,D). The chemical EPSP, in its turn, could have two components caused by activation of the NMDA and non-NMDA subtypes of glutamate receptors.

Labelling of the RS neurons in different reticular nuclei of the brainstem by transmitter-related markers revealed several groups of cells. The most numerous are the RS neurons that utilize L-glutamate as their transmitter (Brodin *et al.* 1985). They can be found in all four reticular nuclei. There are smaller groups utilizing serotonin (5-HT) or other transmitters (Brodin *et al.* 1986, 1988*a*). In addition, there are inhibitory RS neurons utilizing glycine as their transmitter (Wannier *et al.* 1995).

8.4.2   Initiation of swimming

A large body of evidence suggests that the reticulospinal system, and its gluta-matergic subdivision in particular, is responsible for the activation of the spinal locomotor networks:

---

in one of the pairs by applying KYAC. E: Main features of reticulospinal projections: innervation of different parts along the spinal cord, divergence and convergence. C, D are from Ohta and Grillner (1989).

1. Glutamate can act at three types of receptors named after their principal agonists: NMDA, AMPA/kainate, and quisqualate (for review see Watkins and Evans 1981; Davies *et al.* 1982). In the isolated preparation of the lamprey spinal cord, fictive locomotor activity can be induced by pharmacological activation of certain excitatory amino acid receptors—NMDA receptors and the kainate receptors but not the AMPA receptors (Figs. 8.2D and 8.10B) (Grillner *et al.* 1981*b*; Brodin and Grillner 1985*a,b*; Brodin *et al.* 1985). Specific antagonists to these receptors block naturally initiated locomotor activity, both spontaneously occurring or caused by sensory stimulation. Activation of these amino acid receptors thus appears to be a prerequisite for the occurrence of locomotor activity under normal conditions (Brodin and Grillner 1985*a,b*).

2. Electrical or chemical stimulation of many sites within the reticular formation results in activation of the spinal locomotor networks in a stimulus-dependent manner (Figs. 8.12A–C). This activation can be blocked by the excitatory amino acid antagonists.

3. Electrical stimulation of individual Müller cells, which utilize glutamate as their transmitter (Buchanan *et al.* 1987), affects both the amplitude of the segmental motor output and its temporal pattern (Figs. 8.12D–F).

4. The activity of the larger glutamatergic RS neurons (Müller cells and V cells) considerably increases when locomotion is initiated in the intact lamprey. Figure 8.12G shows that illumination of the right eye in a quiescent lamprey initially elicits weak activity in the ipsilateral RS neurons. This activity is then followed by a strong, 'explosive' bilateral activation of the RS system and by swimming (Orlovsky *et al.* 1997). Such a bilateral activation of the RS system always precedes the onset of swimming, irrespective of how the swimming is initiated (spontaneously or by visual, vestibular, somatosensory, or lateral line sensory stimulation). In the intact lamprey, more intensive locomotion is associated with higher levels of activation of the RS system.

5. Activation of the RS neurons is also observed in the *in vitro* brainstem–spinal cord preparation when fictive locomotion is evoked by somatosensory stimuli (Viana Di Prisco *et al.* 1997), vestibular stimuli (Orlovsky *et al.* 1992), or lateral line stimuli (Deliagina *et al.* 1995).

6. Chemical microstimulation of the RS neurons in any of the four reticular nuclei may affect the rhythm of fictive locomotion induced in the spinal cord by NMDA (Wannier *et al.* 1998).

Taken together, these findings support the idea that the summed activity in a population of glutamatergic RS neurons is responsible for the elicitation of locomotion, as well as for the control of its intensity (Brodin *et al.* 1988*b*).

8.4.3   Sensory-motor transformation by the RS system

The reticulospinal system has two important features that considerably simplify the task of the control of locomotion by the CNS. First, activity of this system in the intact lamprey can be maintained at a high level for a long period of time after termination of the stimulus that had elicited swimming. This was demonstrated for stimuli of different modalities: visual (Fig. 8.12G), vestibular, somatosensory (Orlovsky *et al.* 1997), and lateral line (Deliagina *et al.* 1995). A possible explanation for this phenomenon is the specific membrane properties of the RS neurons. In response to a brief stimulus, these neurons are able to generate long-lasting plateau potentials (Viana Di Prisco *et al.* 1997). Figure 8.12H shows that a brief tactile stimulus applied to the head in the semi-intact preparation elicited a long-lasting plateau potential in the RS neuron followed by swimming (monitored as the bursts of EMG recorded from the trunk muscles). These plateau potentials are caused by the reflex pathway that activates NMDA receptors on the membrane of the RS neurons (Viana Di Prisco *et al.* 1995; Dubuc *et al.* 1993). The involvement of NMDA receptors was demonstrated by local application of the NMDA receptor blocker AP5 (2-amino-3-hydroxy-5-phosphonopentanoate) to the surface of the recorded RS cell, which resulted in elimination of the plateau potential response to cutaneous sensory input (Fig. 8.12I,J) (Viana Di Prisco *et al.* 1997). It seems likely that the same mechanism is responsible for the transformation of brief sensory inputs of other modalities into a long-lasting activation of the RS system.

When an RS neuron is generating a plateau potential, it still remains capable of responding to afferent signals and also to the 'efference copy' signals coming from the spinal locomotor CPG. These signals produce rhythmical modulation of the RS neuron discharge (see Fig. 8.12I and Section 8.4.4). Due to the persistent sensitivity to afferent inputs, the RS neurons are able to perform corrections and modifications of the ongoing locomotor pattern (see Section 8.5).

The second important feature of the RS system is that a unilateral sensory input can initiate a bilateral activation of RS neurons, as illustrated in Fig. 8.12G for the case when swimming was evoked by illumination of the right eye. The bilateral, symmetrical activation of the two subdivisions (left and right) of the RS system is a necessary condition for the generation of symmetrical segmental motor output and for rectilinear swimming. Rectilinear swimming is the most common pattern of locomotion in the lamprey; it occurs in different behavioural contexts and can be evoked by different sensory stimuli (Ullén *et al.* 1995*a*,*b*). The principal question is where is a unilateral sensory signal transformed into bilateral activity? One possibility would be that this occurs within the RS system itself. No interconnections between different RS neurons, and between the left and right subdivisions of the RS system in particular, have been reported, however. Thus, the transformation from a unilateral to a bilateral signal takes place at a pre-reticular level. One possibility would be that this occurs in a centre similar to the mesencephalic locomotor region of higher vertebrates (Shik *et al.* 1966*a*; Jordan 1986) (see Section 12.1), or in several centres of this kind. In the lamprey, one of the possible candidates for this role is the area in the brainstem described by Sirota *et al.* (1994), whose microstimulation induces swimming in a semi-intact preparation. Another candidate is the area in the ventral thalamus which also supplies the RS system with drive signals and can elicit symmetrical fictive swimming (El Manira *et al.* 1997*a*).

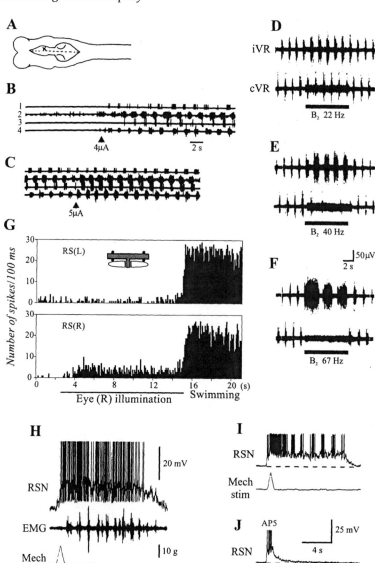

Fig. 8.12 Initiation of swimming by the reticulospinal system. A–C: In the brainstem–spinal cord preparation (A) stimulation of a site in the mesencephalon (marked by a cross) elicits fictive locomotion monitored by alternating bursting activity in the left and right ventral roots at the rostral (1 and 2) and caudal (3 and 4) levels (B,C). With stronger stimulation, the bursting activity increased (C). In B and C, the arrows show the onset of stimulation; the strength of stimulating pulses (µA) is indicated. D–F: In the same type of preparation, intracellular stimulation (shown by bars) of a single RS neuron (the B_2 Müller cell) strongly affects the D-glutamate-induced fictive swimming. The frequency of stimulation is indicated for each trail. G: Histograms of the population activity of the larger RS neurons recorded from the left (L) and right (R) sides of the spinal cord of the intact lamprey by means of

8.4.4 Feedback from the spinal CPG

Experiments on the *in vitro* brainstem–spinal cord preparation (Kasicki *et al.* 1989; Kasicki and Grillner 1986), on the semi-intact preparation (Dubuc and Grillner 1989), and on the intact lamprey (Orlovsky *et al.* 1997) have shown that a considerable proportion of RS neurons exhibit rhythmic modulation of their membrane potential and bursting activity when a locomotory rhythm is generated by the spinal cord. An example of such a modulation is shown in Fig. 8.12I. The peak activity of RS neurons usually coincides with the peak activity of the ipsilateral motor neurons in the rostral spinal segments. A similar pattern of rhythmic modulation is observed during fictive locomotion also in the vestibulospinal neurons (Bussiéres and Dubuc 1992).

The rhythmic modulation of the brainstem neurons is caused by input from the spinal locomotor networks. This was demonstrated for the RS neurons in experiments when NMDA was applied only to the spinal cord but not to the brainstem, and thus only the spinal locomotor networks were activated (Dubuc and Grillner 1989). Influences from these networks were sufficient to produce rhythmical modulation of the RS neurons. It was also found that the modulation is due to both phasic excitatory and inhibitory inputs which affect the RS neurons in opposite phases of the locomotor cycle.

These experiments clearly demonstrated that the spinal networks in the lamprey, responsible for the generation of the locomotor pattern, send signals to higher motor centres (the reticular and vestibular nuclei of the brainstem) about their ongoing activity. Under the effect of these signals, the activity of the brainstem centres and, therefore, the supraspinal commands addressed to the spinal CPG, are dependent on the phase of the locomotor cycle.

Phasic modulation of the activity of the locomotor command systems, caused by efference copy signals from the locomotor CPG, has been observed in different species, from molluscs (see Section 2.3.2) to mammals (see Section 13.4). One of the possible functions of this modulation is to link the descending commands to a certain phase of the locomotor cycle, in which their effect will be most appropriate (the 'gating function'). This idea will be discussed in more detail in relation to the locomotor control system of the cat (see Section 13.5). In the lamprey, this modulation may also play an additional role, that is an induction of higher excitability in the rostral segments (Kasicki *et al.* 1989), which is a necessary condition for

---

implanted electrodes (inset). Illumination of the right eye evoked the moderate activation of the ipsilateral RS neurons followed by the strong bilateral activation and swimming. H–J: Effects of the mechanical stimulation of the skin covering the head region in the semi-intact preparation. H: Brief stimulus elicited a plateau potential and spike activity in the RS neuron accompanied by the rhythmic EMG bursting and undulatory movements of the caudal part of the body. I,J: The plateau potential in the RS neuron evoked by skin stimulation (I) was dramatically reduced by local application of AP5 (blocker of NMDA receptors) to the somata of the neuron (J). Interrupted lines in I,J show the resting membrane potential. A–C are from McClellan and Grillner (1984), D–F are from Buchanan and Cohen (1982), and H–J are from Viana Di Prisco *et al.* (1997), G is from Deliagina, Orlovsky and Grillner (unpublished data).

forward swimming according to the 'trailing oscillator' hypothesis (Matsushima and Grillner 1990, 1992).

8.5   CONTROL OF POSTURAL ORIENTATION AND EQUILIBRIUM

8.5.1   General characteristics of postural control.
Role of vestibular and visual inputs

During steady swimming, the lamprey maintains a horizontal orientation of the body (Fig. 8.13A$_1$), but it can also swim at a certain angle in relation to the horizon (pitch angle β in Fig. 8.13A$_2$). At any pitch angle, the lamprey maintains the dorsal-side-up orientation, with a minimal roll tilt angle α (Figs. 8.13B$_1$,B$_2$) (Ullén *et al.* 1995*a*). It was therefore suggested that there are two postural control systems in the lamprey, relatively independent of each other, one responsible for the orientation in the sagittal (pitch) plane, and the other one for the orientation in the transverse (roll) plane (Orlovsky *et al.* 1992).

In many species of fish, the paired pectoral and pelvic fins are the main effector organs for stabilizing and changing the body orientation in the roll and pitch planes (Harris 1936; Timmerick *et al.* 1990), but the lamprey has no paired fins and is therefore limited to using movements of the body and dorsal fin for this purpose. For changing the orientation in the pitch plane, a flexion of the body in this plane is used. For changing orientation in the roll plane, different motor patterns are used: (1) lateral bending of the body which, due to the downward-deflected tail (Fig. 8.13A$_1$), generates a moment of forces around the longitudinal body axis; (2) twisting of the body, and (3) lateral deviation of the dorsal fin (Ullén *et al.* 1995*a*; Deliagina 1997*a*).

Vestibular input is very important for the systems controlling body orientation in the roll and pitch planes. Blinded animals, as well as intact animals in darkness, orient themselves perfectly with the help of the vestibular apparatus. However, after bilateral labyrinthectomy, lampreys with intact vision cannot maintain any fixed orientation in space and are continuously looping in different planes (Figs. 8.13C$_1$,C$_2$) (de Burlet and Versteegh 1930; Ullén *et al.* 1995*b*). Visual input exerts only a modulatory effect on the body orientation in the lamprey. Illumination of one eye evokes a roll tilt towards the source of light (see inset in Fig. 8.14G) (Ullén *et al.* 1995*b*, 1997). This postural reflex has been described more extensively for bony fish and has been termed 'the dorsal light response' (von Holst 1935; Platt 1983).

8.5.2   Postural control network

The essential components of the postural control network in the brainstem of the lamprey are shown in Fig. 8.13D. Vestibular afferents of the eighth cranial nerve terminate on the neurons of the vestibular (octavomotor) nuclei located in the lateral medulla (Rubinson 1974; Koyama *et al.* 1989). These neurons project to the ipsilateral and contralateral RS neurons in all four reticular nuclei (Wickelgren 1977; Rovainen 1979*a*) which give rise to the main descending spinal projections

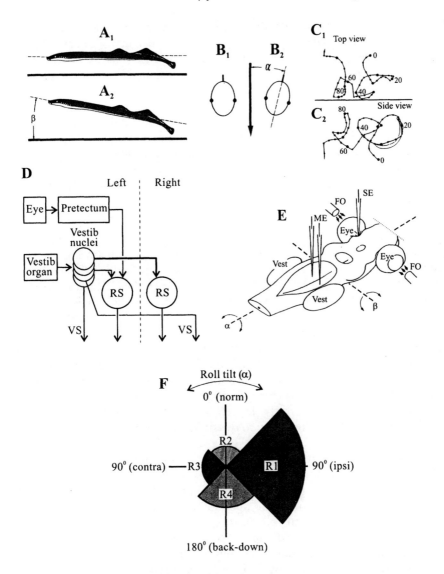

Fig. 8.13 Role of vestibular input in postural control. A_1, A_2: The lamprey swims either horizontally or at a constant angle (pitch, β) in relation to the horizon. B_1, B_2: The lamprey swims with its dorsal side up (B_1), and a deviation from this orientation (roll tilt, α) is rapidly compensated. C_1, C_2: Trajectory of the lamprey (top view, C_1, and side view, C_2) after bilateral labyrinthectomy. The numbers of frames (25 frames/s) are indicated. D: Essential components of the brainstem postural network (RS, reticulospinal neurons; VS, vestibulospinal neurons). E: Experimental arrangement for investigating responses in the brainstem neurons to rotation ($\pm 180°$) in the roll and pitch planes (α and β, correspondingly), and to visual input (illumination of eyes by the fibre optics, FO, or electrical stimulation of the optic nerve, SE). F: Otolith afferents can be classified in four groups (R1–R4) according to their zone of response to roll tilt (α), the radius of the sectors is proportional to the size of the groups. C_1 and C_2 are from Ullén *et al.* (1995a).

from the brainstem. In addition, the neurons of the vestibular nuclei give rise to the bilateral vestibulospinal tract projecting to the rostral spinal segments (Rovainen 1979a; Bussières and Dubuc 1992). The RS neurons receive visual input signalling about the degree of eye illumination; this input is mediated by interneurons located in the pretectal area (Zompa and Dubuc 1996; Ullén *et al.* 1997).

The processing of vestibular and visual information in the postural control network was studied in an *in vitro* preparation consisting of the brainstem isolated with the vestibular organs and, in some experiments, also with eyes (Fig. 8.13E). The preparation could be rotated in space in the roll plane (α) or pitch plane (β), with simultaneous recording from the brainstem neurons. Two classes of neurons were investigated: vestibular afferents and RS neurons (Orlovsky *et al.* 1992; Deliagina *et al.* 1992a,b, 1993).

8.5.2.1 Postural responses in vestibular afferents

The labyrinth of the lamprey consists of the otolith organ (macula) and two semicircular canals, in contrast to three canals in fish and higher vertebrates (Lowenstein *et al.* 1968). The macula primarily supplies the CNS with information about the body orientation in the gravity field, whereas the canals signal about rotation of the lamprey in different planes, including the roll and pitch planes (Lowenstein 1970). The *canal afferents* respond to roll and pitch; the duration of the response is determined by the duration of motion, while the frequency of discharge is related to the speed of motion. Two types of response to movements in the sagittal plane are observed; activation with movements towards nose-down or towards nose-up. These two types correspond to the afferents from the anterior and posterior canals, respectively (Lowenstein *et al.* 1968). All afferents respond to roll towards ipsi-side-down, i.e. to the stimulus activating the receptor cells of both canals.

The *otolith afferents* in the lamprey are both position and motion sensitive in a specific zone of roll and pitch angles, whereas outside this zone of sensitivity the afferents are silent. In the roll plane, four groups of afferents can be distinguished (Fig. 8.13F). The largest group (R1, about 50 per cent of all afferents) is activated around 90° of the ipsilateral roll tilt; the other groups (R2, R3, and R4) have their maxima at 0° (dorsal side up), at 90° of the contralateral roll tilt, and at 180° (ventral side up) respectively. Taken together, these zones cover the whole range of possible orientations of the lamprey in the roll plane. In the pitch plane, there are three groups (P1, P2, and P3) with their maxima at 90° nose-down, 90° nose-up, and at 180° (dorsal side down) positions respectively.

8.5.2.2 Postural responses in reticulospinal neurons

Figure 8.14A shows the response of three RS neurons to rotation in the roll plane. They were recorded simultaneously by means of two microelectrodes in the left (units 1 and 2) and in the right (unit 3) MRRN. The neurons have their zones of activity around 90° contralateral roll tilt. Activation with a contralateral roll tilt is a major characteristic of the RS neurons in all four reticular nuclei, but the neurons from different nuclei differ somewhat in their spatial zones of sensitivity, that is in the angular threshold for their activation, as well as in the angular position of the peak of their response (Fig. 8.14B$_1$). Taken together, the spatial zones of sensitivity of the four nuclei cover the whole range of possible inclinations of the lamprey in the roll plane (Deliagina *et al.* 1992*a*). A similar pattern of the response in RS neurons, that is activation with contralateral roll tilt, was recorded in the intact lamprey by means of implanted electrodes (Deliagina 1997*c*).

Two findings indicate that excitatory input from the contralateral labyrinth, shown by a heavy line in Fig. 8.13D, mediated by the contralateral vestibular nuclei, is the main input driving the RS neurons: (1) The majority of vestibular afferents respond to ipsilateral roll tilt (Fig. 8.13F) whereas the RS neurons respond to contralateral roll tilt (Fig. 8.14B$_1$), and (2) after removal of one of the labyrinths, the responses to roll tilt disappear only in the contralateral RS neurons (Deliagina *et al.* 1992*b*). Since the RS neurons exhibit clear-cut responses to different maintained orientations in the gravity field (Fig. 8.14A), one can conclude that input from the contralateral otolith organ is of primary importance for the generation of a vestibular response in these neurons.

When tested by inclination in the pitch plane, the RS neurons exhibit different patterns of response; some of them respond to nose-up tilt, others to nose-down tilt (Fig. 8.14B$_2$) (Deliagina *et al.* 1992*a*). These patterns of response correspond to those in the different groups of otolith afferents (see Section 8.5.2.1).

An essential common feature of different RS neurons is that they respond to inclination both in the roll and in the pitch planes, within rather wide spatial zones. This is illustrated in Figs. 8.14C$_1$–C$_3$ for an ARRN neuron. One can see that the same level of activity in this neuron can be evoked by different combinations of tilts in the roll and pitch planes. One can thus conclude that (1) the roll control system and the pitch control system share the same descending pathways for transmitting commands to the spinal cord, and (2) by relying only on the activity of a single RS neuron (like the one shown in Figs. 8.14C$_1$–C$_3$), and even on the activity of a population of ipsilateral neurons from different nuclei (Figs. 8.14B$_1$, B$_2$), it is impossible to decide about the true body orientation, and to generate a postural corrective motor response. Evidently, the information required for the generation of postural corrections is coded in the form of population activity of RS neurons, which is decoded in the motor centres at a lower level (in the spinal cord) on the basis of comparing the activities of different groups of RS neurons. A similar organization of the system controlling postural orientation and equilibrium has also been found in invertebrates—molluscs (see Section 1.6), crustacea (see Section 5.5), and insects (see Section 7.5).

8.5.3   A model of the roll control system

A conceptual model for stabilization of the body orientation of the lamprey in the roll plane, based on comparisons of the activities of different RS neuron groups, has been proposed (Deliagina *et al.* 1993; Deliagina 1997*a*,*b*). In Fig. 8.14E, the two antagonistic groups of RS neurons (left and right) are driven by contralateral vestibular input with a maximal response at 90° of contralateral roll tilt (Fig. 8.14F), provided that visual input is absent. Each of the two subpopulations evoke motor responses (rolling) in opposite directions (shown by arrows)

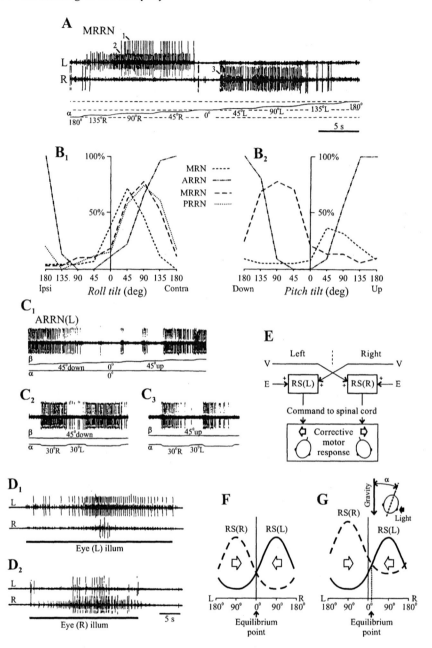

Fig. 8.14 Role of the RS system in postural control. A: Responses to roll tilt in the RS neurons (1–3) recorded extracellularly by two microelectrodes from the left (L) and right (R) MRRN in the *in vitro* preparation (see Fig. 8.13E). The tilt angle of 0° corresponds to the dorsal side up orientation. B_1, B_2: Summary diagrams of responses to roll and pitch in different reticular nuclei. The relative number of neurons active at different positions is presented as a function of roll (B_1) and pitch (B_2). C_1–C_3: Responses of the ARRN neuron to roll (α) and pitch (β)

via the spinal neuronal circuits. These responses are proportional to the degree of activation of the two groups. The model stabilizes the orientation at which the activities of the two groups of RS neurons (left and right) are equal to each other and, therefore, their motor effects compensate for each other, which happens only at the dorsal-side-up orientation; this orientation corresponds to the equilibrium point of the roll control system (Fig. 8.14F).

8.5.4   Stabilization of different postural orientations

Illumination of one of the eyes in the lamprey evokes the dorsal light response, that is an inclination of the animal in the roll plane towards the more illuminated side (inset in Fig. 8.14G). In the *in vitro* preparation (Fig. 8.13E), illumination of one eye or electrical stimulation of the optic nerve results in the excitation of the ipsilateral RS neurons (Deliagina *et al.* 1993; Ullén *et al.* 1996). According to the model (Fig. 8.14E), an additional activation of one group of RS neurons, caused by ipsilateral visual input, results in a shift of the equilibrium point in the roll control system, and the system will now stabilize an orientation differing from the dorsal-side-up orientation, with a tilt towards the illuminated side (Fig. 8.14G). This conclusion was further supported in experiments with an 'artificial' induction of asymmetry in vestibular or visual inputs by means of removal of the sense organs, or electrical stimulation of the corresponding nerves (Deliagina 1997*a,b*).

Thus, in the lamprey a change from one postural orientation to another is based on resetting the equilibrium point in the control system, which occurs under the effect of a tonic drive signal. This principle contrasts to that in *Clione* where a change in the postural orientation is caused by a reconfiguration (change of topology) of the postural control network (see Section 1.6).

8.6   LATERAL TURNS

The lateral turns are part of different forms of behaviour in the lamprey, like steering towards prey, negative phototaxis, escape reaction, etc. (McClellan and Grillner 1983; McClellan 1984; Ullén *et al.* 1993, 1997; McClellan and Hagevik 1997). Most spontaneous turns take place during one single locomotor cycle (McClellan and Hagevik 1997). During the turn, the motor pattern of swimming

---

inclinations presented in different combinations with each other. D_1, D_2: Responses of the RS neurons from the left (L) and right (R) MRRN to illumination of the left (D_1) and right (D_2) eye. E: Conceptual model of the roll control system. Two groups of RS neurons—left (L) and right (R)—receive contralateral vestibular input (V) and ipsilateral visual input (E). They send a command to the spinal cord, where it evokes a corrective motor response (indicated by arrows). F: Activities of the two groups, and the motor responses that they evoke, as a function of the roll tilt for the case when visual inputs are absent. The arrows indicate the direction of motor response evoked by each of the groups. G: The same as in F, but with the tonic input from the right eye caused by its illumination (inset). A,B_1 and B_2 are from Deliagina *et al.* (1992*a*), C_1–C_3 are from Orlovsky *et al.* (1992), D_1 and D_2 are from Deliagina *et al.* (1993), and E–G are modified from Deliagina (1997*a*).

is considerably modified: (1) the cycle duration is increased, (2) the burst intensity and duration increases on the ipsilateral (turn) side, and (3) for large turns, this burst on the ipsilateral side is typically delayed in the cycle (McClellan and Hagevik 1997; Zelenin *et al.* 1997). The changes in timing of the motor pattern imply that the supraspinal command for eliciting a turn is addressed not only to the motor neurons but also to the CPG interneurons.

Recordings of the activity of the left and right populations of RS neurons in the intact lamprey have shown that the turn is associated with some asymmetry in the descending flow of pulses, with a prevalence of the ipsilateral (to the direction of turning) flow (Orlovsky *et al.* 1997). Computer simulations have shown that an asymmetry in descending commands, addressed to the chain of spinal oscillators, can evoke most modifications of the regular swim pattern observed during the turning response in the swimming lamprey (Ekeberg *et al.* 1995; McClellan and Hagevik 1997).

8.7   CONCLUSIONS

1. Swimming in the lamprey is based on caudally propagating periodical waves of lateral body flexions. All components of the locomotor control system in the lamprey have been extensively examined at the behavioural, network, and cellular levels, and their organization and function have been understood to a considerable extent.
2. The motor pattern for swimming is generated by the spinal cord. Motor output in each segment consists of alternating bursts of activity of the left and right motor neuron pools. The onset of activity in each segment is delayed in relation to its rostral neighbour segment. This basic pattern can be generated by the spinal cord deprived of sensory feedback. Small pieces of the spinal cord, at any location along the body, can generate rhythmic oscillations, and the spinal CPG for swimming can thus be viewed as a chain of unitary oscillators.
3. The unitary oscillator consists of two symmetrical parts—the left and right half-centres, which are active in alternation and inhibit each other. The half-centres contain three main classes of interneurons responsible for burst generation and for driving the motor neurons. Both cellular and network properties contribute to the generation of oscillations in this system. First, some of the interneurons are conditional bursters with NMDA-dependent pacemaker properties. Second, the interneurons can be excited upon rebound after termination of the inhibitory input from the contralateral half-centre. Thus, the operation of the unitary oscillator in the lamprey is based on the same general principles as the operation of the swim CPG in *Clione*.
4. The unitary oscillators affect each other through propriospinal connections and form a chain along the spinal cord. The oscillator with the shortest intrinsic period plays the leading role in the chain, and determines the frequency of oscillations in all spinal segments, as well as the direction of propagation of the activity along the spinal cord.

5. Signals from intraspinal mechanoreceptors give rise to the sensory feedback which may affect the locomotor pattern and adapt it to varying environmental conditions.

6. Activation of the spinal locomotor network is produced by an excitatory drive from a population of reticulospinal glutamatergic neurons. This drive increases the excitability of the oscillator interneurons and motor neurons, and transforms the neurons that are conditional bursters from the resting state into the oscillatory state. The reticulospinal system participates in the transformation of brief sensory inputs into a long-lasting response, as well as in the transformation of unilateral sensory input into the bilateral symmetrical activity necessary for rectilinear swimming.

7. The spinal locomotor networks send phasic signals about their rhythmic activity (efference copy) to the brain. These signals cause a periodical modulation of the activity of the neurons that give rise to the reticulospinal and vestibulospinal tracts. A possible function of this modulation is to link the descending commands to a certain phase of the locomotor cycle, in which their effect will be most appropriate.

8. Two postural control systems in the lamprey are responsible for stabilization of the body orientation in the sagittal (pitch) plane and in the transverse (roll) plane respectively. They are driven by vestibular input, whereas visual input exerts only a modulatory effect upon the body orientation. In the roll plane, deviation from the normal, dorsal-side-up orientation activates the otolith afferents on the side facing downward. These afferents excite the contralateral RS neurons which effect the spinal network and evoke a corrective response.

9

Swimming in the toad tadpole

Because of its simplicity, the toad tadpole presents a unique vertebrate animal model for studying the nervous control of locomotion. During the last 20 years it has been used extensively to investigate the spinal mechanisms of undulatory swimming (for reviews see Roberts *et al.* 1983, 1986; Roberts 1989, 1990; Arshavsky *et al.* 1993*c*; Dale and Kuenzi 1997).

9.1   MOTOR PATTERN AND ITS ORIGIN

The main object for studies of the cellular and network mechanisms of undulatory swimming is the embryo of the toad *Xenopus laevis*. The embryos can swim if released from their egg membrane shortly before they normally hatch (Kahn and Roberts 1982). Swimming is due to the waves of lateral body flexion that propagate periodically, at a frequency of 10–25 Hz, from the head towards the tail (Fig. 9.1A). Swimming can be evoked as an escape reaction to different sensory stimuli, for example mechanical stimulation of the skin or dimming the lights (Roberts 1978, 1990). In the whole animal and in the spinal preparation, immobilized by blocking the neuromuscular transmission with α-bungarotoxin, the same stimuli evoke fictive swimming, with alternating activity in the left and right ventral roots in each segment (Figs. 9.1D,E), and with propagation of this activity in the caudal direction (Roberts *et al.* 1981). Thus, the spinal cord contains the CPG that produces the basic motor pattern for swimming.

9.2   CENTRAL PATTERN GENERATOR

As in the lamprey (see Section 8.3.7) the spinal swim CPG in the *Xenopus* embryo can be considered as a chain of unitary oscillators (Tunstall and Roberts 1994; Roberts and Tunstall 1994). Each oscillator generates motor output with rhythmical, alternating activities on the left and right sides. The phase shifts between outputs of neighbouring oscillators determine the propagation of the wave of activity in the caudal direction.

9.2.1 Unitary oscillator

The spinal cord of the late *Xenopus* embryo is small, 100 μm in diameter and a few millimeters in length, and simple in structure (Roberts and Clarke 1982; Roberts *et al.* 1984). There are eight types of spinal neurons in total, but physiological evidence suggests that only two morphological classes of interneurons (commissural and descending, Fig. 9.1B) play an important role in the rhythm generation and in the control of motor neurons. They are termed the inhibitory interneurons (iINs) and the excitatory interneurons (eINs), according to their action on the target cells. There are between 100 and 200 cells in each class on either side of the spinal cord (Clarke and Roberts 1984).

Experiments with pairwise recording revealed principal connections between neurons of different classes (Fig. 9.1C). The eINs produce EPSPs both in the MNs and in the iINs on the ipsilateral side, as well as in other eINs. These EPSPs consist of two components, the fast one mediated by NMDA receptors, and the slow one mediated by AMPA kainate receptors (Dale and Roberts 1985). The iINs produce glicinergic IPSPs in all the cell types on the contralateral side of the spinal cord, and much smaller IPSPs in the cells on the ipsilateral side (Dale 1985).

During fictive swimming, all three types of neurons generate only one spike per swim cycle (Figs. 9.1D–G). The spikes appear almost simultaneously in the neurons on one side (Figs. 9.1F,G), but the spikes in the neurons on the left and right sides alternate (Fig. 9.1E). The spikes are caused by the EPSPs evoked by input from the ipsilateral eINs. When neurons on a given side are active, all types of neuron on the contralateral side receive mid-cycle IPSPs caused by the iINs (Fig. 9.1E) (Soffe *et al.* 1984; Dale and Roberts 1985; Dale 1985; Roberts *et al.* 1985). Thus, the locomotor unitary CPG in the *Xenopus* embryo belongs to a class of generators with two half-centres exerting an inhibitory action on each other. A similar model has been used to explain the rhythm generation in the CPG of *Clione* (see Section 1.2) and lamprey (see Section 8.3). As discussed in relation to *Clione* CPG (see Section 1.3), the operation of the model strongly depends on the properties of each half-centre, specifically, if the half-centres possess spontaneous rhythmic activity or not. The experiments aimed at answering this question brought contradictory results. On one hand, after longitudinal splitting of the spinal cord, each half was able to generate rhythmic activity in response to sensory stimuli (Soffe 1989). On the other hand, no rhythmicity was found in individual spinal neurons in the absence of rhythmical drive from the CPG network as illustrated for a motor neuron in Fig. 9.1H (Arshavsky *et al.* 1993c; Dale and Kuenzi 1997). On the contrary, a very pronounced postinhibitory rebound was found in spinal neurons, as illustrated for a motor neuron in Fig. 9.1I; the ionic mechanisms of this phenomenon have been analysed in detail (Soffe 1990; Dale and Kuenzi 1997). It was therefore suggested that, under normal conditions, the rhythmogenesis is based primarily on the rebound phenomenon, whereas the pacemaker properties of the CPG interneurons only play a secondary role, if any (Roberts *et al.* 1986; Arshavsky *et al.* 1993c). In such a version of the half-centre generator, the main factor determining the cycle period is the duration of the reciprocal IPSPs. The cycle period is effectively the sum of the IPSP durations in each half-centre. This

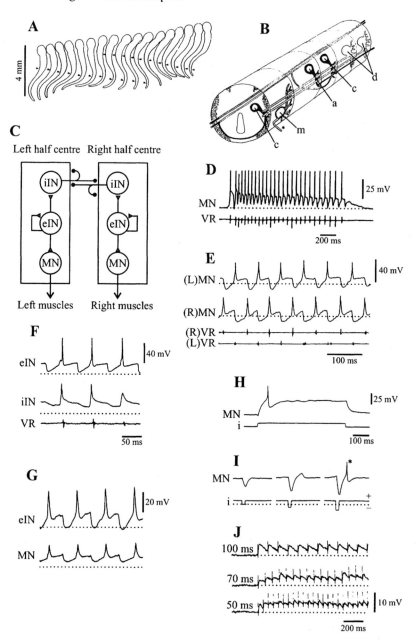

Fig. 9.1 Characterization of swimming in the tadpole (the late *Xenopus* embryo). A: Tracing of swimming movements from a film at 300 frames/s. Arrowheads indicate the points with maximal curvature. B: Diagram of the spinal cord to show neurons of different classes which fire during swimming: m, motor neuron; c, commissural interneurons; d, descending interneurons; a, ascending interneuron; rostral direction to the right. C: Connections between different types of neurons (eIN, excitatory interneuron; iIN, Inhibitory interneuron; MN, motor neuron; triangles, excitatory connections; filled circles, inhibitory

duration in *Xenopus* is typical for vertebrate glycinergic inhibition (25–40 ms), and the sum of the two durations well corresponds to the cycle duration observed during swimming (40–100 ms). Computer simulation of the unitary oscillator network confirmed these intuitive considerations (Roberts *et al.* 1984; Roberts and Tunstall 1990).

Striking similarities but also some differences can be found when comparing the CPGs in *Xenopus* and *Clione* (Arshavsky *et al.* 1993):

1. In both networks, the principal interneurons generate only one spike per cycle and receive one mid-cycle IPSP from the antagonistic interneurons. However, in *Clione* the same interneurons play double roles, that is they both excite the agonistic half-centre and inhibit the antagonistic one, whereas in *Xenopus* these functions are separated between the eINs and the iINs.
2. The rhythm generation in the *Xenopus* CPG is based primarily on reciprocal inhibition between the half-centres and on postinhibitory rebound. The same principle is applied to the *Clione* CPG when it operates in the lower range of locomotor frequencies. At higher frequencies, however, the endogenous rhythmicity of the half-centres plays a significant role.
3. In *Clione*, many motor neurons generate bursts of spikes. By contrast, in *Xenopus* they generate a single spike. This is due to the specific properties of the cell membrane, which make the cell respond by a single spike even to sustained depolarization (Fig. 9.1H) (Soffe 1990; Dale and Kuenzi 1997). Later in ontogenesis, the bursting response to depolarization appears (Sillar *et al.* 1991, 1992).

9.2.2   Coordination of unitary oscillators along the spinal cord

During fictive swimming, the waves of activation of the ventral roots travel along each side of the spinal cord in the rostrocaudal direction, with a time delay of about 1.5 ms mm^{-1} (Tunstall and Roberts 1990, 1994). It has been suggested that the eINs are of prime importance for intersegmental coordination. These neurons

---

connections). D: An episode of fictive swimming evoked in the immobilized preparation by brief sensory stimulus (touch of the skin). The upper trace is an intracellular recording from a motor neuron with rhythmical action potentials superimposed on the ramp depolarization; the lower trace is an extracellular recording from the ipsilateral ventral root. E: Segmental motor output represents rhythmical, alternating discharges in the left and right ventral roots; discharges in the left and right motor neurons and interneurons also alternate. F,G: Simultaneous recording from different neuron types to show that their spikes are synchronized. The dotted lines in D–G indicate the resting potential. H: Injection of a supramaximal depolarizing current (i) into the motor neuron does not elicit repeated firing. I: Injection of a pulse of hyperpolarizing current, on the background of a steady depolarization, elicits rebound firing. J: Intracellular recording from a motor neuron. Stimulation of the axons of presumed eINs at frequencies comparable to the swim frequency causes the EPSPs in the motor neuron to summate and produce a sustained depolarization. The time between the successive stimuli is indicated on the left; the dotted lines indicate the resting potential. A,C–E,H, and I are from Arshavsky *et al.* (1993c), B is from Roberts *et al.* (1986), and F,G, and J are from Dale and Roberts (1985).

are the key elements of the unitary oscillator circuit (Fig. 9.1C), but they also have descending axons (Fig. 9.1B) and, when excited, may activate the interneurons and the motor neurons not only in their own hemisegment but also in more caudal hemisegments. These factors promote the propagation of activity in the caudal direction. Another factor is a longitudinal, rostrocaudal gradient in different characteristics of unitary oscillators. Anatomical evidence shows that there is a rostrocaudal reduction in the numbers per segment of the eINs and of the iINs. It was also found that during fictive swimming, the amplitude of the tonic excitatory synaptic input and mid-cycle inhibition declines in a rostrocaudal direction. It was suggested that, due to these gradients, the caudal segmental networks are less excitable than the rostral ones, which would promote the formation of the 'leading' oscillator in the rostral segments (Tunstall and Roberts 1990, 1991)—a hypothesis similar to the trailing oscillator hypothesis formulated for the intersegmental coordination in the lamprey (see Section 8.3.7). A confirmation of this hypothesis was obtained when pharmacological agents were applied to the caudal spinal segments to change their excitability. This led to changes of the speed of the waves and even to the reversal of the normal direction of spread of motor activity (Tunstall and Roberts 1990, 1991, 1994; Roberts and Tunstall 1994), similar to the results found in the lamprey (see Section 8.3.7).

9.3 INITIATION OF SWIMMING

In the intact and immobilized *Xenopus* embryo, the spinal mechanisms generating the swim motor pattern can be activated by sensory stimuli such as touching the skin or dimming the lights. A body of evidence suggests that this activation is due to the action of excitatory amino acid neurotransmitters upon the spinal neurons:

(1) Bath application of NMDA or kainate to the spinal cord elicits fictive locomotion in immobilized embryos (Dale and Roberts 1984).
(2) Excitatory amino acid antagonists abolish the locomotor response to the sensory stimuli that normally evoke swimming (Dale and Roberts 1984).
(3) The same antagonists also reduce the EPSPs in spinal motor neurons caused by stimulation of presumed eIN axons (Dale and Roberts 1985).

Touching the skin of the *Xenopus* embryo evokes a brief burst of impulses in identified primary sensory neurons and secondary sensory interneurons (Clarke *et al.* 1984; Roberts and Sillar 1990) which drive the CPG networks. Recordings from different types of CPG neurons during swimming episodes evoked by sensory stimuli have shown that, in all CPG neurons, the rhythmic synaptic potentials are superimposed on a ramp depolarization, as illustrated for a motor neuron in Fig. 9.1D. The frequency of swimming is proportional to the amplitude of this depolarization (Sillar and Roberts 1993). In principle, the ramp depolarization may originate in neurons presynaptic to the CPG neurons and/or in the CPG network itself. There is evidence suggesting that this sustained depolarization is generated, at least partly, by the CPG network when it is activated by a brief sensory stimulus. Figure 9.1J shows how a motor neuron responds to repetitive stimulation of the axons of presumed eINs in the range of frequencies comparable to the swim frequencies (Dale and Roberts 1984). One can see an efficient summation of the slow components of the EPSPs, especially at higher frequencies. Computer simulations have shown that, if the eIN evoked EPSPs are sufficiently long-lasting, the half-centre model can generate rhythmic activity superimposed on a sustained depolarization (Roberts and Tunstall 1990).

The duration of the ramp depolarization and of the swimming episodes may depend on many factors, for example on the strength of the triggering stimulus, and on the degree of frequency adaptation in the eINs (Sillar and Roberts 1993). There are also a number of external influences on the CPG network, including those mediated by purinergic neurotransmitters (Dale and Gilday 1996). Termination of swimming can also be evoked by tactile stimulation of the head which excites a specific type of trigeminal pressure receptor (Boothby and Roberts 1992).

9.4 CONCLUSIONS

1. Swimming in the tadpole is based on caudally propagating periodical waves of lateral body flexions controlled by the spinal cord. The spinal networks generating this pattern have been analysed in considerable detail, with identification of the main neuron classes and their interactions.

2. The pattern of fictive swimming in an immobilized animal is very similar to that of normal swimming, which indicates that sensory feedback does not play any significant role in the pattern generation. The spinal CPG can be considered as a chain of unitary oscillators. As in the lamprey, the unitary oscillator in the tadpole consists of two symmetrical parts, the left and right half-centres, which are active in succession and inhibit each other. In contrast to the lamprey, the inter- and motor neurons in each half-centre do not generate bursts but single spikes. Two classes of interneurons play a major role in the unitary oscillators: the excitatory interneurons (eINs) excite each other, the inhibitory interneurons (iINs), and the motor neurons; the iINs produce inhibition of the contralateral half-centre. The postinhibitory rebound is the main factor determining rhythmogenesis and the alternation of activities of the two half-centres.

3. The rostrocaudal propagation of activity along the chain of unitary oscillators is caused by two factors: (i) by the caudally directed projections of the eINs and (ii) by the higher excitability and thus probably, higher intrinsic frequency of the oscillators in the rostral segments.

4. In the escape reaction, the spinal CPG is activated by sensory input. A brief stimulus evokes a long-lasting depolarization in all CPG neurons via the first- and second-order sensory neurons. The depolarization is generated in the CPG network due to the summation of rhythmic EPSPs produced by eINs and underlies the rhythmical activity of the CPG cells.

Part III
Quadrupedal locomotion in mammals

This part is devoted to the locomotor control system of the cat, the most popular object for analysis of different aspects of locomotor control in mammals since the beginning of this century, although some data in other mammals are also reported.

In contrast to the situation with simpler animals like molluscs, the extreme complexity of the cat's locomotor system does not at present allow a sufficiently detailed description of its activity at the neuronal networks level. In the following chapters, we shall primarily consider the functional organization of the system, the role of different subdivisions of the CNS in locomotor control, and the activity of some selected groups of neurons during locomotion. The general principles of organization of the cat's locomotor control system have been discussed in the reviews by Shik and Orlovsky (1976), Orlovsky and Shik (1976), Grillner (1975, 1981), Pearson (1993), Rossignol (1996), Armstrong (1986), and Wetzel and Stuart (1976).

10

General organization of the locomotor control system in the cat

10.1 MOTOR PATTERN IN A SINGLE LIMB

The idea that during locomotion each of the four limbs is driven by its individual control mechanism (the limb controller), which is relatively independent of the controllers for the other limbs, was first formulated by von Holst (1938). This idea emerged from the observation that, under certain conditions, the rhythms of stepping in different limbs may differ from each other. Divergence of rhythms of individual limbs was later observed by other investigators when the animal walked on a treadmill with split belts (Forssberg *et al.* 1980*b*; Halbertsma 1983; Kulagin and Shik 1970). Thus, the basic principle of the control of locomotion in walking animals, that is a considerable autonomy of the individual limb controllers, is common for different species—from crustaceans and insects (see Sections 4.1 and 6.3) to mammals.

Of the three possible descriptions of the motor pattern of the stepping limb, that is kinetics (forces), kinematics (movements), and EMG activity, the latter two are most often used to characterize the activity of the limb controller. A detailed analysis of the motor pattern of the hind limb of the cat was carried out by a number of investigators (Gambarian *et al.* 1971; Abraham and Loeb 1985; Engberg and Lundberg 1969; Loeb 1993; Pratt *et al.* 1991; Pratt and Loeb 1991; Rasmussen *et al.* 1978; reviewed by Rossignol 1996). As in other walking animals (crustaceans, see Section 4.1, or insects, see Section 6.3), the step cycle in the cat consists of two principal parts, the stance (or support) phase and the swing (or transfer) phase. The swing phase starts when the limb reaches the posterior extreme position in relation to the body (Figs. 10.1A$_1$,B). In this phase, the limb is lifted above the ground and moves forward in relation to the body until it reaches the anterior extreme position (Figs. 10.1A$_2$,B). In this position, the paw gets in contact with the ground, and the stance phase starts. Throughout the stance phase, the limb moves backward in relation to the body until it reaches the posterior extreme position. In this phase, the limb is loaded by a part of the body weight, and also develops a propulsive force moving the animal forward.

All the three main joints of the hind limb (hip, knee, and ankle) perform considerable flexion–extension movements during the step cycle, as shown in the stick diagrams of Fig. 10.1B. The temporal pattern of movements at individual joints

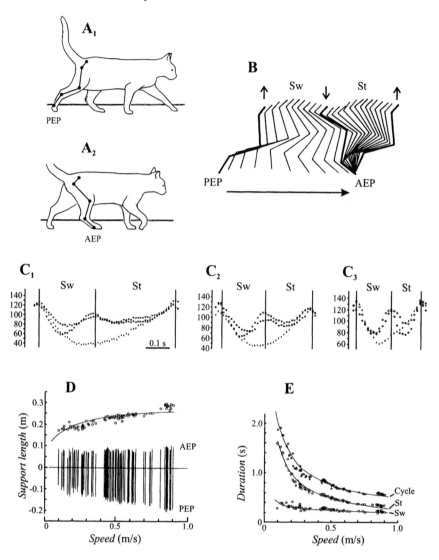

Fig. 10.1 Walking in the cat: kinematic pattern of stepping movements of the hind limb. A_1, A_2: Two extreme positions of the limb—the posterior extreme position, PEP (A_1) and the anterior extreme position, AEP (A_2). B: One complete cycle reconstructed as stick diagrams. The time interval between successive diagrams, 30 ms; the speed of locomotion, $0.6 \, \text{m s}^{-1}$. Arrows indicate switches between stance (St) and swing (Sw) phases. $C_1–C_3$: Angles at the hip (crosses), knee (circles), and ankle (dots) joints plotted against time for three different speeds of locomotion: medium fast walk (C_1), trot (C_2), and gallop (C_3). D: Adjustment of the amplitude of the limb movements—the support length—with speed (circles). The anterior and posterior extreme positions of the toe at different speeds are shown as vertical bars, with zero indicating the vertical hip projection. E: Adjustments of the step cycle with speed. The cycle duration (Cycle), the stance phase duration (St), and the swing phase duration (Sw) are plotted against time. A_1, A_2, and B are from Smith *et al.* (1988), $C_1–C_3$ are from Engberg and Lundberg (1969), and D and E are from Halbertsma (1983).

is presented in the graphs (Figs. 10.1C$_1$–C$_3$) for different speeds of locomotion. Movements around the hip joint are rather simple: this joints is flexing in the swing phase and extending in the stance phase. The maximal hip flexion determines the anterior extreme position of the limb, whereas the maximal hip extension determines the posterior extreme position. Movements at the knee and ankle joints are more complicated: they have two peaks of flexion and two peaks of extension in each step cycle. This is caused by the necessity to shorten the effective length of the limb twice during the cycle. First, the limb must be shortened and lifted above the ground to prevent stumbling in the swing phase. Second, the limb must be shortened when it passes the vertical position to reduce the vertical oscillations of the body in the stance phase.

The essential features of the joint movements and interjoint coordination are preserved over the whole range of locomotor speeds (Figs. 10.1C$_1$–C$_3$). At any speed, there is one peak of flexion and one peak of extension at the hip joint in each step cycle but two peaks of flexion and two peaks of extension at the knee and ankle joints. The swing phase starts with the simultaneous flexion of all joints, and all the joints are simultaneously extended by the end of the stance phase.

To increase the speed of locomotion, there are two principal ways: to increase the frequency of stepping and to increase the amplitude of the stepping movements. In the walking or trotting cat, the latter factor plays only a secondary role. As shown in Figs. 10.1C$_1$–C$_3$, the amplitude of angular hip excursions is relatively constant at different speeds of locomotion. As a result, the amplitude of limb movements—the support length—only slightly increases with the speed in the low-speed range primarily due to the caudal displacement of the posterior extreme position whereas the anterior extreme position remains constant (Fig. 10.1D) (Halbertsma 1983).

By contrast, the temporal characteristics of the step cycle are strongly speed-dependent, and the step cycle at a high speed is much shorter than at a slow speed (Figs. 10.1C$_1$–C$_3$). The shortening of the cycle duration is mainly due to the shortening of the stance phase, whereas the swing phase is much less speed-dependent (Fig. 10.1E). A strong dependence of the stance phase duration on the speed of locomotion, and a relative constancy of the swing phase, are also characteristic of walking in crustaceans (see Section 4.1) and insects (see Section 6.3), suggesting similar functional organizations of the leg controller (for discussion, see Section 11.5).

The kinematic pattern of stepping limb movements shown in Fig. 10.1 is determined by the activity of the very complex muscular apparatus of the limb. Figures 10.2A$_1$–A$_3$ show the anatomy of the hind limb of the cat, with different muscle layers exposed, and Fig. 10.2B shows a simplified kinematic scheme of the limb, as well as the action exerted by different muscles upon the links of the limb. The EMG pattern for some representative hind limb muscles is shown in Fig. 10.2C. The extensor muscles have very similar patterns of activity. The knee extensor vastus lateralis (VL), as well as the ankle extensors gastrocnemius medialis (GM) and gastrocnemius lateralis (GL), become active at the end of the swing phase, shortly before landing the foot, and their activity continues throughout almost the whole stance phase. However, GM and GL have a more abrupt onset than VL.

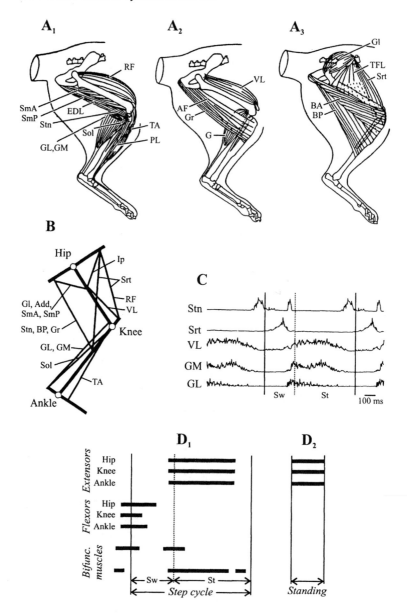

Fig. 10.2 Activity of the hind limb muscles in the step cycle. A_1–A_3: Anatomy of the hind limb of the cat with different layers of muscles exposed. B: Kinematic scheme of the limb. C: EMGs of representative muscles (rectified and filtered). D_1: Phases of activity of the main muscle groups controlling the hip, knee, and ankle joints in the step cycle. D_2: Activity of the same groups during standing. (Abbreviations: AF, adductor femoris; BA, biceps femoris anterior; BP, biceps femoris posterior; EDL, extensor digitorum longus; GM, gastrocnemius medialis; GL, gastrocnemius lateralis; G, gastrocnemius (lateralis and

The pattern of activity of the flexors and the bifunctional muscles (that flex one joint and extend another) are much more diverse. As shown in Fig. 10.2C, the hip flexor sartorius (Srt) is active in the swing phase, whereas the knee flexor–hip extensor semitendinosus (Stn) has two bursts of activity—at the transition from the stance phase to the swing phase, and at the end of the swing phase. These essential features of the EMG pattern in different muscles are emphasized in the diagram (Fig. 10.2D$_1$). The extensors of all the three main joints are active throughout almost the whole stance phase, and thus form a gross extensor synergy.

Due to the forces developed by extensors, the limb becomes rigid enough to bear its part of the body weight. Besides, due to the contraction of extensors, by the end of the support phase the limb joints are vigorously extending, the effective length of the limb increases, and the limb pushes the body forward. The limb extensors form an antigravitational synergy not only during locomotion but also during standing, before stepping movements start or after they finish (this postural activity of the extensors is schematically shown in Fig. 10.2D$_2$). Correspondingly, the extensor activity during locomotion can be considered as a postural component of the stepping movements; this postural activity of extensors is periodically interrupted to let a limb step forward in the swing phase.

As shown in Fig. 10.2D$_1$, flexors and some bifunctional muscles become active shortly before the onset of the swing phase. Contraction of the hip flexors results in a movement of the whole limb forward in relation to the body. Contraction of the knee and ankle flexors results in shortening the limb in the first half of the swing phase. In the second half of this phase, activity of the knee and ankle flexors terminates, and the effective length of a limb increases due to the extension of the knee and ankle joints until the foot touches the ground.

The basic pattern of the flexor and extensor activity (Fig. 10.2D$_1$) persists in the whole range of locomotor speeds and also when the animal walks on an inclined surface (Engberg and Lundberg 1969; Pierotti *et al.* 1989), though some differences can be observed, especially in the muscles of distal joints and bifunctional muscles like Stn, which may have two bursts of EMG per step (Fig. 10.2C) at some speeds but only one burst at different speeds (Perret and Cabelguen 1976, 1980; Wisleder *et al.* 1990; Hensbergen and Kernell 1992; Loeb 1993; Smith *et al.* 1993). Also, the relative contribution of the synergistic muscles with fast-twitch motor units to the force production increases with speed (Walmsley *et al.* 1978; English 1984).

A number of experimental findings strongly suggest that stepping limb movements at different speeds and intensities of locomotion are controlled by the one and the same neuronal network, and that different locomotor patterns can be caused by changing some parameters of this network rather than by its reconfiguration. First, the main temporal characteristics of the step cycle change gradually over a wide range of locomotor speeds (Figs. 10.1D,E), Second, the basic pattern

---

medialis); Gl, gluteus medius; Gr, gracilis; PL, peroneus longus; RF, rectus femoris; SmA, semimembranosus anterior; SmP, semimembranosus posterior; Sol, soleus; Srt, sartorius anterior; Stn, semitendinosus; TA, tibialis anterior; TFL, tensor fasciae latea; VL, vastus lateralis.) A$_1$–A$_3$ are based on Gambarian *et al.* (1971) and C is from Rossignol (1996).

of joint movements (Figs. 10.1C$_1$–C$_3$) and of muscle activity persists at various speeds. Third, as will be shown below (see Section 10.3), the whole range of speeds, intensities, and even gaits of locomotion can be covered by varying only one parameter of the control system.

10.2   INTERLIMB COORDINATION

The controllers for the individual limbs are coordinated with each other due to mutual influences, which results in the establishment of a common rhythm of stepping movements, with definite phase relations between the four limbs determining the gait (von Holst 1938; Shik and Orlovsky 1965). Requirements regarding postural stability are one of the main factors affecting interlimb coordination (Stuart *et al.* 1973). At low and moderate speeds of locomotion, quadrupeds use static equilibrium control, that is the projection of the centre of gravity is positioned between the feet–ground contact points. At high speed, equilibrium becomes dynamic, i.e. in a certain phase of the locomotor cycle the centre of gravity is projected outside the feet–ground contact area.

Two basic types of coordination within the pairs of limbs at the hip and shoulder girdles are observed: (1) strict alternation, when the two limbs of one pair are half a cycle out of phase; (2) in-phase coordination, when the limbs of one pair work in phase with each other so that they extend and flex almost simultaneously. At low and moderate speeds of locomotion, various species use walk and trot (Figs. 10.3A$_1$,A$_2$), with strict alternation of the two limbs of one pair and different phase shifts between the two pairs. If considering the diagonal limbs, the phase shift gradually decreases from 25 per cent of the cycle during slow walking to 0 during trotting and then remains constant at higher speeds (Fig. 10.3B). At the highest speeds, animals are galloping, with in-phase coordination in each pair of limbs. Different forms of gallop are determined by small phase shifts (10–20 per cent of the cycle) between the limbs within a pair (Figs. 10.3A$_3$–A$_5$). According to Goslow *et al.* (1973), cats use a walking gait below 0.7 m s^{-1}, a trotting gait between 0.7 and 2.7 m s^{-1}, and gallop above 2.7 m s^{-1}.

The phase shifts between movements of different limbs, as well as the step length, are determined not only by limb movements relative to the trunk, but also by longitudinal (Figs. 10.3C,D) or lateral (Fig. 10.3E) body movements (Goslow *et al.* 1973; Carlson *et al.* 1979; Ritter 1992). These movements strongly contribute to the locomotor pattern, especially in galloping animals. Thus, in addition to intralimb and interlimb coordination, one more coordinatory problem emerges: the cyclic movements of the trunk must be coordinated with stepping limb movements. Finally, the head also moves cyclically in relation to the trunk, these active movements being most likely aimed at reducing the head oscillations evoked by locomotor limb and trunk movements and at stabilizing the retinal optic image (for a discussion of this problem in humans see, for example, Berthoz and Pozzo (1988)).

To reveal mutual influences between the limb controllers in walking animals, which are responsible for the maintenance of a particular gait, different approaches

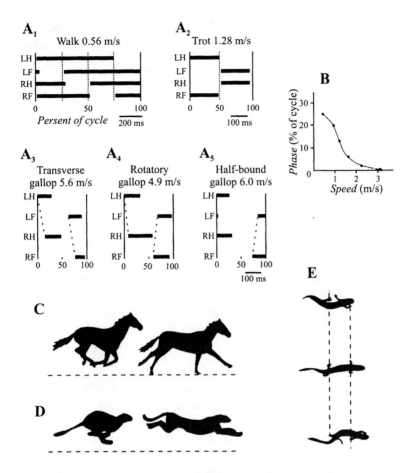

Fig. 10.3 Interlimb coordination. A_1–A_5: Interlimb coordination in the cat exhibiting different gaits. Periods of foot contract are plotted for one step cycle, starting with foot strike of the left hind limb (LH, left hind limb; LF, left fore limb; RH, right hind limb; RF, right fore limb). B: Phase shift between the diagonal limbs in the walking and trotting dog at different speeds of progression. C,D: Longitudinal body movements of horse (C) and cheetah (D) during gallop; note flexion and extension of lower spine. E: Lateral body movements in the walking newt. A_1–A_5 and C–E are from Grillner (1981), B is from Arshavsky *et al.* (1965).

can be used. In experiments on the crayfish (see Section 4.2), the movement of one leg was perturbed, and the effect of this perturbation on the other legs was studied (Cruse and Müller 1986; Cruse 1990). It was found that the multileg system, with individual controllers for each of the legs, is rather stable against perturbations, and the consequences of a perturbation are compensated in one to two cycles. In the dog, the interaction between the limb controllers was studied by measuring the coefficients of correlation between the cycles of different limbs (Shik and Orlovsky 1965). A considerable correlation was found between two to three successive cycles, suggesting that the strength of interactions between the individual limb controllers is similar in the dog and crayfish, and that a distortion of the cycle in one limb is rapidly compensated under the effect of influences from other limb controllers.

Many neural mechanisms may participate in the control of interlimb coordination, both propriospinal (Jankovska and Edgely 1993; Jankovska and Noga 1990; Schomburg 1990; Grillner and Rossignol 1978; Rossignol *et al.* 1993) and with involvement of the spino-brainstem–spinal pathways (English 1980, 1985; Shimamura *et al.* 1991; Matsukawa *et al.* 1982; Udo *et al.* 1982). The relative contribution of these different mechanisms to the maintenance of gait remains unclear, however.

10.3   BRAINSTEM–SPINAL LOCOMOTOR AUTOMATISM

Decerebrate animals are capable of locomotion provided the brainstem is not transected at too low a level. A cut which passes dorsoventrally from the rostral border of the superior colliculus to just in front of the mammillary bodies (transection 1 in Fig. 10.4A) creates a 'pre-mammillary' cat which will walk in the true sense—it can right itself and shows full weight support, maintenance of equilibrium, and normal limb stepping movements almost immediately after operation. By contrast, a 'post-mammillary', or 'mesencephalic' cat (transection 2 in Fig. 10.4A) exhibits neither righting reflexes nor locomotor movements immediately after operation (Hinsey *et al.* 1930), but can restore the ability to stand and walk in one to two weeks (Bard and Macht 1958). With more caudal transections, restoration of this ability has not been reported. Thus, the basic neuronal networks controlling locomotion are located posteriorly to Section 2 in Fig. 10.4A, i.e. in the spinal cord, posterior brainstem (including mesencephalon), and cerebellum (Fig. 10.4A). Governed by this control system, walking in the mesencephalic cat is machine-like in that almost no regard is paid to features of the environment.

A powerful impulse for studying the basic locomotor mechanisms was given in 1965 by discovery of the mesencephalic locomotor region (MLR) (Shik *et al.* 1966*a*, 1967). This is a small area in the midbrain (Fig. 10.4A) partly corresponding to the pedunculopontine and cuneiform nuclei, whose electrical (20–60 Hz, 20–100 µA) or chemical stimulation evokes locomotion in the mesencephalic, pre-mammillary cat. The structure of this area, as well as its input and output connections, will be considered in Chapter 12. The lack of nocisensitivity in decerebrated animals allows one to fix the skull (Fig. 10.4B) and the vertebral column rigidly, which presents a unique opportunity for recording activity of single nerve cells in the brain and spinal cord during walking and running. To have the external mechanical conditions for stepping close to normal, the cat's limbs are put on a treadmill with a moving belt (Fig. 10.4B). In Fig. 10.4C a locomotor sequence evoked by MLR stimulation is shown. All four limbs perform stepping movements and the animal develops a force pushing the treadmill backward.

Stimulation of the MLR in the intact cat also evokes locomotion (Sirota and Shik 1973; Mori 1987; Mori *et al.* 1991). The stronger the stimulation, the higher the speed of progression. During locomotion, the cat passes by or jumps over obstacles (Fig. 10.5). Areas anatomically corresponding to the MLR, the stimulation of which elicits locomotion, were also found in fish, reptiles, and birds (reviewed by Jordan 1991).

Though the MLR is very efficient in initiation of locomotion, destruction of this region does not abolish the ability of the cat to locomote (Orlovsky 1969; Sirota and Shik 1973). These findings strongly suggest that the MLR is one, but not the only one, of the regions through which higher brain centres have access to the locomotor system and can exert a general control of this type of motor activity of the animal (see Section 12.1). Which aspects of the stepping movements are directly regulated through the MLR? Are these the muscular forces, the speed of running, the frequency of stepping, or other characteristics? To answer these questions, the effect of MLR stimulation in the mesencephalic cat was tested under different mechanical conditions for locomotion (Shik *et al.* 1966a). Figure 10.4D shows the stepping movements of the hind limb of the walking cat. During this test, the strength of stimulation was kept constant, but the speed of the treadmill belt was gradually decreased. One can see a corresponding increase in the step cycle duration. Thus, it is not the frequency of stepping that is directly controlled by the MLR. Figures 10.4E_1–E_3 show stepping movements of the left and right hind limbs, and the force developed by the locomoting cat in the same experiment at various strengths of MLR stimulation, while the belt speed was kept constant. The stronger the stimulation, the greater was the propulsive force developed by the cat. In addition, at stronger stimulation, the animal changed the gait from out-of-phase coordination, corresponding to walk and trot (E_1 and E_2), to in-phase coordination, corresponding to gallop (E_3).

Thus, the neuronal mechanisms located in the brainstem, cerebellum, and spinal cord, which are activated by the MLR stimulation, can be called the *automatic system for the control of locomotion* or *locomotor automatism*. The MLR input determines the intensity of muscle contraction, or the power developed by the animal, whereas the speed of progression and the frequency of stepping are not controlled directly, they depend both on the power developed by the muscular system and on the external conditions such as the slope of the road. In the locomoting animal, the automatic system is solving a number of difficult tasks: (1) it activates in a strict succession numerous muscles of each of the four limbs; (2) it coordinates movements of all four limbs with each other; (3) to some extent, the automatic system adapts the stepping movements to external conditions (see Section 11.1); and (iv) it maintains equilibrium. As has been demonstrated by Bard and Macht (1958), the chronic mesencephalic cat exhibits well-coordinated righting and postural reflexes, that is the cat lying on its side is able to assume normal, upright posture, and to maintain this posture during walking. Despite these numerous and complex functions of the automatic system, the system itself can be very easily controlled: it can be activated by exciting a group of MLR neurons, and the level of locomotor activity can be regulated within a wide range by changing the excitatory drive to these neurons. One can suggest that the higher brain centres, which make a decision to locomote, use MLR to exert only a general control of the locomotor activity (see Chapter 12), without directly participating in the control of the stepping limb movements. However, these centres, and the motor

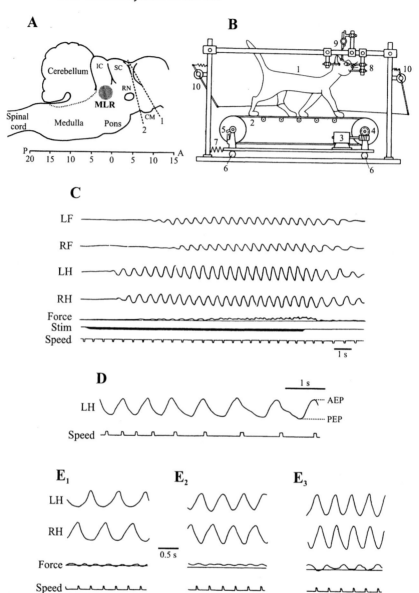

Fig. 10.4 Locomotion in the mesencephalic cat evoked by stimulation of the mesencephalic locomotor region. A: Location of the mesencephalic locomotor region (MLR) in the brain stem. Two levels of decerebration are shown, corresponding to the premammillary preparation (1), and the postmammillary (mesencephalic) preparation (2). (Abbreviations: CM, corpus mammillare; SC, superior colliculus; IC, inferior colliculus; RN, red nucleus.) A and P are the anterior and posterior Horsley-Clark coordinates. B: Experimental arrangement. The mesencephalic cat (1) is fixed in the stereotaxic device (8), with its four legs walking on the belt of treadmill (2) moved by the electrical motor (3,4). The speed of the belt is measured by the contact transducer (5) as 0.5 m displacements of the belt against time.

cortex in particular, will assist the automatic control system when the locomotor task is more complicated, as for example in the case when the foot must be placed on a particular site on the ground and visuo-motor coordination is required. Participation of the visual system and motor cortex in the control of complicated locomotor tasks will be considered in Chapter 14.

10.4 ROLE OF THE SPINAL CORD IN THE GENERATION OF CYCLIC MOVEMENTS

10.4.1 Limb movements for forward stepping

The spinal cord plays a crucial role in locomotor automatism. For a long time it has been known that hind limbs of 'low spinal' cats and dogs (transection of the spinal cord in the thoracic region; Fig. 10.6A$_2$) can perform stepping movements (Freusberg 1874; Sherrington 1906a; Philippson 1905). In cats spinalized as adults, stepping movements of the hind limbs are not well coordinated, and the limbs are sometimes not able to support the body weight. The stepping movements can be considerably improved by suspending the hind quarters, however (Fig. 10.6A$_1$). Activation of the noradrenergic system of the spinal cord may dramatically improve the motor performance (Forssberg and Grillner 1973; Budakova 1973; reviewed by Rossignol 1996) (see Section 11.1), as illustrated in Figs. 10.6B$_1$–C$_3$ for the effect of clonidine (the α_2-noradrenergic receptor agonist) applied directly to the spinal cord. (For a review of pharmacology of stereotypic patterns, see Rossignol 1996) These findings indicate that uncoordinated spinal stepping is caused primarily by insufficient tonic excitatory drive to the neurons of the leg controllers rather than by damage to some specific components of the controller networks.

The locomotor performance is much better in spinal cats subjected to regular daily training on the treadmill (Barbeau and Rossignol 1987; Rossignol *et al.* 1986, 1989), especially if they were spinalized within a few days after birth (Grillner 1973; Forssberg *et al.* 1974, 1980a,b; Smith *et al.* 1982). In the best cases, the kinematics and EMG patterns were close to normal, and the limbs were able to support the hindquarters. The lumbosacral spinal cord can, to some extent, adapt the limb movements to external conditions: the frequency of stepping can vary

---

The treadmill is positioned on two rollers (6); this allows measurement of the force developed by the animal (by means of the transducer, 7). The MLR is stimulated (pulses 20–50 Hz) by the electrode (9). The limb movements are recorded by the transducers (10). C: Locomotor episode evoked by MLR stimulation. D: Movements of the left hind limb during locomotion; the strength of MLR stimulation was kept constant (120 µA), whereas the belt speed was gradually reduced from 1.5 to 0.5 m s^{-1}. E$_1$–E$_3$: Movements of the left and right hind limbs during locomotion; the belt speed was kept constant (1.6 m s^{-1}), whereas the strength of stimulation was different: 100 µA (E$_1$), 150 µA (E$_2$), and 200 µA (E$_3$). (Abbreviations in C–E$_3$: LF, left fore limb; RF, right fore limb; LH, left hind limb; RH, right hind limb; Force, the force developed by the animal and measured by the transducer 7; Speed, the speed of the belt measured by the transducer 5; AEP and PEP, anterior and posterior extreme positions of the foot, respectively.) B,C, and E$_1$–E$_3$ are from Shik *et al.* (1966a) and D is based on Orlovsky *et al.* (1966a).

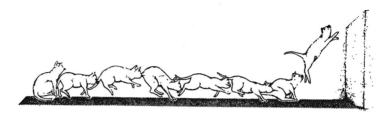

Fig. 10.5 Locomotor activity of the intact cat evoked by electrical stimulation of the mesencephalic locomotor region. Stimulation (current pulses at the frequency 20–50 Hz) was performed through the chronically implanted electrodes. From Mori *et al.* (1991).

in accordance with the speed of the treadmill belt; the interlimb coordination can change from in-phase at low speeds (walk and trot) to counter-phase at high speeds (gallop); when stumbling, the limb can overstep an obstacle (see Section 11.5). The spinal cat is also able to maintain, to some extent, an upright posture of the posterior part of the body, most likely due to the symmetry of the patterns of stepping movements of the left and right limbs (see Section 12.4). It is thus evident that the controllers for the hind limbs, as well as their interconnections responsible for interlimb coordination, are located in the lumbosacral enlargement of the spinal cord. A longitudinal split of the lumbosacral enlargement does not abolish stepping (Kato 1988, 1991). Thus, the controllers for each of the limbs are located in the ipsilateral half of the enlargement.

The motor pattern of fore limb stepping has also been studied in detail (Hoffman *et al.* 1985; Drew and Rossignol 1987; English 1969, 1978*a*,*b*; reviewed by Rossignol 1996). The forelimb step cycle is also subdivided into the stance and swing phases, but the kinematic and EMG patterns are more complex because of the added movement of the scapula relative to the rib cage. However, the organization and function of the fore limb controllers, located in the cervical enlargement of the spinal cord, have been studied to a much lesser extent than those of the hind limbs, mainly because spinalization of an animal at the rostral cervical level presents a difficult problem.

10.4.2   Other cyclic movements

Besides the cyclic movements for forward stepping, the neuronal networks in the lumbosacral enlargement are responsible for the generation of other cyclic movement patterns of the hind limb, which have some features in common with the pattern for forward stepping. They are backward stepping, scratching, paw shaking, and rhythmic limb withdrawal.

10.4.2.1   Backward stepping

Backward stepping (Fig. 10.7) has different kinematic and EMG patterns from forward stepping (Figs. 10.1A$_1$–B) (Buford and Smith 1990; Buford *et al.* 1990). In the swing phase, instead of moving forward in relation to the body, the limb moves backward, whereas in the support phase it moves forward. In contrast to forward

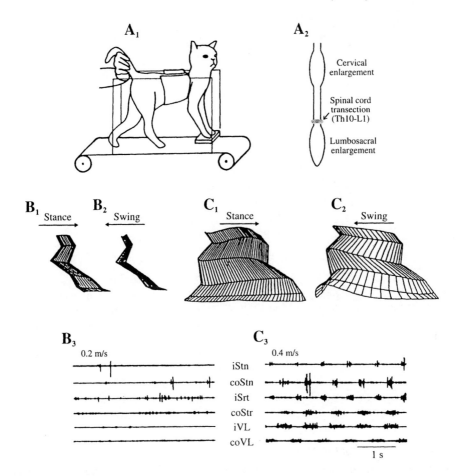

Fig. 10.6 Locomotion in the spinal cat. A_1: The spinal cat (transection of the spinal cord in the thoracic region, as shown in A_2) is able to walk by its hind limbs on the moving belt of the treadmill, especially if the hind quarters are suspended. B_1–C_3: Effect of clonidine on spinal stepping. B_1–B_3: Week and discoordinated stepping movements (B_1, B_2) and EMG activity (B_3) before clonidine application. C_1–C_3: About 30 min after the injection of clonidine (single bolus of 100 μg/100 μl) through the cannula positioned above the L5 segment of the spinal cord. Both the kinematics (C_1, C_2) and EMG recordings (C_3) show a coordinated locomotor pattern. A_1 is from Carter and Smith (1986) and B_1–C_3 are from Rossignol (1996).

stepping, movements at all three main joints of a limb have only one peak of flexion and one peak of extension in each step cycle (Fig. 10.7C). These differences in kinematics are due to a different pattern of muscle activity: in particular, the hip flexor burst is shortened and the hip extensor burst is prolonged, compared with those during forward stepping (compare Figs. 10.9A and B). Since backward stepping is observed also in spinal cats (Rossignol 1996) one can conclude that the

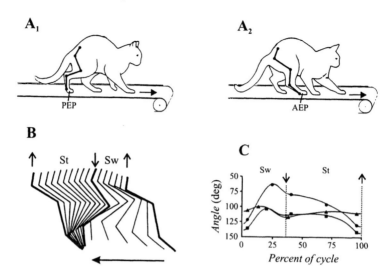

Fig. 10.7 Backward walking in the cat. A_1,A_2: Two extreme positions of the right hind limb—the posterior extreme position (PEP, A_1) and the anterior extreme position (AEP, A_2). B: One complete step cycle of the hind limb is reconstructed as stick diagrams for the swing phase (Sw) and stance phase (St). Intervals between the successive frames, 30 ms. C: Angles at the hip (triangles), knee (dots), and ankle joint (squares) as a function of the phase of the step cycle. From Smith *et al.* (1988).

basic pattern of this type of movement is generated in the lumbosacral enlargement of the spinal cord.

10.4.2.2 *Scratching movements*

In reptiles, birds, and mammals tactile stimulation of a site on the body surface will elicit a site-specific motor response, termed the scratch reflex, in which a limb will reach towards and rhythmically rub against the stimulated site. The task of the scratch reflex is for a limb to exert a force against a site on the body surface that has received tactile stimulation, and to remove an irritating object from that area of the skin (Sherrington 1906*a,b*; Stein 1983).

In the cat, such an area from which the scratch reflex can be evoked (the receptive field) is rather small; it covers only the neck and head (Deliagina *et al.* 1975; Kuhta and Smith 1990). The cat can reach other sites on the body by its mouth and clean them by means of its teeth and tongue. To reach different sites within the scratch reflex receptive field the cat bends its trunk and neck and turns its head so that the irritated area is within reach of the ipsilateral hind limb, that performs the standard oscillatory reflex movements at a frequency of 3–4 Hz (Figs. 10.8A_1–A_3). Figure 10.8B shows the EMG pattern of scratching. Activities of the two groups of limb muscles (flexors and extensors) alternate. The flexor activity prevails both in the duration of bursts and in the burst amplitude; as a result, the limb periodically oscillates around the hemi-flexed, protracted position (Kuhta and Smith 1990; O'Donovan *et al.* 1982).

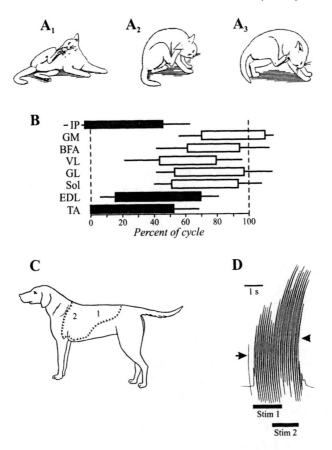

Fig. 10.8 Scratch reflex in the cat and dog. A_1–A_3: Postural adjustments in the cat for scratching different sites on the head. B: EMG pattern for representative muscles during scratching in the cat. For each muscle, the average burst duration is shown, as well as SD for its onset and offset. Flexor muscles are indicated by black bars, and extensor ones by empty bars. (Abbreviations: IP, iliopsoas; GM, gluteus medius; BFA, biceps femoris anterior; VL, vastus lateralis; GL, gastrocnemius lateralis; Sol, soleus; EDL, extensor digitorum longus; TA, tibialis anterior.) C,D: The spinal dog (C) is able to scratch different sites within the receptive field (shown by broken line). The protraction–retraction movements of the hind limb evoked by stimulation of sites 1 and 2 (C) are shown in D. A_1–B are from Kuhta and Smith (1990) and C and D are from Sherrington (1906a).

The rhythm of scratching has a spinal origin. In the classical study of the scratch reflex in dogs with transection of the spinal cord in the thoracic region, Sherrington showed that the basic pattern of scratching persisted, and that the hind limb could reach and scratch different sites within a very wide area (Fig. 10.8C). With stimulation of different sites within the receptive field, the rhythmic component of movements is rather constant, and it is superimposed upon different tonic components, that is the mean values of the hip and knee angles differ for different stimulated sites

(Fig. 10.8D). One can thus conclude that there are some variables in the scratch programme which can be smoothly regulated in accordance with the position of the stimulated site.

In the turtle, the spinal cord is able to generate three different forms of the scratch reflex depending on the location of an irritant. These forms differ in the organization of the employed muscle synergies: some muscles, which contract in phase in one form of scratching, contract in antiphase in other forms (reviewed by Stein 1983).

10.4.2.3   *Paw shaking and limb withdrawal*

In addition to scratching, two more types of rhythmical movement of the hind limb have been described in the cat, both of which can be also observed in spinal animals. Like scratching, both of these movements are aimed at terminating the irritation of the limb:

1. Fast paw shaking can be evoked by making the paw wet (Smith *et al.* 1980, 1985). It consists of rapid (about 10 Hz) oscillations of the limb produced due to the rhythmic flexor and extensor bursts. These bursts alternate in the antagonistic muscles of a single joint, for example in the ankle flexor TA and extensor GM (see Figs. $10.9D_1,D_2$). As regards different joints, their relationships are not so strict, and the phase shift can vary considerably, up to 30 per cent of the cycle (Abraham and Loeb 1985; Smith *et al.* 1980).
2. The rhythmical withdrawal reflex can be observed in the spinal cat if one is squeezing its paw. The animal 'struggles' to get free, and contracts the flexors of the squeezed limb. The bursts of flexor activity are repeated continuously, with a period of about 1 s. No extensor activity is observed in this motor pattern (see Figs. $10.9E_1,E_2$) (Pearson and Rossignol 1991).

Thus, the lumbosacral enlargement of the cat's spinal cord is capable of generating at least five distinct types of rhythmical movements differing in the cycle duration and in the pattern of activity of different muscles within the cycle. In Fig. 10.9, the left column schematically shows, for these five types of movement, the phases of activity of the muscles acting around the hip, knee, and ankle joints, and the right column shows the timing of activity of the flexor and extensor groups in the cycle. Forward stepping (Figs. $10.9A_1,A_2$) is characterized by alternating activity of two main groups, flexors and extensors, whereas the knee flexors can exhibit two periods of activity in a cycle. The cycle duration ranges from 0.5 s to 2 s depending on the speed of locomotion. In backward stepping (Figs. $10.9B_1,B_2$), the hip flexors exhibit a much shorter period of activity than the flexors of other joints, and the two periods of activity in the knee flexors fuse. Muscle synergies utilized in scratching (Figs. $10.9C_1,C_2$) are similar to those of stepping: the activities of the flexors and extensors groups alternate. However, the scratch cycle is much shorter than the step cycle due to a short extensor phase. In the paw shaking reflex (Figs. $10.9D_1,D_2$), the knee extensor is not involved in the extensor synergy (which is characteristic of stepping and scratching) but is coactivated with flexors.

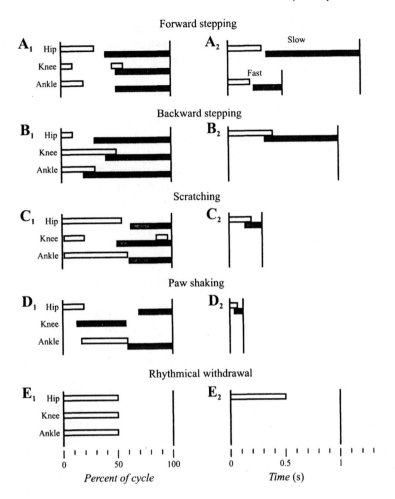

Fig. 10.9 Schematic representation of different types of cyclic hind limb movements. The left column shows the phases of activity of flexor (empty bars) and extensor (black bars) muscles of the main joints within the normalized cycle for different movements. The right column shows the typical time duration of the cycle for different movements, and the periods of flexor and extensor activity. For scratching, two patterns are illustrated—in intact cat (black bars) and in decerebrate cat (black bars plus shaded bars).

Finally, the striking feature of the rhythmical withdrawal reflex (Figs. 10.9E₁,E₂) is the rhythmical activation of only the flexor muscles.

Three of the patterns generated by the spinal cord—forward walking, backward walking, and scratching—have many features in common, and seem to be generated by the same neuronal network which is subjected to moderate modifications for each of the patterns. These modifications may be of two principal types: (1) a change of some parameters of the network, and (2) a change of the connectivity in the network. It seems likely that both types of network modification are used to switch from one pattern to another. Strong evidence in favour of the first type of modification is the gradual transition from the stepping pattern to the scratching pattern observed under certain conditions (Berkinblit *et al.* 1978*b*) (see Section 11.1). On the other hand, a change of the connectivity would give a good explanation for the transition from a single burst pattern to a double burst pattern in some muscles (Figs. $10.9A_1–C_1$). The idea of reconfiguration of the limb control system for different motor patterns ('the mosaic of unit burst generators') was first proposed by Grillner (1981).

As far as the paw shake response is concerned, there is a strong evidence that this motor pattern is generated by a separate neuronal network since it can be observed during stepping, that is both patterns can be generated simultaneously (Smith *et al.* 1985).

10.5   CONCLUSIONS

1. In quadrupedal locomotion, each of the limbs is driven by its individual control mechanisms (the limb controller) which provides the intralimb coordination and determines the major characteristics of the step cycle—the rhythm of stepping, the duration of the stance and swing phases, and the value of muscular activity.
2. The limb controller is located in the spinal cord. It can generate a number of rhythmical movements (stepping, scratching, etc.) differing in the cycle duration and in the pattern of activity of different muscles within the cycle.
3. When controlling stepping movements, the controllers for individual limbs are coordinated with each other by mutual influences, which result in a common rhythm of stepping and definite phase relations between the stepping movements of different limbs—the gait.
4. The motor centres located in the spinal cord, brainstem, and cerebellum constitute a control system—the locomotor automatism—capable of governing locomotion in simple environmental conditions, when visuo-motor coordination is not required. A wide range of locomotor activities, including different speeds of progression, different intensities of stepping movements, and different gaits, can be covered by varying only one parameter in the control system, that is the level of excitation of neurons in a small area of the brainstem—the mesencephalic locomotor region. Via this region, higher brain centres may initiate locomotion and regulate its intensity.

11

Limb controller

In this chapter, we consider in parallel the spinal mechanisms controlling stepping and scratching movements of the cat's hind limb. The reasons for considering scratching are two-fold: First, the stepping and scratching motor patterns have many features in common, suggesting that their control mechanisms share basic elements (see Section 10.4). Second, the mechanisms for scratching are easier to analyse because of their relative simplicity since only one limb performs rhythmic movements, in contrast to stepping where all four limbs participate.

11.1 CENTRAL PATTERN GENERATORS FOR STEPPING AND SCRATCHING

11.1.1 CPG for stepping

It is well established that rhythmic activity with an efferent motor pattern similar to stepping for each of the hind limbs, and with bilateral alternation, can be generated by the spinal cord in the absence of sensory feedback. This was demonstrated in the deafferented cat, that is after transection of all dorsal roots in the lumbosacral enlargement of the spinal cord (Grillner and Zangger 1984). Similar conclusions have been reached in paralysed preparations, with the neuromuscular synapses blocked by curare, so that all phasic afferent feedback is removed, where the motor neuron activity is recorded from the motor axons in the muscle nerves. Such patterns (fictive stepping) have been recorded in various preparations: acute and chronic spinal cats (Baker *et al.* 1984; Grillner and Zangger 1979; Pearson and Rossignol 1991); decerebrate cats with electrical stimulation of the MLR (Fleshman *et al.* 1984; Jordan *et al.* 1979), and thalamic (decorticate) cats (Baev 1978; Perret and Cabelguen 1980). The isolated spinal cord of the newborn rat and chick embryo is also able to generate the efferent locomotor pattern (see Section 11.1.3).

Figure 11.1A shows the activity recorded from three representative muscle nerves—the knee flexor (Stn), hip flexor (Srt), and ankle extensor (GM)—in the paralysed spinal cat; the locomotor CPG was activated by clonidine injection. The activities of the flexor and extensor motor neuron pools alternate; this corresponds to the alternation of the swing and stance phases of a cycle during real stepping (see Section 10.1). With spontaneous fluctuations of the cycle duration the largest changes in duration occurred in the extensor phase, whereas the flexor

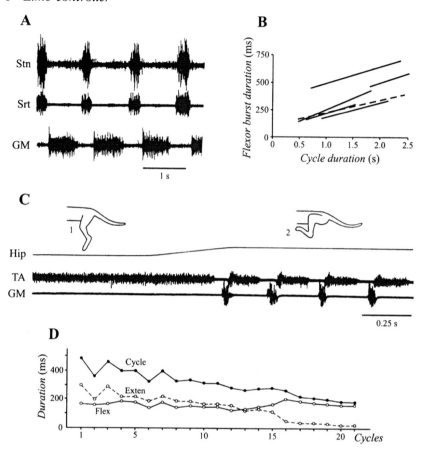

Fig. 11.1 Generation of the efferent pattern for stepping and scratching in the immobilized cat. A: Fictive motor pattern of stepping recorded from hind leg nerves in the immobilized spinal cat treated with clonidine (intravenously). B: Plots of the relationship between the flexor burst duration and the cycle period in five spinal cats. For comparison, the dashed line shows the relationship for the flexor burst in an intact cat walking on the treadmill. C: Fictive motor pattern of scratching recorded from the leg nerves in the immobilized decerebrate cat. The activity in the nerves was elicited by tactile stimulation of the pinna. The leg position (Hip) was changed by an experimenter during the recording (see insets 1 and 2). (Abbreviations: Stn, semitendinosus; Srt, sartorius; GM, gastrocnemius medialis.) D: Spontaneous transition from the stepping pattern to the scratching pattern in the immobilized decerebrate cat. Duration of the cycle (Cycle), extensor phase (Exten), and flexor phase (Flex) are shown in successive cycles. Rhythmic activity was elicited by electrical stimulation of the C_2 spinal segment. A and B are from Pearson and Rossignol (1991), C is from Deliagina *et al.* (1975), and D is from Berkinblit *et al.* (1978*b*).

phase duration changed much less (Fig. 11.1B); similar relations between the cycle duration and the duration of the stance and swing phases are characteristic of real stepping (see Section 10.1). Finally, some motor neuron pools that exhibit a more complicated pattern of activity—two bursts per cycle—in the intact animals (see

Section 10.1), could generate a similar pattern during fictive stepping and during stepping in deafferented animals (Grillner and Zangger 1975, 1979, 1984; Perret 1983). Thus, some essential features of the motor pattern for stepping—bilateral alternation, shorter and less variable flexor bursts than the extensor bursts, two bursts per cycle in some muscles—can be seen in the efferent motor pattern generated by the spinal CPG under open-loop conditions. When the feedback loop is closed, the pattern is considerably modified, however (see Section 11.5).

A stepping-like efferent pattern of the fore limbs can also be generated in immobilized preparations (Viala and Vidal 1978; Terakado and Yamaguchi 1990; Cabelguen *et al.* 1984; Yamaguchi 1991).

11.1.2 CPG for scratching

Experiments on the cat with deafferented hind limbs and on the paralysed cat have shown that a rhythmic efferent motor pattern similar to scratching can be evoked by tactile stimulation of the scratch reflex receptive field, or by electrical or chemical stimulation of the cervical spinal cord (Sherrington 1910; Jankowska 1959; Feldberg and Fleischhauer 1960; Deliagina *et al.* 1975, 1981). Figure 11.1C shows the activity recorded from the muscle nerves supplying the ankle flexor (TA) and extensor (GM) in the paralysed decerebrate cat. Tactile stimulation of the ipsilateral pinna elicited tonic activity in TA, but the rhythmic activity was absent until the limb was flexed by the experimenter and put in a normal position for scratching. Thus, the rhythm generator for scratching can be activated by signals delivered by a command propriospinal system (see Chapter 12) provided the generator also receives a 'confirmation' that the limb is in the appropriate position for scratching, i.e. protracted forward. The rhythm of fictive scratching (Fig. 11.1C) has approximately the same frequency (about 4 Hz) as the rhythm of real scratching (see Section 10.4.2.2). The flexor bursts are formed due to the interruptions of the tonic flexor activity. Thus, under open-loop conditions, the spinal CPG can produce the efferent motor pattern with some essential features of scratching movements. When the feedback loop is closed, the pattern is modified to some extent, however (see Section 11.5).

The pattern of fictive scratching differs from the pattern of fictive stepping in that the scratch cycle is much shorter, and the extensor burst constitutes a smaller portion of the cycle than the flexor burst (compare Figs. 11.1A and C). In some cases, however, a motor pattern with a spontaneous gradual transition from the cycle characteristics for stepping to the cycle characteristics for scratching was observed (Fig. 11.1D) (Berkinblit *et al.* 1978*b*). This transition was due to a gradual shortening of the extensor burst, whereas the flexor burst remained nearly constant. This observation strongly suggests that the same neuronal network, with one changeable parameter, is responsible for the generation of both motor patterns.

Two other rhythmical motor patterns—paw shake and limb withdrawal (see Section 10.4.2.3)—can also be generated by the spinal cord deprived of sensory feedback, that is they are generated by the spinal CPGs (Pearson and Rossignol 1991).

11.2   LOCALIZATION OF THE RHYTHM GENERATOR

The neuronal mechanisms controlling stepping and scratching movements of the hind limb—the hind limb motor centre—are located in the hind limb enlargement of the spinal cord. In the cat, the hind limb enlargement includes the segments L3–S1 (Fig. 11.2A); in the rat it includes the segments T12–L6. Experiments with longitudinal splitting (Kudo and Yamada 1987), unilateral destruction (Berkinblit *et al.* 1978*a*), and unilateral pharmacological activation (Kjaerulff and Kiehn 1997) of the hind limb enlargement have shown that the basic neuronal mechanisms for generating the rhythm of stepping and scratching are located in the ipsilateral half of the enlargement.

The motor neuron pools of the hind limb are distributed over the length of the enlargement: in the cat the pools of the hip muscles are located mainly in the L4–L5 segments, those of the knee muscles in L5–L6, and those of the ankle and digit muscles in L7–S1 (Fig. 11.2A) (Romanes 1964). During stepping and scratching, all these pools exhibit rhythmic activity. A great number of interneurons, situated over the whole length of the enlargement, also exhibit rhythmic activity related to that of the motor neurons. Mapping of the spinal cord during fictive scratching has shown that the majority of the rhythmically modulated neurons are located in the medial and lateral parts of the intermediate area of the spinal grey matter, as well as in the ventral horn, that is in laminae VI and VII according to the Rexed's nomenclature (Rexed 1954) (Fig. 11.2B) (Berkinblit *et al.* 1978*a*; Baev *et al.* 1981). A corresponding location of active neurons has been found for stepping (Baev *et al.* 1979; Orlovsky and Feldman 1972).

In a number of studies, activity-dependent markers were used to try to localize neurons involved in the generation of stepping or scratching rhythm (Viala *et al.* 1988; Dai *et al.* 1990; Barajon *et al.* 1992). These studies have shown that interneurons with increased activity during rhythm generation are more concentrated in the intermediate grey matter of the spinal cord. It remains unclear, however, if they are involved in rhythmogenesis.

Using a slice preparation of the rat spinal cord, neurons that are located ventrolateral to the central canal in medial laminae VII have been found to have pacemaker-like properties induced by NMDA. These conditional bursters may constitute a part of the rhythm generator (Hochman *et al.* 1994).

A major question concerning the location of the rhythm generating network is if the oscillatory neurons are concentrated in a limited area of the spinal cord enlargement, or if they are distributed over the whole length of the enlargement? Experiments with lesions or functional inactivation of different areas along the enlargement have shown that rather small parts of the spinal cord can generate both stepping and scratching rhythms. Figures 11.2C_1–F_2 illustrate an experiment with localization of the rhythm generating segments for scratching (Deliagina *et al.* 1983). In Fig. 11.2C_1 is shown the efferent activity in the flexor (Srt) and extensor (G) nerves during fictive scratching, as well as the activity of the spinal interneuron (IN) from the L4 segment. Then, by cooling L5 (the location of the cooling probe is shown in Fig. 11.2C_3), the caudal part of the spinal hind limb centre,

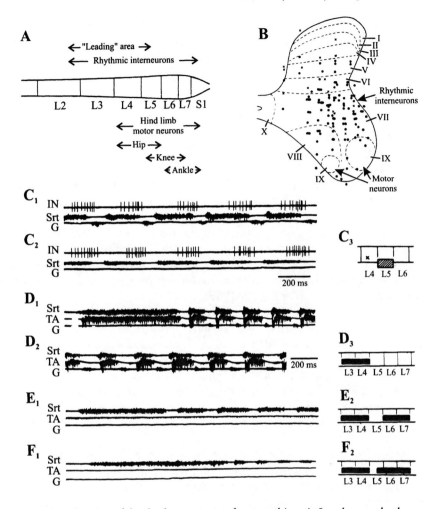

Fig. 11.2 Localization of the rhythm generator for scratching. A: Lumbosacral enlargement of the spinal cord of the cat. Locations of the motor neuron pools controlling muscles of different joints are indicated. The interneurons which are rhythmically bursting during fictive scratching can be found in all segments of the enlargement. B: The distribution of rhythmically bursting neurons over the cross section of the spinal cord grey matter (dots); neurons with weaker modulation are indicated with crosses. Numbers of Rexed's layers (I–X) are indicated. C_1–F_2: Generation of fictive scratching by the spinal cord a part of which was destroyed or functionally inactivated. Rhythmic activity in the spinal cord was elicited in the immobilized decerebrate cat by pinna stimulation. C_1–C_3: Effect of cooling (10°C) of the L5 segment. C_1: Activity of the muscle nerves and of the interneuron (IN) from the segment L4 before cooling. C_2: The same during cooling. Position of the cooling probe on the lateral surface of L5 and the site of IN recording is shown in C_3. D_1–D_3: Effect of destruction of the grey matter in the L3 and L4 segments. D_1: Activity of three muscle nerves before destruction. D_2: The same after destruction. The extent of the lesion is shown in D_3. E_1: Generation of the scratching rhythm by the isolated L5 segment. The grey matter in L3, L4 and L6, L7 was destroyed (E_2). F_1: With additional destruction of the grey matter in the caudal L5 (shown in F_2), the rhythmic pattern was considerably changed. (Abbreviations: Srt, sartorius; TA, tibialis anterior; G, gastrocnemius). B is from Berkinblit *et al.* (1978*a*) and C_1–F_2 are from Deliagina *et al.* (1983).

starting from L5, was functionally disconnected from its rostral part, which was demonstrated by the termination of activity in the G motor neuron pool located caudal to the cooling probe, in L7–S1 (Fig. 11.2C_2). Nevertheless, the L3 and L4 segments continued to generate the normal scratch rhythm monitored by the rhythmic activity of the Srt motor neurons from L4, as well as by rhythmic bursts in the interneuron from L4.

The L3 and L4 segments are not the only rhythm generating segments. After destruction of the grey matter in those segments (Fig. 11.2D_3), the rhythmical generation in L5 and more caudal segments (Fig. 11.2D_2) remained almost unchanged compared with control (Fig. 11.2D_1). After destruction of the grey matter both rostral and caudal to L5 (Fig. 11.2E_2), the single L5 segment was also able to generate the rhythm (Fig. 11.2E_1). With further reduction of the volume of grey matter (Fig. 11.2F_2), a normal scratch rhythm could not be evoked, however (Fig. 11.2F_1). There is indirect evidence that the most caudal segments, L6–S1, are also capable of rhythm generation, but to a lesser extent than the rostral segments L4 and L5 (Deliagina *et al.* 1983). In the turtle, the anterior segments of the enlargement also have a greater capacity for generating the rhythmic pattern for scratching than the posterior segments (Mortin and Stein 1989).

The local oscillatory networks are unified into one single rhythm generator for the limb, with a common rhythm for all segments, due to the connections between the local oscillators. There is evidence that the local oscillators are not equipotent in the united system. As one can see in Figs. 11.2D_1,D_2, rhythmical bursts in the two flexor nerves, Srt and TA, are not completely synchronized, but rather TA motor neurons, located caudally to Srt motor neurons, start to fire with a delay of about 20 ms in relation to Srt motor neurons in each cycle. This suggests that the rostral segments play a leading role and determine the rhythm of the whole system.

Similar results have been obtained for stepping. In chronic experiments on adult cats it was shown that the spinal cord could generate stepping movements of the hind limbs provided that the cord was transected rostral to the L4 segment. More caudal transections abolished the movements (Afelt *et al.* 1973). In acute experiments, using L-DOPA (L-dihydroxyphenylalanine) to elicit locomotor activity (Budakova 1973), rhythmic oscillations in the lower part of the spinal cord could be evoked provided the transection was not performed lower than in the L5 segment (Grillner and Zangger 1979).

In the isolated spinal cord of the newborn rat, locomotor-like efferent rhythmic activity can be evoked by applying NMDA (see for example Kudo and Yamada 1987), or a mixture of NMDA and 5-HT (serotonin). Lesion studies on this preparation have shown that the capacity for generation of the locomotory rhythm is also distributed over the spinal cord enlargement (segments T11–L4) (Kjaerulff and Kiehn 1996), with a maximal capacity in the most rostral segments (Kjaerulff and Kiehn 1996; Cazalets *et al.* 1995). A similar distribution has been found in the chick embryo spinal cord (Ho and O'Donovan 1993). It seems likely that the oscillatory mechanism in the rostral segments has a higher frequency and determines the rhythm of oscillations in the whole spinal hind limb centre. A similar idea was advanced for the lamprey spinal cord (see the trailing oscillator hypotheses, Section 8.3). The dominance of the rostral ('leading') segments over the caudal ones fits well with the fact that it is in these segments that the neuronal networks controlling the hip muscles, i.e. the muscles of the joint that determines the limb position (see Section 11.5) are located.

Three experimental findings, namely: (1) the existence of a number of local oscillators distributed along the spinal cord enlargement, (2) the somatotopic representation of the limb muscles along the enlargement (see Fig. 11.2A), and (3) the supply of the motor neurons with input signals generated, to a large extent, by local oscillators (see Fig. 11.2E$_1$), speak in favour of the idea that different joints, and even different muscle groups, may have their own rhythm generating networks (Grillner 1981). It seems likely that these networks are not identical to each other. Simple alternation of flexor and extensor activity is characteristic of the hip muscles, whereas some of the knee, ankle, and digit muscles can exhibit more complicated patterns (see Section 10.1 and Figs. 10.2C,D$_1$). The possible arrangement of the spinal networks generating these different patterns are considered in the next section.

11.3   MODELS OF THE RHYTHM GENERATOR

11.3.1   Generation of basic pattern for stepping and scratching

The neuronal networks in the spinal cord generating the rhythms for stepping and scratching have not yet been identified despite extensive efforts (see for example Burke and Fleshman 1986; Berkinblit *et al.* 1978*a,b*; Shefchyk *et al.* 1990; Baev *et al.* 1979). Two main models have been proposed to explain generation of these rhythms—a biphasic generator and a three-phasic generator.

The *biphasic generator*, usually termed the half-centre generator, was proposed by Brown (1911) and was considered in detail to explain the generation of the locomotory rhythm in *Clione* (see Section 1.3) and lamprey (see Section 8.3). Briefly, bursts in two groups of interneurons constituting the flexor half-centre (F) and the extensor half-centre (E) (Fig. 11.3A), alternate due to mutual inhibitory influences between the half-centres. Some factors, like spike frequency adaptation, limit the burst duration in each group and promote transitions of activity from one half-centre to the other. The two half-centres perform activation of the corresponding, flexor or extensor, motor neurons and inhibition of the antagonistic motor neurons. Strong evidence in favour of the half-centre hypothesis has been obtained by Lundberg and his colleagues (Jankowska *et al.* 1967*a,b*; Lundberg 1981). Though the two groups of interneurons constituting the half-centres have not been directly identified, their effects on the motor neurons and on each other have been demonstrated. In the immobilized spinal cat treated with DOPA, electrical stimulation of high-threshold cutaneous or muscle afferents (termed 'flexor reflex afferents', FRA) of the ipsilateral limb resulted in a long-lasting activation of the flexor motor neurons (Fig. 11.3B) and in inhibition of the extensor motor neurons (Fig. 11.3F). Stimulation of the contralateral FRA resulted in a long-lasting activation of the extensor motor neurons (Fig. 11.3E) and inhibition of

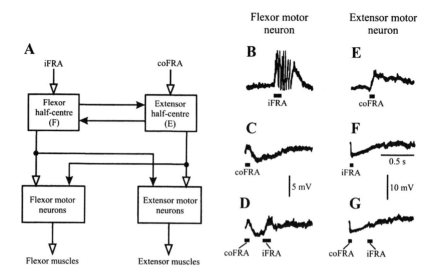

Fig. 11.3 Half-centre model of the locomotor rhythm generator and the experimental evidence in its favour. A: The half-centre model. White and black triangles represent the excitatory and inhibitory connections, respectively. B–G: Responses in the flexor and extensor motor neurons to stimulation of the flexor reflex afferents in the ipsilateral and contralateral limbs (iFRA and coFRA). Recordings were performed in the spinal cat treated with L-DOPA. Based on Jankowska *et al.* (1967*a,b*).

the flexor motor neurons (Fig. 11.3C). Two observations support the hypothesis that the FRA stimulation responses are mediated by neural mechanisms that also participate in the generation of stepping:

1. The excitatory responses resemble, in their amplitude and duration, the activity of the flexor and extensor motor neurons in the swing and stance phases of the step cycle, respectively.
2. FRA stimulation could sometimes evoke a series of locomotor-like alternating bursts in flexor and extensor motor neurons.

The inhibitory interaction between the premotor (F and E) groups of interneurons becomes evident with successive stimulation of the ipsi- and contralateral FRA: an excitatory response could be abolished by a preceding activation of the antagonistic group of interneurons (Figs. 11.3D,G).

As was discussed in Section 1.3, the rhythmic activity in a half-centre model may be caused by two factors, that is by network properties (mutual inhibition between the two half-centres), and by endogenous rhythmicity in each of the half-centres. In the latter case, each of the half-centres can itself produce the rhythm, without participation of the antagonistic half-centre. Neurons with NMDA-dependent pacemaker properties (conditional bursters) have been found in spinal cord slice preparations (Hochman *et al.* 1994). The relative contribution of the two factors in the rhythmogenesis in the spinal cord remains unclear, however.

Thus, the half-centre model of the spinal rhythm generator (Fig. 11.3A), proposed by Brown (1911), now has support from a large body of experimental evidence. This model well explains the generation of the basic pattern of stepping, that is alternation of bursts in the flexor and extensor motor neuron pools. More complicated patterns, like double bursts in some flexor muscles (see Section 11.1) are difficult to explain without modifications of the original version of the model (see Section 11.3.2), however.

The *three-phasic generator*, usually termed the generator with a switch-off mechanism (Fig. 11.4A), was originally proposed to explain the generation of the respiratory rhythm (Bradley *et al.* 1975; Cohen and Feldman 1977) and experimentally identified in the feeding system of the snails *Lymnae* and *Planorbis* (Rose and Benjamin 1981; Benjamin 1983; Elliot and Benjamin 1985; Arshavsky *et al.* 1988*a–c*). Some aspects of this model were discussed in relation to the locomotor CPG of *Tritonia* (see Section 2.1.2). This model well explains the generation of the scratching rhythm. The model is derived from the analysis of the activity of spinal interneurons during fictive scratching (Berkinblit *et al.* 1978*a,b*). Figure 11.4B shows the phases of activity of 120 unidentified interneurons from the leading area of the hind limb centre (L4–L5 segments) in the normalized scratch cycle, that is the phase distribution of neurons. The neurons were subdivided into three groups according to the phase of their activity in the cycle. Group 1 neurons are firing in the flexor phase of the cycle, and the profile of their population activity (Fig. 11.4C_1) is very similar to that of flexor motor neurons (FMN, Fig. 11.4B). Group 3 neurons are firing at the end of the cycle, and the profile of their activity (Fig. 11.4C_3) resembles that of the extensor motor neurons (EMN, Fig. 11.4B). It seems likely that groups 1 and 3 are responsible for activation of the flexor and extensor motor neurons, respectively. However, the pattern of population activity in group 2 has no correlates with the efferent pattern. This activity gradually increases towards the end of the flexor phase (Fig. 11.4C_2) due to the continuous recruitment of new neurons (Fig. 11.4B), as well as due to acceleration of their firing rate in the course of a burst. The peak of group 2 activity coincides with the transition from the flexor to the extensor phase. It was suggested (Berkinblit *et al.* 1978*a,b*) that groups 1–3 have the following functions. Group 1 receives a tonic excitatory drive from an external source—the propriospinal pathways responsible for elicitation of the scratch reflex (see Section 12.2), and phasic inhibitory input from group 3. Group 2 is a central component of the network: when activated by the excitatory drive from group 1, group 2 starts to generate a ramp-shaped activity. The growing activity in group 2 may be caused by mutual excitation of the neurons in this group, and/or by specific membrane properties in individual neurons (see for example Arshavsky *et al.* 1988*a–c*). When group 2 reaches a definite level of activity, it excites group 3. Some of the group 3 neurons are inhibitory, they produce inhibition of group 1 and thus deprive group 2 of the excitatory drive, thereby terminating its activity. Groups 1 and 3 produce activation of the flexor and extensor motor neurons, respectively, and inhibition of the antagonistic groups. Computer simulation of the generator with switch-off mechanism (similar to that shown in Fig. 11.4A) reproduced the patterns of activity of the three neuron groups (Fig. 11.4D) (Shadmehr 1989).

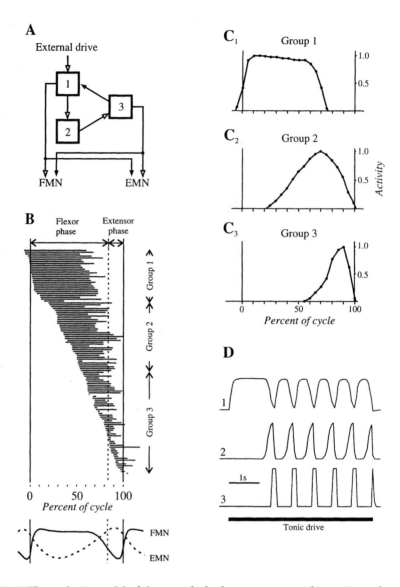

Fig. 11.4 Three-phasic model of the scratch rhythm generator, and experimental support of this model. A: Three-phasic model of the rhythm generator. Excitatory connections between the neuronal groups are shown by white arrows, inhibitory connections by black arrows. B: Phase distribution of spinal interneurons in the scratch cycle. The burst position of each neuron in the normalized scratch cycle is shown by a bar. The profiles of activity of the flexor and extensor motor neurons are shown below the graph. All neurons have been divided into three groups (1–3) according to the phases of their activity. C_1–C_3: Population activity of the groups 1–3 as a function of the phase of the cycle (arbitrary units). D: Computer simulation of the network largely similar to that shown in A. Activity of groups 1–3 is presented as a function of time (arbitrary units). The network was activated by a tonic drive to group 1 and 2 neurons. B and C are from Berkinblit *et al.* (1978*a*) and D is from Shadmehr (1989).

Analysis of the phase distribution of unidentified spinal interneurons during stepping (Bayev *et al.* 1979; Orlovsky and Feldman 1972*b*) has shown that the pattern of their activity is much more complex than a mere alternation of flexor and extensor bursts, which was predicted by the half-centre model. In particular, many neurons are gradually recruited and start firing during the flexor phase. This finding suggests that a group of neurons with a function similar to that of group 2 in the rhythm generator for scratching (Fig. 11.4A), also participates in the generation of the rhythm for stepping. It thus seems likely that the basic mechanisms of both models—the biphasic, half-centre model and the three-phasic model with the switch-off mechanism—are utilized in the spinal rhythm generator. An attempt to formulate a synthetic model was made by Gelfand *et al.* (1988). Figure 11.5 shows their synthetic model designed to explain the generation of both stepping and scratching patterns. In addition to the rhythmical component, the model can also generate a postural component of motor output, that is a tonic flexor activity for scratching and a tonic extensor activity for stepping. The principal sensory influences on the transitions between the flexor and extensor phases of a cycle, which have been demonstrated experimentally (see Section 11.5) are also incorporated into the model. The model consists of flexor and extensor units, F and E. The flexor unit consists in its turn, of two subunits, F_1 and F_2. In the scratching mode of operation (Figs. 11.5A,C), the flexor unit F receives tonic excitatory input. This input determines the postural component of a movement. The subunit F_1 inhibits the extensor unit E. The subunit F_2, when activated by F_1, starts to generate ramp output, and produces excitation of the extensor unit E. When excitatory input to E from F_2 overcomes the inhibitory input from F_1, the extensor unit E becomes active and inhibits F_1, and thereby F_2. In the scratching mode, the only excitatory input to the extensor unit E is provided by F_2, and with termination of this input the activity of the extensor unit E also terminates; the extensor burst is, therefore, very brief which is characteristic of scratching (see Fig. 11.1C). An inhibitory sensory input S from limb mechanoreceptors is addressed to the subunit F_2 and does not allow the activity to transit from F to E except for at the very rostral position of the limb (a white sector in Fig. 11.5A). This may explain the finding that the scratch rhythm is generated only at the protracted position of the hind limb (Fig. 11.1C).

In the stepping mode of operation (Figs. 11.5B,D), not the flexor unit but the extensor unit E receives a tonic excitatory drive. This input determines the postural component of a movement, that is the activity of the antigravitational, extensor muscles. When active, the extensor unit E inhibits the flexor unit. Due to the sensory feedback, a backward deflection of the limb causes inhibition of the extensor unit E, and thereby disinhibition of the flexor unit F. This explains the crucial role of afferent input signalling the hip position (see Section 11.5). Without sensory influences (open-loop conditions), a termination of the extensor phase is caused only by the internal processes in the network, that is by the burst-terminating factors in the extensor unit E. The flexor phase is generated according to the same principle as in scratching (see above).

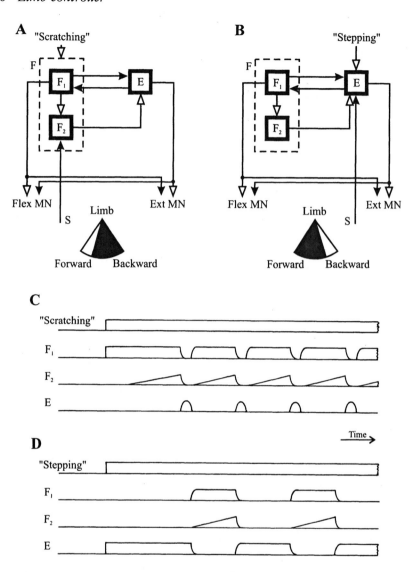

Fig. 11.5 A synthetic model capable of generation of both scratching and stepping rhythms. The mode of operation of the model depends on the tonic excitatory drive, 'Scratching' (A) or 'Stepping' (B). The temporal patterns for the two modes are shown in C and D respectively. The model consists of the flexor (F) and extensor (E) units; the flexor unit in its turn consists of two subunits (F_1 and F_2). There are reciprocal inhibitory interactions between F_1 and E. F_1 also exerts a delayed excitatory action on E via F_2. The flexor motor neurons (Flex MN) receive an excitatory drive from F_1 and an inhibitory drive from E. The extensor motor neurons (Ext MN) receive an excitatory drive from E and an inhibitory drive from F_1. An inhibitory sensory input (S) signals the limb position. In the scratching mode of operation of the generator (A), S comes at any limb position (black sector) except for the most protracted position (white sector); it is addressed to F_2. In the stepping mode (B), S comes at any limb position (black sector) except for the caudal one (white sector); it is addressed to E. C,D: Activity of the F_1, F_2, and E functional blocks of the generator

11.3.2 Transformation of the basic pattern

A simple, basic pattern with alternating activity of flexors and extensors in each of the joints is characteristic of the majority of the motor neuron pools both in stepping and in scratching. However, some pools exhibit patterns differing from the basic one. These pools may have two bursts of activity per cycle, or they may generate a burst with a phase shift in relation to the majority of pools. It has been suggested that most of these complicated patterns can be explained by interactions of excitatory and inhibitory inputs, coming from the flexor and extensor units of the rhythm generator, and converging on the target motor neurons. It has also been suggested that these central influences on the motor neurons are mediated by special groups of premotor interneurons, and that these interneurons are under powerful sensory influences (Perret 1983). Figures 11.6A,B show that the phases of activity of two motor neuron pools, RF and Stn, during fictive stepping can be dramatically changed under the effect of sensory input. When the ipsilateral paw was mechanically stimulated (Fig. 11.6A) the Stn activity was in phase with the activity of most flexor pools monitored by the Srt motor neurons, whereas the RF activity was in antiphase. With stimulation of the contralateral paw (Fig. 11.6B), the RF burst phase was shifted to the flexor phase, while the Stn burst now occurred in the extensor phase. Experiments of this kind suggested a rather complicated pattern of convergence of excitatory and inhibitory inputs from the flexor and extensor subdivisions of the rhythm generator, not only on the motor neurons of bifunctional muscles like RF and Stn, but also on pure flexor and extensor motor neurons. For example, motor neurons of bifunctional muscles PB–Stn receive, from the extensor unit of the rhythm generator, a direct excitatory input as well as an inhibitory input mediated by the afferent-dependent interneurons (Fig. 11.6F); these interneurons have not been identified yet, however. An excitatory input from the flexor unit is presumably also mediated by the afferent-dependent interneurons. Pure flexor and extensor motor neurons also receive a portion of their excitatory drive via afference-dependent interneurons (Figs. 11.6D,E) (Perret and Cabelguen 1976, 1980; Perret 1983). However, the temporal profiles of the discharges in some motor neuron pools differ so strongly from the pure flexor and extensor profiles that they can hardly be explained on the basis of the convergence of inputs from the flexor and extensor subdivisions of the rhythm generator. As shown in Fig. 11.6C, the flexor digitorum longus (FDL) motor neurons receive two excitatory inputs, one in the extensor phase and one in the flexor phase (Burke and Fleshman 1986). The flexor phase input, however, has an extremely short duration, and is most likely generated by a special network (F* in Fig. 11.6G). This network is presumably triggered at the moment of transition from the flexor phase to the extensor phase, and generates a brief burst.

In real movements, some further complications of the basic, centrally generated pattern for each of the joints can be caused by the different classes of neurons

---

evoked by an excitatory tonic drive. In C, the drive ('Scratching') is addressed to the F unit; in D, the drive ('Stepping') is addressed to the E unit. See text for further explanations. Modified from Gelfand *et al.* (1988).

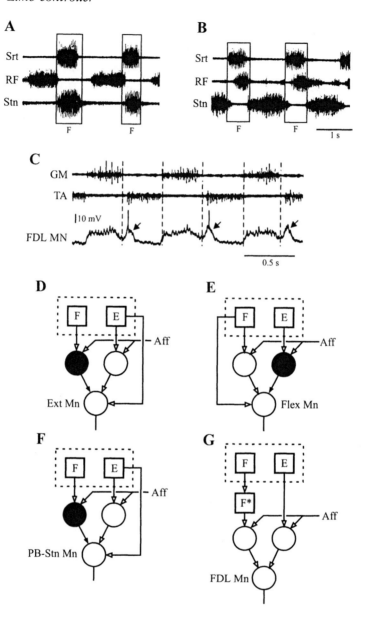

Fig. 11.6 Convergence of outputs from the rhythm generator on motor neurons. A,B: Efferent activity recorded from three limb nerves (sartorius, Srt; rectus femoris, RF; and semitendinosus, Stn) during fictive locomotion in curarized cat. Tonic stimulus (paw pinching) was applied to the ipsilateral (A) or contralateral (B) limb. Flexor phases of the cycle are indicated by rectangles. C: Efferent activity in the leg nerves (gastrocnemius medialis, GM; and tibialis anterior, TA), and the intracellular activity of the flexor digitorum longus (FDL) motor neuron recorded during fictive locomotion. Note the additional bursts in FDL MN activity (marked by arrows). D–G: Four examples of the convergence of inputs from the flexor (F) and extensor (E) subdivisions of the rhythm generator on different motor

constituting the output motor stage of the limb controller (see Section 11.4) and by different afferent influences (see Section 11.5). Active properties of the motor neuron membrane can also contribute, to some extent, to shaping the output motor pattern (Hounsgaard *et al.* 1988).

11.4 OUTPUT MOTOR STAGE AND OTHER TARGETS OF THE RHYTHM GENERATOR

The spinal rhythm generator performs a number of functions:

1. It supplies motor neurons with rhythmical input, thus producing the basic motor pattern of stepping and scratching.
2. It informs other limb controllers about its activity, which is necessary for inter-limb coordination.
3. It informs different motor centres of the brain about its activity. This is critical for the organization of their interaction with the spinal limb controllers. This problem will be considered in Chapter 13.
4. It modulates its own sensitivity to descending signals coming from various brain centres (see Chapter 13).
5. It modulates the efficiency of transmission of signals in different spinal pathways in a phase-dependent manner, thus reconfiguring the spinal network during the course of the step or scratch cycle. This modulation is partly due to phasic influences of the rhythm generator on the output motor stage of the limb controller.

Several groups of spinal neurons, that is alpha motor neurons, gamma motor neurons, and interneurons activated by Ia spindle afferents and mediating reciprocal inhibition between the antagonistic muscles (Ia interneurons), comprise a functional unit—the output motor stage (Fig. 11.7A). This unit exercises control over the activity of synergistic muscles of a given joint, and coordinates the activity of antagonistic muscles (for a review, see Baldissera *et al.* 1981). The initial reason for regarding the above mentioned groups as a functional unit was the remarkable fact that the supraspinal inputs to alpha motor neurons, gamma motor neurons, and Ia interneurons were found to be basically the same. In other words, by sending an impulse to alpha motor neurons via a certain input, the experimenter inevitably activated gamma motor neurons and Ia interneurons as well; this led to the concept of 'alpha–gamma-linked reciprocal inhibition' (Hongo *et al.* 1969*a,b*).

neurons: pure extensor (D), pure flexor (E), double-joint muscles posterior biceps and semitendinosus, PB–Stn (F), and flexor digitorum longus, FDL (G). The inputs are mediated by the interneurons that are also under afferent influences (empty circles, excitatory interneuron; filled circles, inhibitory interneurons). See text for further explanations. A,B are from Perret and Cabelguen (1980) and C is from Burke and Fleshman (1986).

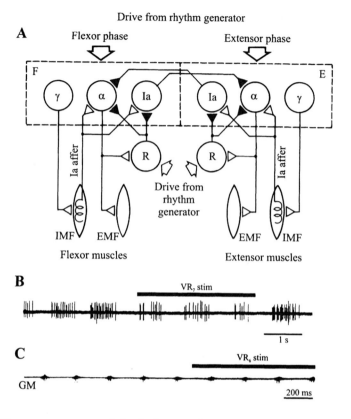

Fig. 11.7 Output motor stage of the limb controller. A: Two subunits controlling a single joint—the flexor subunit (F) and the extensor subunit (E). Each subunit includes three groups of neurons—alpha motor neurons (α), gamma motor neurons (γ), and Ia interneurons of the system reciprocal inhibition (Ia). Mutual connections, connections with Renshaw cells (R), and connections with intrafusal (IMF) and extrafusal (EMF) muscle fibres are shown. B: Electrical stimulation (25 Hz) of the seventh ventral root (VR$_7$ stim) did not affect the rhythm of fictive locomotion monitored by the activity in the axons of motor neurons from the filament of VR$_7$. C: Electrical stimulation (50 Hz) of the sixth ventral root (VR$_6$ stim) did not affect the rhythm of fictive scratching monitored by the activity in GM nerve. B is from Pratt and Jordan (1980) and C is from Orlovsky and Feldman (unpublished data).

The output motor stage functions as a unit not only in the motor acts generated by the brain but also in those generated by the spinal cord, in particular in stepping and scratching. The output motor stage is driven by the spinal rhythm generator and does not take a part in rhythmogenesis. This was demonstrated in experiments with stimulation of the ventral roots during fictive stepping or scratching (Pratt and Jordan 1980; Feldman and Orlovsky 1975). It was found that an intense high-frequency stimulation did not affect the stepping and scratching rhythms generated by the spinal cord (Figs. 11.7B,C), although the activity of a great proportion of alpha motor neurons and Ia interneurons was inevitably affected by the antidromic stimulation of the motor axons, according to the scheme of interconnections shown in Fig. 11.7A. Below, the activity of different neuron groups constituting the output motor stage, as well as the activity of the closely associated Renshaw cells will be considered during stepping and scratching.

11.4.1   Alpha motor neurons

Figures $11.8A_1-A_4$ show the activity of a flexor (TA) motor neuron during fictive scratching, and Figs. $11.8B_1,B_2$ show the activity of an extensor (G) motor neuron. In the initial, postural stage of the scratch reflex, the TA motor neuron is strongly depolarized and firing, while the membrane potential of G motor neuron is not affected. With the beginning of rhythm generation, the TA motor neuron exhibits periodical pauses in its firing due to repolarization down to the resting membrane potential. These pauses correspond to an extensor phase of the scratch cycle, in which the G motor neuron is depolarized and firing. The extensor phase (E) is followed by a flexor phase (F) in which the TA motor neuron depolarizes again up to the level reached in the postural stage, and begins to fire. In this phase, the G motor neuron repolarizes down to the resting potential. These findings suggest that, during scratching, the flexor and extensor motor neurons are controlled primarily by excitatory inputs from the corresponding subdivisions of the rhythm generator, whereas inhibitory inputs only play a secondary role.

Figures $11.8C_1,D_1$ show the activity of the flexor (Srt) and extensor (Sm) motor neurons during fictive locomotion (Orsal *et al.* 1986). They are depolarized and firing in the flexor and extensor phases of the step cycle, respectively, and hyperpolarized between their phases of activity. The hyperpolarization is caused by an inhibitory synaptic input as demonstrated by injection of Cl^- ions into the motor neurons (Figs. $11.8C_2,D_2$). Thus, during stepping, the flexor and extensor alpha motor neurons are driven by alternating excitatory and inhibitory inputs from the rhythm generator (see also Chandler *et al.* 1984).

11.4.2   Gamma motor neurons and rhythmic modulation of the stretch-reflex

Gamma motor neurons innervate intrafusal muscle fibres and affect the sensitivity of the stretch receptive muscle spindle afferents (Granit 1950; Hunt 1952; for a review see Matthews 1972). Rhythmic central modulation of the discharge frequency of gamma motor neurons in phase with alpha motor neurons was initially revealed by recording activity of the Ia muscle spindle afferents during locomotion in the decerebrate cat (Severin *et al.* 1967). Figure 11.9A shows a response of the Ia afferent from the ankle extensor G to stretching of this muscle caused by a passive flexion of the joint. The response to stretching decreased during locomotion (Fig. 11.9B) and even completely disappeared with more intense stepping (Fig. 11.9C). Instead, the afferent was firing in the stance phase of the step cycle, when its parent muscle was shortening. Similar 'gamma-modulation' of Ia spindle afferents was observed in the walking decorticate cat (Perret and Buser 1972; Perret 1976; Cabelguen 1981; Cabelguen *et al.* 1984). In the intact walking cat, the modulation was expressed to a lesser extent, however (Prochazka

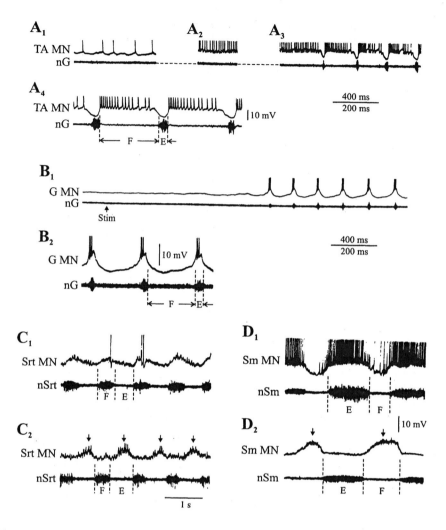

Fig. 11.8 Activity of motor neurons in the immobilized cat. A,B: Intracellular recording from the tibialis anterior motor neuron (TA MN, A_1–A_4) and gastrocnemius medialis motor neuron (GM MN, B_1,B_2) during fictive scratching. Scratching was evoked by pinna stimulation (onset of stimulation is indicated by arrow, Stim). The scratch rhythm was monitored by the activity in gastrocnemius nerve (nG). C_1–D_2. Intracellular recordings from the sartorius motor neuron (Srt MN, C_1,C_2) and semimembranosus motor neuron (Sm MN, D_1,D_2) during fictive locomotion. The locomotory rhythm was monitored by the activity in sartorius nerve (nSrt, C_1,C_2) and semimembranosus nerve (nSm, D_1,D_2). Recordings were performed before (C_1,D_1) and after (C_2,D_2) injection of chloride ions into the motor neurons. The injection resulted in a shift of the peak of depolarization to the opposite phase of the step cycle (indicated by arrows). In A_1–D_2, flexor (F) and extensor (E) phases of the cycle are indicated. A_1–B_2, are from Berkinblit *et al.* (1980) and C_1–D_2 are from Orsal *et al.* (1986).

et al. 1976; Prochazka and Gorassini 1998*a,b*; Loeb and Duysens 1979; Loeb and Hoffer 1981), suggesting that the degree of 'alpha–gamma coupling' can be regulated under the effect of corticospinal influences (Cabelguen 1986). Gamma-modulation was also found in the fore limb spindle afferents during locomotor activity (Cabelguen *et al.* 1984).

Powerful influences of the gamma motor neurons on the spindle receptors, overcoming the action of the muscle shortening, were also found during scratching, both in the postural and in the rhythmical stages of the scratch reflex (Fig. 11.9D) (Feldman *et al.* 1977).

Direct recordings from the gamma motor neurons (Murphy *et al.* 1984) revealed two different patterns of behaviour during locomotion: (1) tonic activation, that is an increase of the firing rate (Fig. 11.9E), and (2) phasic modulation, that is an increase of the firing rate in phase with the alpha motor neurons, and inhibition in the opposite phase (Fig. 11.9F). The first pattern was observed in the static gamma motor neurons, the second one in the dynamic motor neurons; the neurons were classified according to their effect on the muscle spindles (Crowe and Matthews 1964).

One of the main effects produced by the Ia afferents in the spinal cord is the monosynaptic excitation of alpha motor neurons of the parent muscle and its synergists. This effect underlies the stretch reflex (for a review see Matthews 1972). The stretch reflex in extensor muscles is very important in the stance phase of the step cycle: due to this reflex, loading the limb will lead to an increase of the extensor activity (see Fig. 11.12A). The larger the contribution of the stretch reflex to the muscle activity is relative to the central contribution, the smaller are the distortions of the kinematic pattern in the stance phase caused by changes of load applied to the limb. In the swing phase the extensors are passively stretched due to the contraction of the flexor muscles, on the other hand, and the reflex excitation of extensors would be harmful. From this point of view, the rhythmical modulation of the gamma motor neurons in-phase with the alpha motor neurons, and the corresponding modulation of the response of Ia afferents to muscle stretch, seems very reasonable.

The other cause for the rhythmic modulation of the stretch reflex is the step cycle-related changes of the responses of alpha motor neurons to synaptic inputs. The sensitivity of the extensor motor neurons increases in the stance phase, when they are depolarized, and decreases in the swing phase, when they are hyperpo-larized (Figs. $11.8C_1,D_1$). Due to these two factors, the gain of the stretch reflex is strongly dependent on the phase of the step cycle, and changes with the EMG activity and the force developed by the muscle (Figs. 11.9G,H) (Akazawa *et al.* 1982).

11.4.3 Ia interneurons and the system of reciprocal inhibition

The Ia interneurons mediate an inhibitory action of the Ia afferents of a given muscle upon the motor neurons of the antagonistic muscle(s) (Jankowska and Roberts 1971,1972; Hultborn *et al.* 1971; Hultborn 1972) (Fig. 11.7A), and are thus responsible for the well-known phenomenon of inhibition of the

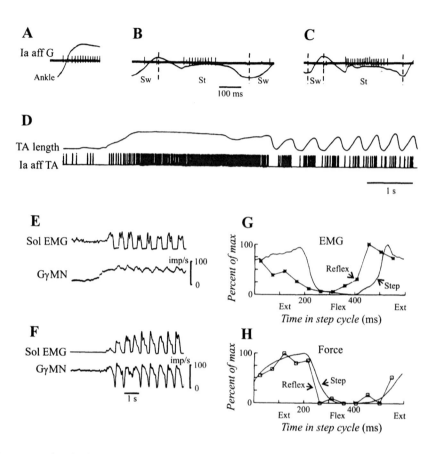

Fig. 11.9 The rhythmic central drive to gamma motor neurons and its functional role. A–C: Response of a Ia spindle afferent from m. gastrocnemius (Ia aff G) to passive movement of the ankle joint (Ankle, flexion up, A), and its activity during weak (B) and more intense (C) locomotion of the decerebrate cat. D: Activity of the Ia spindle afferent from m. tibialis anterior (Ia aff TA) during scratching in the decorticate cat. Upper trace (TA) shows the muscle length (contraction up). Note that the afferent is active during muscle contraction. E,F: Activity of the tonic (E) and phasic (F) gastrocnemius gamma motor neurons GγMN during locomotion of the decerebrate cat. The recordings were made from the axons of motor neurons in the nerve of m. gastrocnemius. Upper trace is EMG of m. soleus. G,H: Rhythmic modulation of the stretch reflex (Reflex) during locomotion of the decerebrate cat recorded as an additional (in relation to undisturbed steps) EMG (in G) or force (in H) evoked in different parts of the step cycle by brief stretching of the m. soleus. The profile of the ongoing EMG (in G) or force (in H) is also shown (Step). Approximate positions of the extensor (Ext) and flexor (Flex) phases of the step cycle are indicated. A–C are from Severin *et al.* (1967), D is from Feldman *et al.* (1977), E,F are from Murphy *et al.* (1984), and G is from Akazawa *et al.* (1982).

antagonistic muscles when a given muscle is passively stretched (Liddell and Sherrington 1924). During real stepping, Ia interneurons are rhythmically bursting in-phase with their parent muscle, i.e. the muscle supplying them with Ia afferent input (Fig. 11.10A). This bursting activity of the Ia interneurons is caused by two inputs, from the spinal rhythm generator and from the Ia muscle spindle afferents. Periodical input from the rhythm generator has been demonstrated in the experiments with fictive locomotion (Feldman and Orlovsky 1975; Jordan 1983; McCrea *et al.* 1980). Figure 11.10C shows rhythmical bursting of the Ia interneuron of the knee extensor quadriceps (Q = Vast + Add) during fictive stepping. The neuron is firing in the extensor phase of the step cycle. On the contrary, Ia interneurons of the flexors Pb–Stn muscles were active in the flexor phase of the cycle. Similar results, that is a central modulation of Ia interneurons, have been obtained for scratching (Deliagina and Orlovsky 1980). Thus, in each of the subunits—flexor or extensor—of the output motor stage (Fig. 11.7A), the rhythm generator produces co-activation of the alpha motor neurons, gamma motor neurons, and Ia interneurons.

Due to the rhythmical central drive, the Ia interneurons perform a gating function for their input signals (Feldman and Orlovsky 1975; Deliagina and Orlovsky 1980). As shown in Fig. 11.10C, during fictive stepping the Ia interneuron responds to electrical stimulation of the Ia afferent fibres only in the extensor phase of the cycle, when the interneuron is excited by the rhythm generator, and does not respond in the flexor phase. Compare this modulation with the consistent responses at rest (Fig. 11.10B). When excited, the Ia interneurons perform inhibition of the alpha motor neurons of the antagonistic muscles. In stepping, the activity of flexor and extensor subunits of the output motor stage alternate under the effect of the spinal rhythm generator. This means that the Ia inhibition is delivered to the antagonistic motor neurons in that phase of the step cycle in which they must not fire. Thus, by inhibiting the antagonistic motor neurons, the Ia interneurons contribute to the generation of the basic locomotor pattern, i.e. the alternating activity of flexors and extensors. It was found that input from Ia interneurons is the main source of inhibition of the motor neurons in between their bursts. This was demonstrated by injection of strychnine (antagonist of glicine, the 1a interneuron transmitter) which effectively decreased the hyperpolarization phase in the motor neurons (Pratt and Jordan 1987).

11.4.4   Renshaw cells

Collaterals of the alpha motor neuron axons form excitatory synapses on the Renshaw cells (Fig. 11.7A) (Renshaw 1941). Via these synapses, Renshaw cells receive excitatory input in-phase with the corresponding motor neurons. It was found that Renshaw cells fire rhythmically during fictive locomotion; they are activated somewhat after the respective motor neurons and Ia interneurons (Jordan 1983; McCrea *et al.* 1980; Pratt and Jordan 1987). Experiments with fictive scratching have shown that Renshaw cells not only receive input from the motor axon collaterals but also from the spinal rhythm generator. The central drive is most

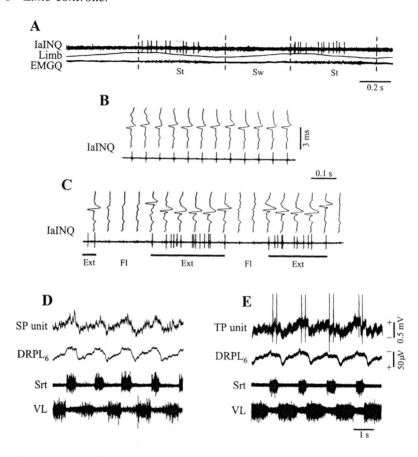

Fig. 11.10 Central modulation of the transmission of signals in reflex pathways. A: Activity of the Ia interneuron that receives Ia input from m. quadriceps (IaINQ). The interneuron was recorded in the walking decerebrate cat along with the m. quadriceps EMG (EMGQ) and limb movement (Limb, protraction up). Stance (St) and swing (Sw) phases of the cycle are indicated. B,C: Responses of IaINQ to stimulation of the Q nerve at rest (B) and during fictive locomotion (C). The lower trace is a continuous recording of the activity of the neuron, and the upper traces show the responses to repetitive nerve stimulation (1.3 threshold for Ia afferents). The neuron is bursting in the extensor phase (Ext) and silent in the flexor phase (Fl). D,E: Rhythmic modulation of the dorsal root potential recorded from the L_6 dorsal root (DRPL$_6$) and of the membrane potential in the cutaneous afferents (superficial peroneal, SP unit, and tibialis posterior, TP unit) during fictive locomotion of the decerebrate cat. The locomotor rhythm was monitored by recording from the sartorius (Srt) and vastus lateralis (VL) nerves. A–C are from Feldman and Orlovsky (1975) and D,E from Gossard and Rossignol (1990).

pronounced in the flexor-coupled Renshaw cells whose pattern of activity drastically differs from that of the flexor motor neurons (Deliagina and Feldman 1981).

The Renshaw cells have two targets in the output motor stage, the alpha motor neurons and the Ia interneurons (Fig. 11.7A). Strong electrical stimulation of a ventral root results in a depression of both motor neurons (Renshaw 1941) and

Ia interneurons (Hultborn *et al.* 1971; Feldman and Orlovsky 1975). However, under ordinary conditions, the inhibitory effects produced by the Renshaw cells are much weaker. It has been shown that, during fictive scratching, a multiple increase of the activity of flexor-coupled Renshaw cells towards the end of the flexor phase correlates with only a minor decrease of the activity of the flexor motor neurons (Deliagina and Feldman 1981).

11.4.5   Phase-dependent reconfiguration of the spinal networks

Phasic excitatory and inhibitory influences of the rhythm generator upon different spinal neurons results in a phase-dependent reconfiguration of the spinal networks. Two examples of such a reconfiguration have already been considered—the modulation of the stretch reflex and the modulation of the reciprocal inhibition:

1. The stretch reflex is enhanced in one part of the cycle and almost completely inhibited in another part (Fig. 11.9H); this modulation is caused by the phasic action of gamma motor neurons on the muscle spindles (Figs. 11.9B–F), as well as by the phase-dependent changes of the membrane potential of alpha motor neurons (Figs. 11.8C_1,D_1).
2. The inhibitory effect of Ia afferents on the antagonistic alpha motor neurons drastically changes in the course of the cycle due to the phase-dependent modulation of the response of Ia interneurons to sensory input (see Fig. 11.10C).
3. A striking example of the modulation of reflexes was presented by Forssberg *et al.* (1977) (see Section 11.5). Stimulation of the dorsum of the foot in the walking cat, applied in the swing phase, leads to an additional activation of flexors, and in overstepping the obstacle. The same stimulus applied in stance phase elicits additional activation of extensors.

There are many other examples of phasic modulation of the signal transmission in reflex pathways both in the hind and in the fore limb during stepping (see for example Andersson *et al.* 1978; Rossignol and Gauthier 1980; Rossignol and Drew 1985; Arshavsky *et al.* 1986; Rossignol *et al.* 1988; Edgley *et al.* 1988; Shefchik *et al.* 1990; Gossard *et al.* 1994; Rossignol 1996).

The spinal rhythm generator performs a phase-dependent modulation of the membrane potential and the membrane conductance and, therefore, of the excitability of motor neurons and interneurons. This is a primary cause of the phasic modulation of signal transmission in reflex pathways. Presynaptic inhibition of the primary afferent terminals is a second source of this modulation. It is well established that depolarization of afferent terminals results in a decrease of the synaptic transmission (Rudomin *et al.* 1998). The degree of depolarization can be easily monitored by recording a dorsal root potential. This potential exhibits a phase-dependent rhythmical modulation both in stepping (Baev 1980; Gossard and Rossignol 1990; Baev and Kostyuk 1982) and in scratching (Baev and Kostyuk 1981). Figures 11.10D,E show oscillations of the dorsal root potential, as well as directly recorded oscillations of the depolarization in the axon terminals of two cutaneous afferents (from the superficial peroneal nerve, SP, and tibialis posterior nerve, TP) during fictive locomotion (Gossard and Rossignol 1990). Two waves of depolarization can be distinguished: a smaller one in the extensor phase of the cycle and a larger one in the flexor phase. In some afferents, the depolarization can be so large that it evokes spike discharges (Fig. 11.10E) (Dubuc *et al.* 1985; Gossard and Rossignol 1990). The antidromic spike discharges caused by presynaptic depolarization of afferent terminals were observed also in the walking intact cat (Beloozerova and Rossignol 1994). These results led to the conclusion that the efficiency of synaptic transmission in the cutaneous reflex pathways is cycle-dependent, with a minimum in the flexor phase (Gossard and Rossignol 1990). Transmission in the terminals of muscle afferents is also subjected to presynaptic modulation (Gossard *et al.* 1991).

11.5   SENSORY FEEDBACK

11.5.1   Different roles of sensory feedback in stepping and scratching

Deafferentation of the hind limb causes a dramatic impairment of stepping movements (Shik *et al.* 1966*b*; Grillner and Zangger 1975, 1984; Wetzel *et al.* 1976) whereas scratching movements are less affected (Deliagina *et al.* 1975). The difference in importance of sensory feedback corresponds well to the different functional roles of these two types of movement:

1. Scratching movements are performed under invariable external conditions— the limb oscillates in the air and touches the skin only slightly. This contrasts to stepping in which the limb strongly interacts with the ground throughout the stance phase of the cycle.
2. Demands concerning accuracy are very different in scratching and stepping. For example, during locomotion even a small mistake, for example lifting a foot before the contralateral limb has been landed, or an improper positioning of the foot at the end of the swing phase, can lead to loss of balance. Comparable distortions of the pattern of scratching movements will not have such dramatic consequences.
3. Stepping movements of an individual limb are a part of the gross locomotor synergy which includes interlimb coordination, maintenance of equilibrium, etc, and numerous motor centres interact to coordinate various aspects of locomotion. This contrasts to the scratch reflex in which only one limb is involved in the rhythmic activity.

It was found that the rhythm generator of the CPG for stepping is very sensitive to different sensory inputs (Shik *et al.* 1966*b*; Andersson *et al.* 1978; Rossignol *et al.* 1981; Andersson and Grillner 1983; Conway *et al.* 1987). Figures 11.11A$_1$–A$_3$ show that the ongoing rhythm of fictive stepping can be easily entrained by imposed periodical passive movements of a limb, either towards lower frequencies or higher frequencies (Figs 11.11A$_2$,A$_3$) (Andersson and Grillner 1983). Limb movements with an amplitude of only a few degrees are sufficient to entrain the rhythm (Fig. 11.11B) (Andersson *et al.* 1978). These findings strongly suggested that, in real stepping, the timing of different events in the step cycle is determined not by the internal processes in the spinal limb centre—that is not by the CPG activity—but rather by afferent signals about the limb movement. Experiments on walking cats with intact sensory feedback loops have shown that afferent signals from the limb mechanoreceptors play a crucial role in the control of different aspects of stepping movements.

11.5.2 Stance–swing and swing–stance transitions

The transition from the stance phase to the swing phase is under powerful sensory influences, especially from the afferents signalling hip position (Andersson and Grillner 1981, 1983; Kriellaars *et al.* 1994). As was shown in Fig. 10.4D, the swing phase starts at approximately the same posterior extreme position both at a low and at a high speed of walking. One can suggest that the nervous mechanism for transferring the limb forward cannot be triggered until a definite posterior limb position has been reached. In other words, the step cycle duration is determined, to a large extent, by the time needed to reach the posterior extreme position, as has already been discussed for stepping in the invertebrates (see Sections 4.6.1 and 6.3.2). The role of signals about hip position was studied in experiments on the spinal cat walking on the treadmill (Fig. 11.11C) (Grillner and Rossignol 1978). An experimenter kept the foot of the right hind limb on his palm and gradually deflected it backward. The animal did not try to perform a step forward by the manipulated limb despite the fact that the contralateral limb was stepping regularly. However, when the hip extension reached 90°, the transfer mechanism was triggered, the limb left the palm of the experimenter and stepped forward. The posterior hip position, at which the swing phase starts, depends to some extent on the current position of the contralateral limb. By repeating this experiment, the dependence of the swing phase onset on the phase of the contralateral hind limb was revealed (Fig. 11.11D). The curve has two peaks: one peak in the stance phase and one in the swing phase. Such a pattern of interlimb influences can be responsible for the counter-phase coordination of stepping movements of the two limbs during walk, and in-phase coordination during gallop (see Section 10.2).

There is also one more factor affecting the swing phase onset—unloading of the limb (Duysens and Pearson 1980). Figure 11.11E shows that an additional force applied to the tendon of one of the extensor muscles of the hind limb in the walking cat prevented the limb controller from generating the flexor burst; the swing phase did not start, and the controller continued to activate the extensor muscles. The flexor activity started immediately, however, when the extensor muscle was unloaded, and the flexor burst was followed by a normal rhythmical locomotor pattern. In real locomotion, extensors of a limb are loaded under the effect of the body weight. In alternating gaits (walk and trot), extensors get unloaded by the end of the stance phase since the contralateral limb takes upon itself a part of the body weight at the moment when it touches the ground. This experiment (Fig. 11.11E) shows that unloading the extensors is an important condition for triggering the nervous mechanism transferring the limb forward. Thus, sensory feedback signalling about the limb position (Fig. 11.11C) and about the load applied to the limb (Fig. 11.11E), together with the influences from the contralateral

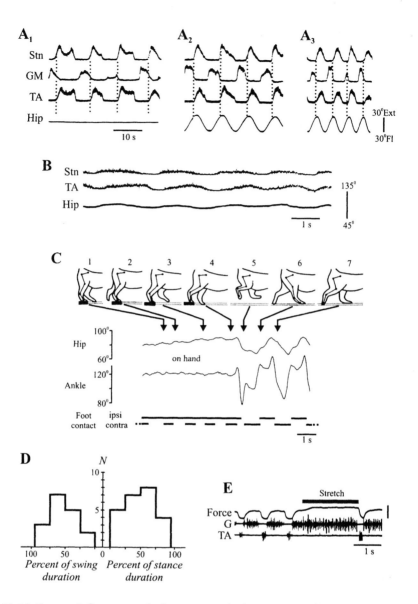

Fig. 11.11 Sensory influences on the locomotory rhythm. A_1–A_3 and B: Entrainment of the fictive locomotor activity by sinusoidal hip movements of different frequencies and amplitudes. Fictive locomotion was evoked in low spinal cats by Nialamid and DOPA injection. The CPG activity was monitored by recording from the semitendinosus, gastrocnemius medialis, and tibialis anterior nerves (Stn, GM, and TA). Dotted lines indicate onset of the Stn activity in the locomotor cycle. A_1, no hip movement; A_2, low-frequency hip movements; A_3, higher-frequency hip movements; B: hip movements of a very small amplitude. C: Lift-off response in the walking spinal cat. The ipsilateral limb was positioned on the hand of the experimenter (symbolized by a block under the foot) and gradually moved backwards. The limb started stepping upon reaching a certain posterior hip position. There are shown: hip and ankle angles (Hip, Ankle), and ground contact of the ipsi- and contralateral foot. Stick diagrams show the limb position at different moments of the locomotor sequence (indicated by arrows). D: Interlimb coupling during lift-off responses. There is shown a distribution of lift-off responses (similar to that in C) in the swing phase and stance phase of the cycle of the contralateral limb. E: Effect of stretching the extensor, m. gastrocnemius

limb controller (Fig. 11.11D), promote the interlimb coordination, which is a necessary condition for the maintenance of equilibrium during locomotion (see Section 10.2).

The transition from swing to stance phase is less affected by sensory feedback than the stance–swing transition. It was demonstrated that the onset of extensor activity precedes (by 20–50 ms) the foot contact with the ground and, therefore, is not triggered by signals about foot landing (Engberg and Lundberg 1969). Also, the flexor bursts generated by the locomotor CPG are much less variable than the extensor bursts (Pearson and Rossignol 1991) (see Figs. 11.1A,B) suggesting that the flexor bursts are generated by a more rigid central programme.

In conclusion, the functional organization of the limb controller for stepping in the vertebrates (cat) and invertebrates (crustacea, insects) has many features in common (see Chapters 4 and 6). In both types of animal, the intrinsic rhythm of the CPG is completely suppressed by afferent influences which determine the timing of principal events in the step cycle (see Fig. 4.4A). The basic function of the locomotor CPG in both types of animal is the formation of the muscle synergies for the stance and swing phases, as well as the phasic modulation of the transmission of signals in different sensory and central pathways.

11.5.3 Modification of the motor pattern within the stance and swing phases

Besides the influences on the temporal characteristics of the locomotor pattern considered above (i.e. the influences on the duration of the stance phase and on the timing of transition from stance phase to swing phase), afferent signals also produce a modulation of the intensity of muscle contraction in the stance phase of the step and thus adapt the limb to the load applied at different moments during this phase. A major role in this adaptation is played by the stretch reflex. Due to this reflex, the muscle activity becomes dependent not only on the central drive to the alpha motor neurons but also on the muscle length, and considerably increases with additional stretch of the muscles (Fig. 11.12A). Selective block of the gamma motor axons in motor nerves significantly reduces the EMG amplitude (Severin 1970). One can also suggest that by varying the gain in this reflex pathway (for example, by increasing activity of the gamma motor neurons) the elasticity of the limb in the support phase can be regulated (see for example Grillner 1972).

In contrast to the stance phase, in which the limb is continuously affected by the body weight, the external conditions for limb movement in the swing phase do not usually change since the limb is freely moving in the air. However, the motor programme for limb transfer can be modified to some extent, and the limb controller will immediately react to any external influences upon the moving limb. For instance, a contact of the limb with an obstacle drastically changes the locomotor

during locomotion of decerebrate cat. The EMGs of m. gastrocnemius (G) and m. tibialis anterior (TA), and the force developed by G are shown. A_1–A_3 are from Andersson and Grillner (1983), B is from Andersson *et al.* (1978), C and D are from Grillner and Rossignol (1978), and E is from Pearson and Duysens (1976).

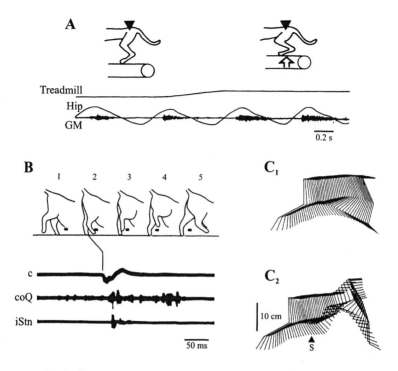

Fig. 11.12 Role of afferent input in the stance and swing phases of the step cycle. A: Effect of loading the hind limbs. The decerebrate cat, with its hind quarters rigidly fixed, was walking on the treadmill. Lifting the treadmill (indicated by the upward deflection of the upper trace, and symbolized by the arrow in the right inset) led to an increase of EMG of m. gastrocnemius medialis (GM). B: Contact reaction during swing in the walking spinal cat (filming at 64 frames/s). The obstacle is shown as a black rectangle. In lower record, the contact (c) was followed by a short latency bursts in the ipsilateral m. semitendinosus (Stn) and contralateral m. quadriceps (Q). C_1,C_2: Kinematic analysis of the contact reaction (filming at 80 frames/s). The successive stick diagrams for the swing phase in normal step (C_1) and in disturbed step (C_2) are shown. The limb position at the moment of stimulation is indicated by an arrow (S). A is from Orlovsky (1972d) and B–C_2 are from Forssberg *et al.* (1977).

pattern to prevent the animal from stumbling and from a loss of equilibrium (Forssberg *et al.* 1977). Figure 11.12B shows successive limb positions during stepping in the spinal cat. In frame 2, the dorsum of the foot hits an obstacle (the black square). This happened at the end of the swing phase, before the foot would normally have reached the ground. The stimulus elicited a flexion of the knee, which brings the foot backward and upward (frame 3). The subsequent flexion at all joints, as well as an extension of the contralateral knee, brings the foot well above the obstacle (frame 4). In frame 5, the limb extends to contact the ground again. Thus, both a decrease of the effective length of the affected limb, and an increase of the effective length of the contralateral limb which is supporting the hindquarters at the moment of disturbance, considerably raises the foot of the affected limb above the ground (compare Figs $11.12C_1$ and C_2). This reaction starts with a very short latency, about 10 ms (Fig. 11.12B), and can be evoked only in the swing phase, while in the stance phase the same stimulus results in additional activation of the ipsilateral knee extensors (Forssberg *et al.* 1974). Thus, the spinal control system not only performs phase-dependent modulations of reflex responses (see Section 11.4), but also a switch from one type of motor response to a completely different type.

These modifications of the motor pattern in the stance and swing phases, elicited by sensory feedback in the walking cat, are very similar to those observed in the walking insects where both the sensory modulation of the activity of antigravity muscles in the stance phase, and reflexive overstepping an obstacle in the swing phase are observed (see Section 6.3).

11.6 CONCLUSIONS

1. When deprived of sensory feedback, the limb controller can operate as a CPG and generate efferent patterns closely resembling stepping, scratching, and other rhythmical movements of the limb.
2. The networks generating the rhythms for stepping and scratching are distributed in the hind limb enlargement of the spinal cord, with the most rostral segments playing a leading role in rhythmogenesis.
3. The rhythm generating network has not been identified yet. Two models, biphasic and three-phasic, have been proposed to explain the rhythm generation in the spinal cord. It was also proposed that each joint has its own rhythm generating network, and that the networks for different joints interact to produce a common rhythm.
4. The rhythm generator performs four principal functions: (i) It supplies the motor neurons with alternating excitatory and inhibitory inputs. (ii) It informs other limb controllers about its activity, which is necessary for interlimb coordination. (iii) It informs different motor centres in the brain about its activity, which is necessary for organization of their interaction with the spinal limb controllers. (iv) It performs a phase-dependent modulation of the efficiency of signal transmission in different reflex pathways.
5. All identified cell types, constituting the output motor stage of the limb controller (alpha motor neuron, gamma motor neurons, and Ia interneurons of the system of reciprocal inhibition), are driven by the rhythm generator and exhibit rhythmic bursting.
6. The relatively simple output pattern of the rhythm generator is transformed into a more complicated pattern of activity of the motor neurons due to the convergence of excitatory and inhibitory influences from the rhythm generator.
7. Under closed-loop conditions, the timing of different events in the step cycle is largely determined not by the internal processes in the spinal limb centre, that is not by the CPG activity, but by afferent signals about limb movement.

A crucial role in determining transition from the stance to the swing phase is played by the signals about the hip position and unloading of the limb.

8. Several reflex mechanisms adapt the limb movements to external conditions. In the stance phase, the extensor activity is modulated largely by the stretch reflex. In the swing phase, external stimuli can evoke modifications of the motor pattern of the limb transfer.

12

Initiation of locomotion

In the cat, signals from the brain to the spinal cord are transmitted through several descending pathways—the reticulospinal, vestibulospinal, rubrospinal, and corticospinal tracts, as well as the propriospinal pathways. Of these pathways, the reticulospinal tract and the propriospinal pathways are directly related to the initiation of locomotion. Their roles will be considered in the following sections. The problem of the initiation of locomotion in mammals has been reviewed by Armstrong (1986, 1988), Jordan (1986, 1991), Jordan *et al.* (1992), Garcia-Rill (1986), Garcia-Rill and Skinner (1986), Gelfand *et al.* (1988), Shik (1983), Mori (1987), and Mori *et al.* (1991).

12.1 ROLE OF THE RETICULOSPINAL SYSTEM IN INITIATION OF LOCOMOTION

Different areas along the medial reticular formation of the pons and medulla give rise to numerous spinal projections. There is ample evidence to suggest that the reticulopinal (RS) neurons from the nucleus reticularis gigantocellularis (NRGC) and nucleus reticularis magnicellularis (NRMC) (Fig. 12.1A) constitute a command system for activation of the spinal locomotor mechanisms. Axons of neurons from these nuclei descend in the ventrolateral funiculi of the spinal cord and branch in the fore limb and hind limb enlargements as well as in the thoracic region. It has been demonstrated that individual reticulospinal neurons may project to one, two, three, or even four spinal limb centres (Peterson *et al.* 1975; Wolstencroft 1964; Matsuyama *et al.* 1997) and thus may present neural substrate for the control of gross locomotor and postural synergies.

12.1.1 Different inputs eliciting locomotion converge on the RS neurons and excite them

There are several areas in the brainstem and cerebellum which, when stimulated, elicit locomotion in the intact animal or in the reduced preparation. Inputs from most of these areas converge on the RS neurons and excite them. One of these areas is the mesencephalic locomotor region, MLR (Figs. 12.1A,B$_2$) considered earlier (see Section 10.3) as input to the locomotor automatism. Anatomical studies have shown that neurons of the MLR project to a wide area in the medial

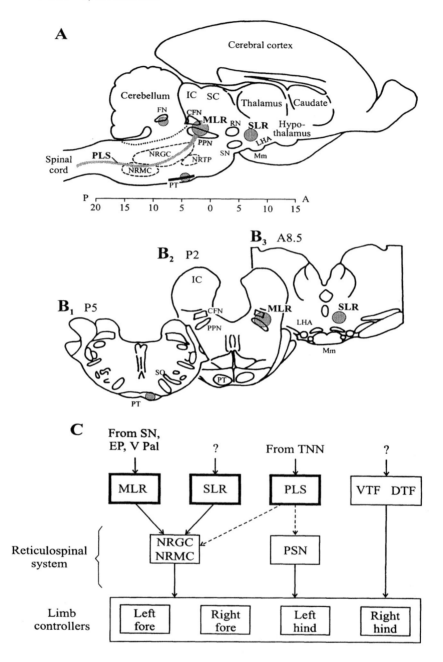

Fig. 12.1 Command systems for the initiation of locomotion. A–B₃: Areas in the brain stem and cerebellum eliciting locomotion. Parasagittal (A) and frontal (B₁–B₃) presentation of the effective areas (shaded). The anterior/posterior (A/P) Horsley-Clark coordinates are indicated. C: An overview of the structures involved in the initiation of locomotion (see text). (Abbreviations: CFN, cuneiform nucleus; DTF, dorsal tegmental field; EP, entopeduncular nucleus; FN, fastigial nucleus; FF, fields of Forel; IC, inferior colliculus; LHA, lateral hypothalamic area; MLR, mesencephalic locomotor region; Mm, mammillary bodies; NRGC, nucleus reticularis gigantocellularis; NRMC, nucleus reticularis magnocellularis;

reticular formation but largely to the NRGC and NRMC (Baev *et al.* 1988; Steeves and Jordan 1984; Garcia-Rill *et al.* 1983*a*). Stimulation of the MLR in the mesencephalic cat results in activation of a large proportion of the RS neurons (Orlovsky 1970*a,b*). Figures 12.2A$_1$,A$_2$ show that a prolonged MLR stimulation (pulse frequency 30 Hz) causes activation of an RS neuron and evokes locomotion. With stronger stimulation, the firing frequency of the neuron increases further, and the intensity of locomotor movements increases as well (Figs. 12.2A$_3$,A$_4$). During stimulation, short latency (presumably monosynaptic) EPSPs are seen in the RS neuron in response to each stimulus applied to the MLR (Fig. 12.2B$_1$). With stronger stimulation, the action potentials in the RS neuron become phase-locked to the stimuli (Fig. 12.2B$_2$).

A different area in the brainstem eliciting locomotion when stimulated is the sub-thalamic locomotor region, SLR (Figs. 12.1A,B$_3$) (Orlovsky 1969; Waller 1940). The SLR also projects to the medial reticular formation (Baev *et al.* 1988), and a large number of the RS neurons receive excitatory input from the SLR (Orlovsky 1970*a*).

The fastigial nucleus of the cerebellum (FN in Fig. 12.1A) projects to a wide area in the medial reticular formation (Walberg *et al.* 1962). Stimulation of this nucleus also elicits locomotion in the mesencephalic cat and similarly activates a large proportion of RS neurons (Mori *et al.* 1997).

It was found that locomotion in the mesencephalic cat also can be evoked by stimulation of the pyramidal tract in the medulla (PT in Figs. 12.1A,B$_1$) (Shik *et al.* 1968). In these experiments, the tract was transected a few millimeters caudal to the stimulated site. The effect of stimulation is presumably mediated by numerous cortico-reticular fibres terminating on the RS neurons (Magni and Willis 1964).

Finally, experiments on the thalamic cat, with a transection of the brainstem at the precollicular-premammillar level (see Fig. 10.4A) have shown that spon-taneous bouts of locomotor activity, or the locomotor activity elicited by a brief sensory stimulus (Orlovsky 1969), are associated with a considerable increase in the activity of RS neurons (Orlovsky 1970*b*). Chronic recordings from the RS neurons in intact cats have also shown that their activity during locomotion is considerably higher than at rest (Drew *et al.* 1986).

12.1.2 Integrity of the RS pathways is essential for the initiation of locomotion

Experiments with impairment of signal transmission in the RS pathways have presented further support for the idea that the RS system plays a crucial role in the initiation of locomotion. It has been found that inactivation of the medial reticular

---

NRTP, nucleus reticularis tegmenti pontis; PLS, pontomedullary locomotor strip; PPN, pedunculopontine nucleus; PSN, propriospinal neurons; PT, pyramidal tract; RN, red nucleus; SC, superior colliculus; SLR, subthalamic locomotor region; SO, superior olive; SN, substantia nigra; TNN, nucleus of the trigeminal nerve; V. Pal, ventral pallium; VTF, ventral tegmental field.)

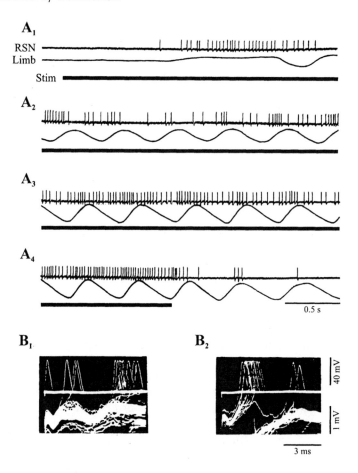

Fig. 12.2 Activity of a reticulospinal neuron during locomotion. Locomotion was evoked in the mesencephalic cat by MLR stimulation (30 Hz) and the neuron was recorded intracellularly. A_1–A_4: Activity of the neuron (RSN) and movements of the ipsilateral hind limb (protraction, up). Stimulation in A_3 and A_4 was stronger than in A_1 and A_2. B_1,B_2: Responses of the reticulospinal neuron during locomotion to the stimuli applied to the MLR. The oscilloscope sweep was triggered by the stimulating pulses. Stimulation was stronger in B_2. From Orlovsky (1970*b*).

formation by cooling reversibly blocks locomotion evoked by MLR stimulation (Shefchyk *et al.* 1984). Some of the cells in the MLR are cholinergic, and it has been found that injection of a cholinergic antagonist in the area of NRGC and NRMC abolishes an MLR-evoked locomotion (Garcia-Rill and Skinner 1987*a*,*b*). Finally, it is known that axons of RS neurons from NRGC and NRMC descend in the ventrolateral funiculi of the spinal cord, and it has been found that these funiculi must be intact for a coordinated locomotor pattern to be elicited from the brainstem (Steeves and Jordan 1980; Eidelberg 1981).

All these findings taken together strongly suggest that the RS neurons from the NRMC and NRGC represent a command system for initiation of locomotion.

Direct stimulation of the medial reticular formation, however, evoked stepping movements with different distortions, or produced only tonic effects on the limb and body musculature (Garcia-Rill and Skinner 1987*a*; Noga *et al.* 1988). A possible explanation for these negative findings is that the RS neurons in the NRGC and NRMC do not represent a homogeneous population, and that only some of them are responsible for the elicitation of locomotion whereas others may participate in modifications of the pattern of stepping (see Section 13.4) or perform other motor functions. With massive stimulation of the reticular formation, the RS command system cannot be activated properly and selectively.

12.1.3 Role of the mesencephalic and subthalamic locomotor regions

Location of the MLR corresponds to two anatomical structures in the brainstem—the cuneiform nucleus (CFN) and the pedunculopontine nucleus (PPN, Figs. 12.1A,B$_2$). The SLR is located in medial and posterior areas of the hypothalamus, partly coinciding with the field of Forel (Figs. 12.1A,B$_3$). A number of lines of evidence suggest that the locomotor effects produced by stimulation of these two brainstem areas are not experimental artifacts but rather are the reflections of the functional role of the MLR and SLR in the initiation of locomotion. It seems most likely that both MLR and SLR represent two independent inputs to the reticular formation, and that these inputs are responsible for a specific activation of those RS neurons which constitute the locomotor command system:

1. Stimulation of the MLR or SLR results in activation of RS neurons (see Section 12.1.1). A unilateral stimulation elicits bilateral activity, which is necessary for symmetrical activation of the left and right limb controllers and for rectilinear walking (Orlovsky 1970*a,b*).
2. Stimulation of the MLR or SLR elicits locomotion not only in a reduced preparation, but also in the intact cat. In the latter case, the locomotor activity is well coordinated with the postural adjustments and with the visually-guided steering control (see Fig. 10.5 for the MLR-evoked locomotion) (Sirota and Shik 1973; Mori *et al.* 1991).
3. The activity of the MLR neurons increases during locomotion (Garcia-Rill *et al.* 1983*b*).
4. Bilateral destruction of the MLR in otherwise intact cats does not prevent voluntary or reflexive initiation of locomotion, neither does it prevent the initiation of locomotion by SLR stimulation. Bilateral destruction of the SLR, in contrast, for a few days deprives the animal of the capability to voluntarily initiate locomotion, but locomotion can still be induced by MLR stimulation (Sirota and Shik 1973).

Thus, the MLR and SLR can be considered as two independent inputs exerting a control over the locomotor automatism (Fig. 12.1C) (see also Section 10.3). The functional significance of double input to the RS neurons constituting the locomotor command system—through the MLR and through the SLR—is not clear, however. One may suggest that these two inputs are used for eliciting locomotion in different behavioural contexts. For instance, the SLR-evoked locomotion may be associated with 'searching behaviour' (Mori *et al.* 1989). Apart from the MLR or SLR stimulation, locomotion in a reduced preparation can also be evoked by stimulation of the pyramidal tract transected a few millimeters below the stimulated site (Shik *et al.* 1968) and by stimulation of the fastigial nucleus of the cerebellum (Mori *et al.* 1997) (see Section 12.1.1). In both cases, the stimulation presumably results in a direct activation of a large number of fibres passing the stimulated sites and projecting onto the RS neurons (Magni and Willis 1964). It remains unclear, however, if the initiation of locomotion from these two sites is an experimental artifact caused by massive, unspecific activation of inputs to the RS neurons, or if it is a reflection of the functional role of cortical and cerebellar projections onto the reticular formation.

12.1.4   Effects of the reticulospinal command system on the spinal cord

A precise identification of the RS neurons constituting the locomotor command system has not been accomplished. It is presumed that glutamatergic RS neurons play the major role in activation of the spinal limb controllers for stepping, because direct application of NMDA to the lumbosacral spinal cord elicits stepping movements of the hind limbs (Douglas *et al.* 1993). Similarly, activation of NMDA receptors in an isolated spinal cord preparation from the neonatal rat can produce locomotor activity in a dose-dependent manner (Kudo and Yamada 1987). Furthermore, the initiation of locomotion from the brainstem can be blocked by excitatory amino acid antagonists (Fenaux *et al.* 1991; Douglas *et al.* 1993).

Activation of the excitatory amino acid receptors on the spinal neurons is not the only way to substitute the effect of the RS system and to initiate locomotion in mammals. Some other neurotransmitters, norepinephrine and serotonine in particular, can elicit locomotor activity in the spinal cord but they are not necessary for initiating locomotion via different routes (Steeves *et al.* 1980). These findings suggest that different components of the RS system may supplement each other when initiating locomotion (for a review of the pharmacology of descending control see Jordan *et al.* (1992) and Rossignol and Dubuc (1994)).

Spinal targets of the RS fibres responsible for the elicitation of locomotion have not yet been identified. It seems likely that the majority of interneurons receiving descending RS drive are located in the dorsomedial area of the spinal grey matter (laminae V–VII), where the maximal early field potentials, synchronized with the pulses stimulating the MLR, have been recorded (Jordan 1991; Noga *et al.* 1995).

12.2   ROLE OF THE POLYSYNAPTIC PATHWAYS IN THE INITIATION OF LOCOMOTION

The medial area of the MLR represents a rostral part of a narrow strip ($\sim$200 µm in diameter) passing through the lateral tegmentum of the brainstem and reaching the first cervical segments of the spinal cord (the pontomedullary locomotor strip, PLS in Fig. 12.1A). Stimulation at points along this strip elicits locomotion in the mesencephalic cat (Mori *et al.* 1977; Shik and Yagodnitsyn 1977; Gelfand *et al.* 1988). The strip seems not to be a continuous tract: after a local lesion to one region of the strip, locomotion can still be elicited by stimulating other sites. Somas of neurons sending axons in the PLS are situated medial to the strip. It has been suggested that the PLS represents a chain of polysynaptically interacting neurons 'conducting' excitation in the caudal direction (Kazennikov *et al.* 1987). The close anatomical and functional proximity of the PLS to the mesencephalic nucleus of the trigeminal nerve suggests that the PLS mediates a sensory-associated triggering of locomotion (Noga *et al.* 1988; Beresovskii and Baev 1988; Baev *et al.* 1988).

Another strip has been found in the spinal cord. Stimulation of a certain site in the dorsal part of the lateral funiculus elicits well-coordinated stepping of the ipsilateral hind limb. It has been suggested that this spinal strip, like the strip in the brainstem, represents a chain of polysynaptically interacting propriospinal neurons (Kazennikov *et al.* 1983; Shik 1983; Gelfand *et al.* 1988). It has also been suggested that excitation of neurons in the chain is 'conducted' from the brain to the spinal limb controllers (Fig. 12.1C). No experimental evidence in favour of the idea that the activity propagates along the PLS and then along the spinal strip has been presented, however. By contrast, it is well established that a different rhythmical motor pattern, scratching, can be evoked in the hind limb centre via propriospinal pathways (Sherrington 1906*a,b*; Deliagina 1977; Berkinblit *et al.* 1977), without involvement of the RS system (Pavlova 1977).

12.3 INPUTS TO THE LOCOMOTOR REGIONS OF THE BRAINSTEM

Anatomical studies have shown that the cuneiform and pedunculopontine nuclei which correspond to the MLR (Figs. 12.1A,B$_2$), and the fields of Forel which correspond to the SLR (Figs. 12.1A,B$_3$), receive projections from numerous areas of the mid- and forebrain (Garcia-Rill and Skinner 1986). Three inputs to the MLR from the output nuclei of the basal ganglia, that is from substantia nigra, the entopeduncular nucleus, and ventral pallidum (Fig. 12.1C), are GABAergic and inhibitory. Local injection of GABA antagonists (bicuculline or picrotoxin) into the pedunculo-pontine nucleus resulted in the initiation of locomotion (Garcia-Rill *et al.* 1985, 1990) whereas spontaneous locomotion could be observed after injection of GABA and its agonists into the MLR area (Garcia-Rill *et al.* 1985; Pointis and Borenstein 1985).

The involvement of the structures directly projecting on the MLR, that is substantia nigra, the entopeduncular nucleus, and ventral pallidum, in the initiation of locomotion has been demonstrated by both injection of different neurotransmitters and their antagonists into the corresponding areas and by stimulating them electrically (Garcia-Rill and Skinner 1986; Garcia-Rill 1986; Garcia-Rill *et al.* 1981*a,c*). On the basis of these findings a hypothesis was formulated that the MLR is normally controlled by inhibitory structures, and that the initiation of locomotion is associated with a process of disinhibition (Grillner *et al.* 1997). Excitatory inputs to the MLR from the forebrain are no less important than inhibitory ones, however. This follows from the finding that after removal of most of the influences from the forebrain by means of decerebration, the spontaneous locomotor activity is absent (see Section 10.2).

Similar experiments have shown that some other structures of the forebrain, which do not project directly on the MLR, can strongly affect the locomotor activity. In particular, it has been found that an excitatory effect on locomotion can be obtained by injection of dopamine and amphetamine in the nucleus accumbens, injection of picrotoxin in the ventral tegmental area, and injection of NMDA in the hippocampus (Mogeston 1991). The complexity of the forebrain neuronal mechanisms, however, does not allow us at present to estimate the real contribution of these different structures in the initiation of locomotion.

12.4 CONTROL OF POSTURAL TONE

An upright body orientation during locomotion is maintained due to the activity of the postural control system. This system is located in the brainstem, cerebellum, and spinal cord, which is demonstrated by the fact that the chronic mesencephalic cat is able to maintain equilibrium when it is freely walking on the floor (Bard and Macht 1958).

Postural control includes two aspects: the control of body orientation, and the control of equilibrium (Horak and Macpherson 1995). Postural orientation implies a maintenance of the horizontal position of the trunk, which is most appropriate for the forward progression in four-legged animals like the cat. This postural orientation is due to a coordinated control of the tone in the antigravity (extensor) muscles of the four limbs. Some aspects of equilibrium control were considered earlier (see Section 10.2).

In the brainstem, two areas have been found that strongly affect the postural tone and therefore the trunk orientation when stimulated. The area located in the dorsal tegmental field of the caudal pons (DTF, Figs. $12.3A_1,A_2$) exerts an inhibitory action upon the muscle tone in all four limbs (Figs. $12.3B_1–B_3$), while the area in the ventral tegmental field (VTF, Figs. $12.3A_1,A_2$) exerts an excitatory action. A striking peculiarity of both these effects is that they considerably outlast the stimulus, and different values of the force can be 'set up' by applying brief stimuli to the DTF or VTF (Fig. 12.3C) (Mori *et al.* 1982).

Stimulation of the DTF and VTF affects the postural tone both when an animal is standing and when it is walking (Mori 1987; Mori *et al.* 1991, 1992). As shown in Fig. 12.3D, stimulation of the inhibitory pontine area (DTF) during locomotion terminates the locomotor activity. Stimulation of the excitatory area (VTF) strongly enhances the locomotor activity (Fig. 12.3E). Similar results have been obtained both in decerebrate and in intact animals. These experiments have shown that the DTF and VTF affect not only the output motor stage of the limb controllers, but also the rhythm generator. In this sense inputs to the spinal locomotor networks from the locomotor and postural brainstem centres supplement each other: inputs from the areas affecting the postural tone, under some conditions, can initiate and terminate locomotion. It seems likely, however, that only a combined action of the postural tone centres and the locomotor centres may

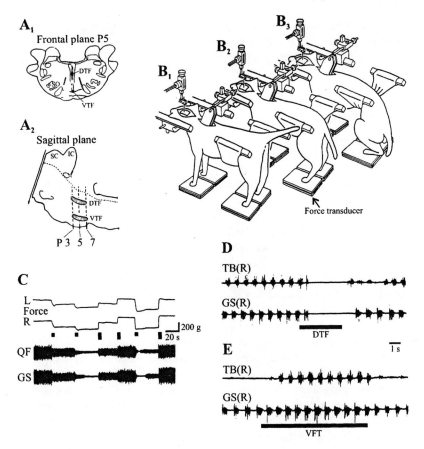

Fig. 12.3 Stimulation of two pontine areas affect the postural tone. A_1, A_2: Location of the effective sites in the dorsal tegmental field (DTF) and ventral tegmental field (VTF) as viewed in the frontal Horsley-Clark plane P5 (A_1) and sagittal plane (A_2) (SO, superior olive; SC, superior colliculus; IC, inferior colliculus). $B_1–B_3$: Schematic depiction of postural changes induced in the decerebrate cat by stimulation of the DTF. B_1: Before stimulation, the cat maintains a standing posture. B_2, B_3: The DTF stimulation gradually decreases the antigravitational muscular tone. C: Setting and resetting of the level of force developed by the hind limbs. The EMGs from m. quadriceps femoris (Q) and m. gastrocnemius/soleus (GS) of the left hind limb were recorded along with the forces developed by the left and right limbs (L and R). Stimulation (50 Hz) of the DTF is indicated by single bars, stimulation of the VTF by double bars. D,E: Suppression and augmentation of the MLR-evoked locomotion by concomitant stimulation of the DTF (50 Hz, 10 µA) and VTF (50 Hz, 20 µA) respectively. The EMGs were recorded from the right fore limb (triceps brachial muscle, TB) and right hind limb (gastrocnemius-soleus muscles, GS). From Mori (1987).

provide a wide range of specific characteristics of the locomotor pattern like fast running with half-flexed limbs or slow walking with extended limbs. In this sense, the mechanisms controlling the tone in the antigravity muscles can be considered a part of the system for initiation of locomotion (see Fig. 12.1C). The influences of the postural tone mechanisms on the spinal limb controllers are, at least partly, transmitted through the RS system (Takakusaki *et al.* 1989). It remains unclear, however, to what extent the two systems interact at the brainstem level and at the spinal level.

12.5 CONCLUSIONS

1. Activation of the spinal locomotor networks is produced primarily by an excitatory drive from a population of reticulospinal neurons located in the pons and medulla—the locomotor command system. This effect is most likely mediated by the excitatory amino acid receptors.
2. The locomotor command system can be activated via two inputs—the mesencephalic locomotor region (MLR) and the subthalamic locomotor region (SLR). Both MLR and SLR project bilaterally to the RS neurons and thus transform a unilateral input into the bilateral activity of the RS system necessary for symmetrical activation of the spinal limb controllers.
3. The MLR receives inputs from the output nuclei of basal ganglia—substantia nigra, entopeduncular nucleus, and ventral pallidum. Via the MLR, these structures may initiate and terminate locomotion.
4. Locomotion can also be initiated via polysynaptic pathways in the brainstem and spinal cord, most likely without involvement of the RS system.
5. A necessary condition for the normal locomotor performance is a sufficient tone in the antigravity (extensor) muscles of all four limbs. This tone can be decreased or increased by stimulating two areas located in the dorsal and ventral tegmental fields of the pons, respectively. These two areas also affect the rhythm generating spinal networks and are thus supplementary to the main locomotor command system.

13

Role of the cerebellum in locomotor coordination

Apart from initiating locomotion (see Chapter 12), supraspinal motor centres perform a number of other functions related to locomotor control, including maintenance of equilibrium, visuomotor coordination, coordination of locomotor movements with other types of movements, etc. An important role in these functions is played by the cerebellum. Some aspects of the involvement of the cerebellum in the control of locomotion are considered in this chapter. This problem has been reviewed by Arshavsky *et al.* (1983, 1986) Armstrong (1986*b*, 1988), and Orlovsky (1991).

13.1 STRUCTURES INVOLVED IN THE SUPRASPINAL CONTROL OF HIND LIMB MOVEMENTS

Different brain motor centres participate in the correction and modulation of the motor patterns generated by the spinal limb controllers. The cerebellum plays an important role in the organization of supraspinal influences on the spinal mechanisms. As shown in numerous studies, removal of the cerebellum, lesions to its parts, or their temporary functional inactivation results in discoordination of stepping movements, both in otherwise intact animals and in humans (see for example Chambers and Sprague 1955*a,b*; Udo *et al.* 1979*b*; Tsukahara *et al.* 1983; Orlovsky *et al.* 1966; for a review of older studies see Dow and Moruzzi 1958) and in reduced (decerebrate) preparations (Orlovsky 1970*c*; Udo *et al.* 1979*a*, 1980). The decerebrate, mesencephalic cat, with its 'locomotor automatism' (see Section 10.3), presented a good model for studies of the role of cerebellum in locomotor coordination. In this chapter, we consider the contribution of the cerebellum in the control of stepping movements of the hind limb. The scratch reflex, with only one limb involved in rhythmic activity, was also used as a simpler model to enhance the analysis of signal processing in the cerebellum.

Figure 13.1 shows the gross anatomy of the cerebellum (A) (Larsell 1953), the principal types of cerebellar neurons and their interconnections (B) (for a review, see Eccles *et al.* 1967), and the interactions between the cerebellum and related structures of the brainstem and spinal cord which participate in the control of hind limb movements (C) (for a review see Armstrong 1986, 1988; Arshavsky *et al.*

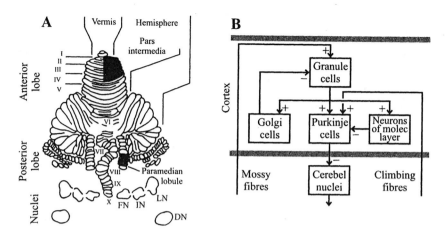

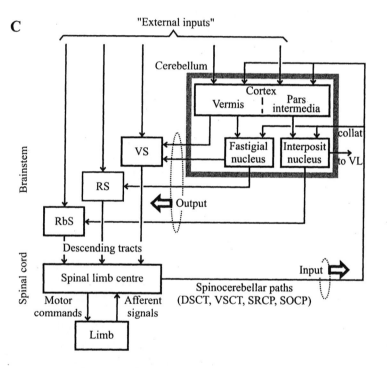

Fig. 13.1 A: Schema of the cerebellar cortex and its target nuclei. Roman numerals indicate the lobules according to Larsell (1953). Hind limb areas in the anterior lobe and paramedian lobule are shown in black. IN, FN, LN, and DN are interpositus, fastigial, lateral and Deiters' nuclei respectively. B: Interaction between different types of cerebellar neurons, and their afferent inputs (plus, excitatory synapse; minus, inhibitory synapse). Grey lines delineate the cerebellar cortex. C: The spino-cerebellar loop comprises the cerebellum and related structures involved in the control of the hind limb movements in the decerebrate cat. (Abbreviations: VS, RS, and RbS, vestibulospinal, reticulospinal and rubrospinal neurons; VL, the ventrolateral nucleus of thalamus; DSCT, dorsal

1986). All these elements constitute a nervous mechanism termed the spinocere-bellar loop (Arshavsky *et al.* 1983, 1986) (see below).

The hind limb of the cat has two areas of representation in the cerebellar cor-tex, a large one in the anterior lobe, and a smaller one in the paramedian lobule (Fig. 13.1A) (Chambers and Sprague 1955a,b). Both these areas belong to the spino-cerebellum, that is the subdivision of the cerebellum closely interacting with to the spinal cord, in contrast to the cerebro-cerebellum (the hemispheres) and vestibulo-cerebellum (a small portion of the vermal part).

The anterior lobe consists of two parts differing in their efferent projections (Fig. 13.1C) (Larsell 1953). The Purkinje cells are the only 'output' neurons of the cerebellar cortex (Fig. 13.1B). The Purkinje cells from the lateral, paravermal part (pars intermedia) project to the interposite nucleus of the cerebellum. This nucleus, in its turn, projects to the red nucleus which gives rise to the rubrospinal tract. The Purkinje cells from the medial part (vermis) have two projections, one to the lateral vestibular nucleus of Deiters which gives rise to the lateral vestibulospinal tract, and another one on the fastigial nucleus of the cerebellum. The fastigial nucleus, in its turn, projects to the reticular nuclei of the brainstem which give rise to the reticulospinal tract, and also to Deiters' nucleus (Chambers and Sprague 1955a,b).

Influences of the hind limb subdivision of the cerebellum on the cerebral cortex are mediated by the interposite nucleus projecting to the ventrolateral nucleus of thalamus which, in turn, projects to the cerebral cortex (Rispal-Padel 1979).

In addition to inputs from the cerebellum, the neurons giving rise to spinal descending tracts receive numerous inputs from the forebrain and midbrain struc-tures, including the cortico-rubral (see for example Fanardjan and Gorodnov 1983; for a review see Massion and Sasaki 1979; Massion 1967) and cortico-reticular (for a review, see Brodal 1957) projections, vestibular input to the Deiters' nucleus (for a review, see Brodal 1974; Brodal *et al.* 1962), etc. Besides, the cere-bellum itself receives input from the cerebral cortex mediated by the pontine nuclei (for a review, see Evarts and Thach 1969; Allen and Tsukahara 1974). All these inputs are designated as 'external inputs' in Fig. 13.1C. As a consequence of decere-bration, most of these inputs do not function in the mesencephalic cat. In this preparation, the hind limb subdivisions of the cerebellum receive their main affer-ent input from the spinal cord.

13.2   SIGNALS COMING FROM THE SPINAL CORD TO THE CEREBELLUM

Four pathways transmit signals from the spinal hind limb centre to the cerebellum—the dorsal and ventral spinocerebellar tracts, as well as the spino-reticulocerebellar and spino-olivocerebellar pathways (Fig. 13.1C).

---

spinocerebellar tract; VSCT, ventral spinocerebellar tract; SRCT, spino-reticulocerebellar pathway; SOCP, spino-olivocerebellar pathway). A grey contour delineates the cerebellar structures. Based on Arshavsky *et al.* (1986b).

13.2.1 Dorsal spinocerebellar tract

The dorsal spinocerebellar tract (DSCT) originates in the upper lumbar segments, ascends in the dorsolateral funiculus of the spinal cord, and terminates as mossy fibres in the lateral part (pars intermedia) of the hind limb projection zone of the cerebellar cortex (Figs. 13.2F–H). The main afferent input to the majority of DSCT neurons is excitatory and formed by the Ia fibres coming from the primary spindle receptors of a single limb muscle or of a few synergists. Some DSCT neurons are activated by Ib fibres from the Golgi tendon organs (muscle force receptors), by joint receptors, or by tactile receptors of the foot (Lundberg and Oscarsson 1956, 1960; Lundberg and Winsbury 1960; for a review, see Oscarsson 1965, 1973).

During locomotion, DSCT neurons fire in bursts in a definite phase of the cycle (Arshavsky *et al.* 1972*a,d*). Figure 13.2A shows activity of a DSCT neuron receiving input from the ankle extensors. The neuron was activated by passive flexion of the ankle joint, along with the excitation of the ankle extensor gastrocnemius caused by the stretch reflex. During locomotion, both Ia and Ib afferents of the ankle extensors fire in the stance phase of the step cycle, when the extensors are active (Severin *et al.* 1967). For the Golgi tendon organs, this is because the extensors develop a maximal force in the stance phase; for the Ia afferents this is due to the gamma drive to the muscle spindles (see Section 11.4). Correspondingly, the DSCT neuron receiving input from the ankle extensors, is firing during the stance phase, and its activity is proportional to the muscle activity (Figs. 13.2B,C).

The activity of DSCT neurons is completely determined by their peripheral afferent inputs, and they are not subject to any influences from the spinal rhythm generator (Arshavsky *et al.* 1972*d*, 1986). As shown in Fig. 13.2D, the DSCT neuron in the walking cat exhibited no rhythmical modulation of its discharge rate after the hind limb has been deafferented. Similarly, the DSCT neuron was not modulated during fictive scratching in the immobilized cat (Fig. 13.2E). Thus, the DSCT can be considered as a pathway supplying the cerebellum with information regarding the activity of the peripheral motor apparatus. One should note, however, that the DSCT neurons are not pure mechanical sensors in the sense that their main input—the Ia afferents—is subject to the central gamma drive.

13.2.2 Ventral spinocerebellar tract and spino-reticulocerebellar pathway

The ventral spinocerebellar tract (VSCT, Figs. 13.3I–L) originates from two groups of cells in the L3–L6 segments, ascends in the contralateral lateral funiculus of the spinal cord, and terminates as mossy fibres in the hind limb projection zone of the cerebellar cortex (Burke *et al.* 1971; Hubbard and Oscarsson 1962; Lundberg and Oscarsson 1962*a*). In contrast to the DSCT, the VSCT neurons have no specific peripheral sources for their excitation (Oscarsson 1957; Lundberg and Weight 1971; Arshavsky *et al.* 1972*e*); they rather respond by a weak excitation to different stimuli applied not only to the ipsilateral but also to the contralateral hind limb (Figs. 13.3A–D). During locomotion, however, the VSCT neurons exhibit an intense cycle-related bursting activity (Fig. 13.3E) (Arshavsky *et al.* 1972*b,e*). Deafferentation of the hind limbs did not abolish this bursting activity of the VSCT neurons (Fig. 13.3F), thus demonstrating the existence of input to these neurons

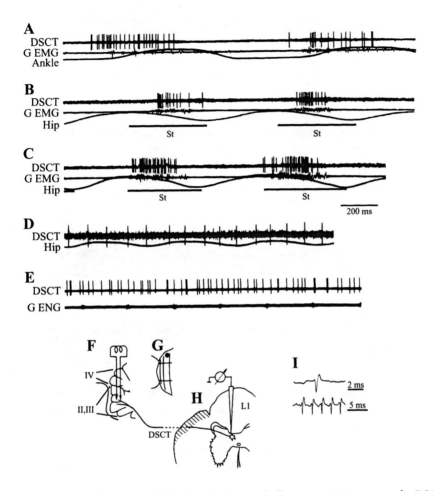

Fig. 13.2 Activity of neurons of the dorsal spinocerebellar tract. A: Response of a DSCT neuron to passive flexion of the ipsilateral ankle joint. B,C: Activity of the same neuron during weak (B) and intense (C) locomotion. The neuron was recorded along with the EMG of gastrocnemius muscle and limb movement (flexion upward). D: Activity of a DSCT neuron during locomotion of the cat with deafferented hind limbs. E: Activity of a DSCT neuron during fictive scratch reflex recorded along with the gastrocnemius ENG. F–H: Identification of a DSCT neuron. The neuron was recorded in the L1 segment and identified by the antidromic response to stimulation of the hind limb area in the pars intermedia of the cerebellar anterior lobe. The site of insertion of the stimulating electrode is shown in G (black dot), its position in the cortex (in the lobes II, III) is shown in F. Position of the recording electrode near a DSCT neuron and location of the DSCT in the spinal cord (hatched area) are shown in H. I: Antidromic response of the neuron to a single stimulus and to a train of pulses applied to the cerebellum. A–D and F–I are from Arshavsky *et al.* (1972*a,d*). E is from Arshavsky *et al.* (1986*b*).

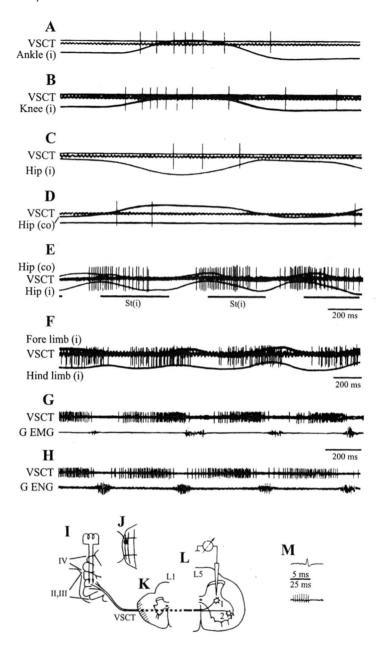

Fig. 13.3 Activity of neurons of the ventral spinocerebellar tract. A–D: Responses of a VSCT neuron to passive flexion of the ipsilateral hind limb at different joints (A–C) and to flexion of the contralateral hind limb (D). E: Activity of the same neuron during locomotion. F: Activity of a VSCT neuron during locomotion of a cat with deafferented hind limbs. G,H: Activity of a VSCT neuron recorded initially during actual scratching (G) and then during fictive scratching. Note that in G the neuron was recorded along with the gastrocnemius EMG, and in H, with the ENG. I–M: Identification of VSCT neurons. The neurons were recorded from the intermediate zone of the

from the spinal rhythm generator (Arshavsky *et al.* 1972*f*). Moreover, this input plays a crucial role in the rhythmical bursting of the VSCT neurons. This was shown by comparing activity of individual neurons during real (Fig. 13.3G) and fictive scratching (Fig. 13.3H) (Arshavsky *et al.* 1975, 1978*b*). Thus, the VSCT conveys information to the cerebellum not about the peripheral events but rather about the activity of the spinal networks generating stepping and scratching. The idea that some spinocerebellar pathways, including the VSCT, convey information on intraspinal processes, was first formulated by Lundberg (1971) and Oscarsson (1973).

The spino-reticulocerebellar pathway (SRCP, Figs. 13.4C–E) is not a direct spinocerebellar tract. Axons of the first-order spinal neurons ascend on both sides of the cord and terminate on the second-order neurons located in the lateral reticular nucleus (LRN) of the medulla. In their turn, the LRN neurons project as mossy fibres to a wide area of the cerebellar cortex including the hind limb projection zone (Lundberg and Oscarsson 1962*b*; Morin *et al.* 1966; Grant *et al.* 1966). When tested in a quiescent animal, the LRN neurons have even wider receptive fields than the VSCT neurons: they respond to stimulation of the nerves of three or even four limbs (Lundberg and Oscarsson 1962*b*; Clendenin *et al.* 1974*a*–*c*). During locomotion and scratching, the LRN neurons exhibited cycle-related bursting activity which was much stronger than that evoked by any exteroceptive or proprioceptive stimuli (Arshavsky *et al.* 1977, 1986), thus suggesting that the SRCP informs the cerebellum not about peripheral events but rather about central events. Comparison of the activity of individual LRN neurons during real (Fig. 13.4A) and fictive scratching (Fig. 13.4B) has shown that their firing patterns practically did not change after cessation of the rhythmical afferent inflow (Arshavsky *et al.* 1978*a*). Thus, the SRCP like the VSCT conveys information about the activity of the spinal network (CPG) controlling stepping and scratching movements.

This network consists of two principal parts—the rhythm generator and the output motor stage (see Sections 11.3 and 11.4). There is evidence that both VSCT and SRCP transmit information about the activity of the rhythm generator part. As shown in Section 11.2, a crucial role in the rhythmogenesis is played by the rostral part of the lumbosacral enlargement of the spinal cord ('leading area', Fig. 11.2A). The VSCT and SRCP were found to reflect the activity just in this leading area. Experiments with inactivation of the caudal spinal cord by means of cooling—similar to those shown in Fig. 11.2C—have demonstrated (Arshavsky *et al.* 1984*a*) that the patterns of bursting in the VSCT and LRN neurons observed before cooling (Figs. 13.5A,C) changed only slightly after inactivation of the L6–S1 segments

---

grey matter (1) or from the border zone of the ventral horn (2) in the L5 (or L4) segment (L), and identified by stimulation of the hind limb area in the vermus (marked in J) or in the pars intermedia of the anterior lobe. Location of the VSCT in the contralateral part of the spinal cord at L1 level is shown in K (hatched area). M: Antidromic responses of a neuron to a single stimulus and to a train of pulses applied to the cerebellum. A–E and J–M are from Arshavsky *et al.* (1972*e*), F is from Arshavsky *et al.* (1972*f*), and G,H are from Arshavsky *et al.* (1978*b*).

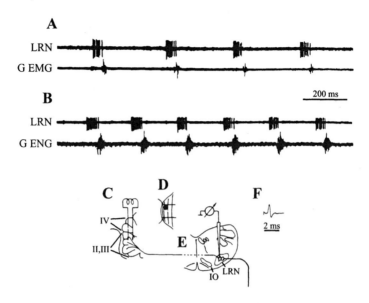

Fig. 13.4 Activity of neurons of the spino-reticulocerebellar pathway. A,B: Activity of a neuron of the lateral reticular nucleus recorded initially during actual scratching (A) and then during fictive scratching (B). Note that in A the neuron was recorded along with the gastrocnemius EMG, and in B, with the ENG. C–E: Identification of an LRN neuron. The neuron was recorded from the lateral reticular nucleus (LRN in E; IO, inferior olive) and identified by the antidromic response (F) to stimulation of the hind limb area in the vermis of the cerebellar anterior lobe (C,D). A,B are from Arshavsky *et al.* (1978*a*).

(Figs. 13.5B,D), which contain the majority of neurons controlling limb movements, especially the neurons constituting the output motor stage (see Fig. 11.2A).

Which aspects of the activity of the rhythm generating network are reflected in the signals conveyed by the VSCT and SRCP? A likely answer to this question was obtained when the phase distribution within the scratch cycle of the spinal interneurons recorded from the 'leading area' (Fig. 13.5E) (see Section 11.3) was compared with the phase distribution of the VSCT and SRCP neurons (Fig. 13.5F) (Arshavsky *et al.* 1986). In these two graphs, each neuron was characterized not only by the phase of its bursting in the scratch cycle but also by the frequency profile in the burst, and by the response to pinna stimulation preceding the bursting activity. A striking similarity can be found between the two populations of neurons characterized by these variables.

In Section 11.3.1, all rhythmic spinal interneurons were subdivided into three groups (1–3 in Fig. 13.5E) presumably differing in their functional role in the rhythm generating network (Berkinblit *et al.* 1978*a*). By comparing Figs. 13.5E and F one can see that these three groups of interneurons have their counterparts in the population of VSCT and LRN neurons. It thus seems likely that the VSCT and SRCP convey to the cerebellum the information about activity of the main groups of spinal interneurons of the 'leading area' responsible for the rhythm generation. Of the two pathways, the VSCT neurons (thin lines in Fig. 13.5F) monitor activity mainly of the first and second groups of interneurons (1 and 2 in Fig. 13.5E), whereas the LRN neurons (thick lines in Fig. 13.5F) monitor activity of the third group (3 in Fig. 13.5E).

13.2.3   Spino-olivocerebellar pathway

The spino-olivocerebellar pathway (SOCP) has first-order neurons in the spinal cord, and second-order neurons in the inferior olives of the medulla; the latter ones project to the cerebellar cortex as climbing fibres (Oscarsson and Sjolund 1977*a–c*; Eccles *et al.* 1968). Since climbing fibre input produces a characteristic response in the Purkinje cells ('complex spike') (Eccles *et al.* 1966), the activity of the SOCP pathway is easy to study by observing complex spikes in the Purkinje cells. It was found that SOCP input is weakly, if at all, correlated with the rhythm of stepping (Armstrong *et al.* 1982, 1988*b*; Orlovsky 1972*b*; Udo *et al.* 1981) or the rhythm of scratching (Arshavsky *et al.* 1984*b*). Thus, it seems likely that the SOCP does not play any significant role in informing the cerebellum about the cycle-related events either on the periphery or in the spinal cord, and therefore does not contribute to the operative control of stepping movements. However, climbing fibre input to Purkinje cells was found to be sensitive to certain 'extraordinary' peripheral stimuli caused by considerable perturbations of the step cycle (Matsukawa and Udo 1985; Lou and Bloedel 1992; Andersson and Armstrong 1985; Yanagihara and Udo 1994). It was suggested that SOCP input contributes to the cerebellar-induced plastic modifications of the locomotor programme (Lou and Bloedel 1992) (see also Ito (1984) for an extensive discussion of this problem).

Thus, the studies of the cerebellar input signals during locomotion and scratching have shown that the cerebellum receives information about the activity of the spinal networks controlling limb movements (via the VSCT and SRCP)—the efference copy, and information about performance of these movements (via the DSCT). Below we shall consider how the cerebellum utilizes these two types of signal.

13.3   FORMATION OF THE OUTPUT CEREBELLAR SIGNALS

13.3.1   Cerebellum performs modulation of the descending tract neurons

The cerebellar output signals affect numerous targets, both in the brain and in the spinal cord. The spinal cord can be affected via the descending spinal tracts—the vestibulospinal (VS), rubrospinal (RbS), and reticulospinal (RS) ones (Fig. 13.1C). Neurons giving rise to these tracts are located in the brainstem, and their activity during stepping and scratching in the mesencephalic cat was recorded. It was found that during stepping or scratching, in the absence of influences from the forebrain, the cerebellum is practically the only source of rhythmic, cycle-related drive signals coming to the neurons giving rise to descending tracts (Orlovsky 1970*b,c*, 1972*d,e*). Figure 13.6A shows the activity during locomotion of an RbS

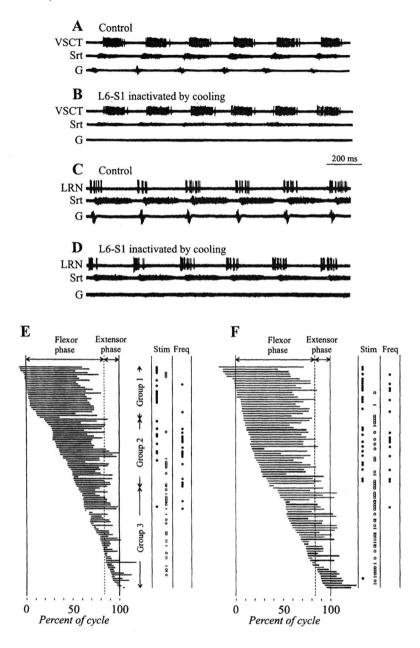

Fig. 13.5 Origin of signals transmitted by the ventral spinocerebellar tract and spino-reticulocerebellar pathway. A–D: Effects of cooling of the L5 segment upon activity of a VSCT neuron (A,B) and an LRN neuron (C,D) during fictive scratching. Activity of the neurons is shown before cooling (A,C) and 60 s after beginning of cooling (B,D) when the caudal part of the spinal cord is inactivated as monitored by cessation of the rhythmical activity in n. gastrocnemius (lower trace). The middle trace is the sartorius ENG. For methods, see Figs. 11.2C₁–C₃. E,F: Comparison of the behaviour of spinal interneurons

neuron from the red nucleus, with its axon projecting to the spinal hind limb centre (Figs. 13.6E–G). The neuron has its peak activity in the swing phase of the step cycle when the flexor muscles were active. Decerebellation of the animal resulted in cessation of the rhythmical modulation in the majority of RbS neurons, as illustrated in Fig. 13.6B. The same conclusion relates to the activity of RbS neurons during scratching—they are active in the flexor phase of the cycle (Fig. 13.6C), and this phasic activity disappears after removal of the cerebellum (Fig. 13.6D) (Arshavsky *et al.* 1988*d*).

A clear-cut rhythmical modulation is also characteristic of the majority of VS and RS neurons provided the cerebellum is intact. Decerebellation resulted in a cessation of this modulation. The only change in the activity of the RbS, RS, and VS neurons in the decerebellated animals, associated with the locomotor activity of the animal, is an increase of their tonic firing rate during locomotion as compared with the resting conditions (Figs. 13.6H–J) (Orlovsky 1970*b,c*, 1972*d,e*).

13.3.2 Role of different inputs in formation of the output cerebellar signals

During locomotion and scratching, the cerebellum receives two types of signals from the spinal cord—signals about activity of the spinal rhythm generator (via the VSCT and SRCP) and signals about actual limb movements (via the DSCT) (see Section 13.2). The output cerebellar signals cause a rhythmical modulation of the VS, RbS, and RS neurons. It was found that the output cerebellar signals are formed almost exclusively on the basis of information sent to the cerebellum by the spinal rhythm generator, whereas the signals about the motor performance play a secondary role. Evidence in favour of this conclusion was obtained in three types of experiments:

1. The pattern of rhythmical modulation, observed during real movements both in individual neurons of descending tracts and in their population activity, changed only slightly after the animal had been immobilized. This was demonstrated for the VS neurons (Figs. 13.7A,B) (Arshavsky *et al.* 1978*c*) and for the RbS neurons (Arshavsky *et al.* 1978*e*).
2. Perturbing the stepping movements when they involved only distal joints (knee and ankle) and did not disrupt the locomotory rhythm, only slightly affected the pattern of modulation of the RbS neurons (Fig. 13.7C), despite that such perturbations presumably caused considerable changes in the afferent signals. In contrast, the perturbation of hip movement, which affected the rhythm

---

and neurons of the spino-cerebellar pathways during fictive scratching. E: The phase distribution of spinal interneurons from L4 and L5 segments (repetition, with some additional data, of Fig. 11.4B). F: The phase distribution of VSCT neurons (thin lines) and LRN neurons (heavy lines). In E,F, the Stim column shows the behaviour of neurons during the latent period of scratching (filled circles, neurons are activated; open circles, neurons have no resting discharge and are not activated; minuses, resting discharge of neurons is inhibited). In the Freq column, filled circles indicate the neurons whose discharge frequencies increase in the course of the burst. A–D are from Arshavsky *et al.* (1984*a*) and E,F are from Arshavsky *et al.* (1978*b*).

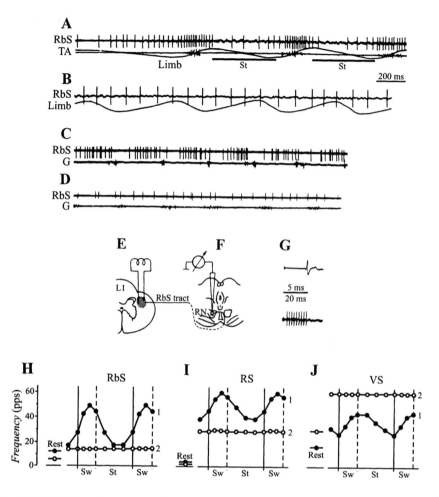

Fig. 13.6 Activity of neurons of rubro-, reticulo-, and vestibulospinal tracts and the role of the cerebellum in their modulation. A–D: Activity of rubrospinal (RbS) neurons. A: Activity of a RbS neuron during locomotion of the cat with intact cerebellum, recorded along with the EMG of m. tibialis anterior and the movement of the contralateral hind limb (protraction up). B. Activity of an RbS neuron during locomotion of the decerebellate cat. C: Activity of an RbS neuron during scratching of the cat with intact cerebellum. D: Activity of an RbS neuron during scratching of the decerebellate cat. In C and D the lower trace is the m. gastrocnemius EMG. E–G: Identification of a RbS neuron. The neuron was recorded from the red nucleus (RN in F) and identified by its antidromic response to stimulation of the RbS tract on the contralateral side of the spinal cord in the L1 segment (hatched area in E). G: Antidromic responses of the neuron to a single stimulus and to a train of pulses applied to the RbS tract. H–J: Relationship between the discharge frequency of the 'average' neurons of the rubrospinal tract (H), reticulospinal tract (I), and vestibulospinal tract (J), and the phase of the step cycle of the hind limb (ipsilateral in I and J, and contralateral in H). Curves with filled circles (1) correspond to the animals with intact cerebellum, with empty circles (2), to decerebellate animals. For both preparations, the average frequency of the background activity in the descending tracts is also indicated (Rest). A, B, and H are from Orlovsky (1972*e*), C–G are from Arshavsky *et al.* (1978*e*), I is from Orlovsky (1970*b*), and J is from Orlovsky (1972*d*).

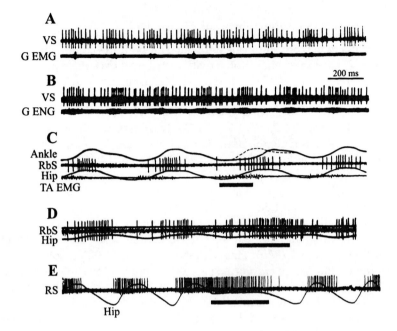

Fig. 13.7 Role of sensory information and efference copy signals in the modulation of neurons of descending tracts. A,B: Activity of a vestibulospinal (VS) neuron recorded initially during actual scratching (A) and then during fictive scratching (B). In A, the lower trace in the gastrocnemius EMG; in B, the ENG. C: Disturbances of the hind limb stepping movement at the ankle joint produce no effects on the activity of the rubrospinal (RbS) neuron. D,E: Perturbation of the hip movement strongly affects the activity of the same RbS neuron (D) and the activity of the reticulospinal (RS) neuron (E). The periods of external action on the limb are shown by bars. A,B are from Arshavsky *et al.* (1978*c*), C,D are from Orlovsky (1972*e*), and E is from Orlovsky (1970*b*).

generator and caused a break (resetting) of the locomotory rhythm, caused a change in the cerebellar output signals which was reflected in a considerable change of the pattern of modulation of the RbS and RS neurons (Figs. 13.7D,E) (Orlovsky 1970*b*, 1972*e*).

3. Recording of cerebellar neurons during locomotion of intact cats has shown that their modulation pattern was almost independent on the vigour of locomotion when comparing walking on a horizontal surface and uphill, or walking at different speed, despite that the different intensities of stepping movements were presumably related to considerable changes in the afferent inflow to the cerebellum (Armstrong and Edgley 1988).

Of the two pathways transmitting signals from the spinal rhythm generator to the cerebellum (the VSCT and the SRCP), the VSCT plays a more significant role in the formation of the cerebellar output signals: this has been demonstrated by separate transections of the VSCT and the SRCP (Arshavsky *et al.* 1978*c*,*e*).

13.3.3   Processing of information in the cerebellum

Signals arriving to the cerebellum via individual mossy fibres comprising the VSCT and the SRCP, have their phases of activity distributed over the whole step cycle (Arshavsky *et al.* 1972*e,f*, 1974) or scratch cycle (Arshavsky *et al.* 1978*a,b*), as was illustrated in Fig. 13.5F. On the other hand, the mossy fibre input to the Purkinje cells in the cerebellar cortex is characterized by a very extensive divergence and convergence (Palkovits *et al.* 1971*a–c*, 1972). Nevertheless, this input produces a clear-cut rhythmical modulation of the Purkinje cells activity both during stepping (Figs. 13.8A,D) (Orlovsky 1972*b*) and scratching (Fig. 13.8F) (Arshavsky *et al.* 1984*b*), thus indicating that individual Purkinje cells are driven by mossy fibres firing in-phase with each other. A similar modulation was observed in the walking intact cat (Armstrong and Edgley 1988).

The Purkinje cells in the hind limb projection zone of the cerebellar cortex have their phases of activity distributed over the whole step or scratch cycle (Orlovsky 1972*b*; Arshavsky *et al.* 1984*b*). This is illustrated in Figs. 13.8D,F for the Purkinje cells recorded from the pars intermedia of the anterior lobe. By averaging the activity of these cells over the whole recorded population, a relatively weak phase-dependent modulation can be revealed for the step cycle (Fig. 13.8E), and almost no modulation for the scratch cycle (Fig. 13.8G). Besides, projections of the Purkinje cells on the cerebellar nuclei neurons are characterized by a wide convergence and divergence (Palkovits *et al.* 1977). Nevertheless, the cerebellar nuclei neurons exhibit a clear-cut rhythmical modulation both during locomotion (Fig. 13.9A) (Orlovsky 1972*e*) and during scratching (Antziferova *et al.* 1980), thus indicating that individual neurons of the cerebellar nuclei are driven by Purkinje cells firing in phase with each other. In addition to an inhibitory input from the cerebellar cortex (via the axons of Purkinje cells), neurons of the cerebellar nuclei also receive an excitatory input from the spinal cord via the collaterals of fibres of the spinocerebellar pathways (Fig. 13.1C) (see for example Eccles *et al.* 1974). The relative contribution of these two inputs—from Purkinje cells and from afferent collaterals—to the rhythmical modulation of the activity of cerebellar nuclei neurons during locomotion remains unknown.

Driven by the Purkinje cells and by the collaterals of cerebellar afferents, neurons of the cerebellar nuclei exhibit a rather uniform pattern of modulation: both in the fastigial nucleus and in the interpositus nucleus, they fire preferentially in the flexor phase of the step cycle (Orlovsky 1972*c*) or scratch cycle (Antziferova *et al.* 1980; Arshavsky *et al.* 1980), as illustrated for a neuron from the fastigial nucleus in Fig. 13.9A. Figures 13.9B–E show the phase distribution and the population activity of the interpositus neurons during stepping (Figs. 13.9B,C) and scratching (Figs. 13.9D,E). A pronounced modulation of the cerebellar nuclear neurons was also observed during locomotion of intact cats (Armstrong and Edgley 1988).

Excitatory input from the interpositus neurons (Figs. 13.9B,C) is responsible for the rhythmical modulation of the RbS neurons with their peak of activity in the flexor phase of the step cycle (curve 1 in Fig. 13.6H); without this input, the rhythmical modulation is absent (curve 2 in Fig. 13.6H). Correspondingly, excitatory input from the fastigial nucleus, which is also maximal in the flexor phase of the cycle (Orlovsky 1972*e*), is responsible for the rhythmical modulation

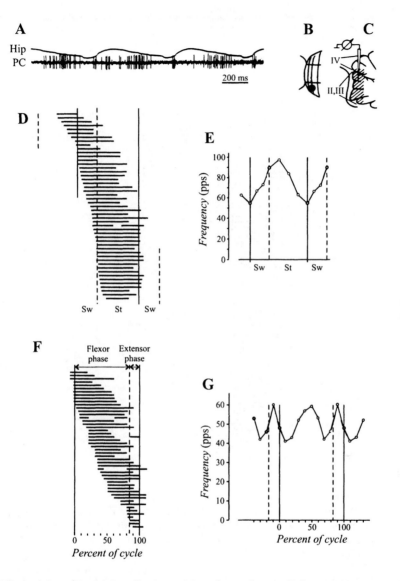

Fig. 13.8 Activity of Purkinje cells. A: Activity of a Purkinje cell during locomotion. The cell was recorded from the hind limb zone in the pars intermedia of the anterior lobe (B,C). D: The phase distribution of Purkinje cells (recorded from the area shown in B,C) in the step cycle. E: The discharge frequency of the 'average' Purkinje cell as a function of the phase of the step cycle. F: The phase distribution of Purkinje cells (recorded from the area shown in B,C) in the cycle of fictive scratching. G: The discharge frequency of the 'average' Purkinje cell as a function of the phase of the scratch cycle. A–E are from Orlovsky (1972*b*) and F,G are from Arshavsky *et al.* (1984*b*).

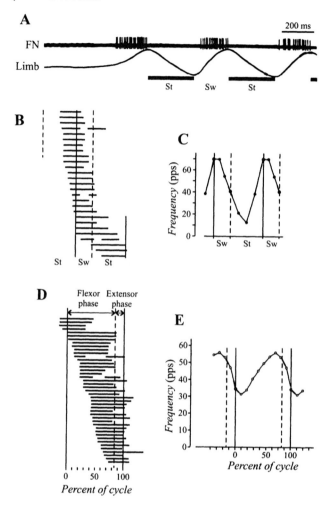

Fig. 13.9 Activity of neurons of the cerebellar nuclei. A: Activity of a neuron of the fastigial nucleus (FN) during locomotion. B,C: Relationship between the activity of neurons of the interpositus nucleus (IN) and the phase of the step cycle of the ipsilateral hind limb. B: The phase distribution of IN neurons. C: The discharge frequency of the 'average' IN neuron as a function of the phase of the step cycle. D,E: Relationship between the activity of IN neurons and the phase of the cycle of fictive scratching. D: The phase distribution of IN neurons. E: The discharge frequency of the 'average' IN neuron as a function of the phase of the scratch cycle. A–C are from Orlovsky (1972c) and D,E are from Arshavsky *et al.* (1980b).

of RS neurons, most of which have their peak of activity also in the flexor phase (curve 1 in Fig. 13.6I). For the VS neurons, direct monosynaptic inhibitory input from the Purkinje cells (Ito and Yoshida 1964) presents the main source of both tonic and rhythmic influences during locomotion and scratching in decerebrate cats. This follows from the findings that (1) decerebellation results in a dramatic increase of the tonic firing of VS neurons, and in termination of their rhythmical modulation (compare curves 1 and 2 in Fig. 13.6J), and (2) most neurons of the fastigial nucleus, also projecting on the VS neurons (Fig. 13.1C) and supplying them with excitatory input (Brodal *et al.* 1962) have their peak of activity in the flexor phase of the cycle (Orlovsky 1972*c*) while most of the VS neurons are firing later in the cycle, that is at the beginning of the extensor phase (curve 1 in Fig. 13.6J) (Orlovsky 1972*d*).

13.4   SIGNALS TRANSMITTED VIA DESCENDING TRACTS AND THEIR INFLUENCES ON THE LOCOMOTOR PATTERN

The results presented above have shown that the activity in the RS, VS, and RbS descending tracts in the mesencephalic cat increases during walking, and that this activity is rhythmically modulated by the cerebellum (see Figs. 13.6H–J). The role of activity in the descending tracts was examined in the experiments with stimulation of these tracts during locomotion in the mesencephalic cat (Orlovsky 1972*a*) and, for the RS tract, also in the intact cat (Drew 1991*b*; Drew and Rossignol 1984).

13.4.1   Vestibulospinal tract

Experiments with stimulation of the Deiters' nucleus, which gives rise to the VS tract, in non-locomoting preparations have shown that the VS tract exerts a rather uniform action on spinal motor output—it excites the ipsilateral extensor motor nucleus (see for example Wilson 1972; Grillner *et al.* 1970). In the walking cat, the principal effect of stimulation, that is excitation of the extensor motor neurons, persists but becomes strongly phase-dependent (Orlovsky 1972*a*). Figure 13.10A shows the effect of stimulation of the Deiters' nucleus on the flexor (TA) and extensor (G) muscles of the ipsilateral hind limb in the walking mesencephalic cat. The stimulation was performed in different phases of the step cycle. The first train of stimuli was applied in the stance phase, when the extensors are active. The stimulation resulted in a considerable increase of the extensor activity but, as in the cycles without stimulation, the extensor burst was timed to the stance phase. The second train was applied earlier in the cycle, that is in the swing phase and at the beginning of the stance phase. This stimulation also resulted in a considerable increase of the extensor activity, but again this activity remained tightly linked to the stance phase. The third train was applied even earlier in the cycle, during the transition from stance phase to swing phase, and again it affected only the amplitude of the extensor burst but not its timing. None of the stimulations affected the phase or amplitude of the flexor burst. These experiments have shown that, during locomotion, the brain motor centres can regulate, via the VS tract, the level of extensor activity. They have also shown that there is a powerful gating mechanism in the spinal cord that allows the brain centres to affect the extensor activity only during the stance phase of the step cycle. The gating mechanism is based, at least partly, on the periodical modulation of the sensitivity of the extensor motor

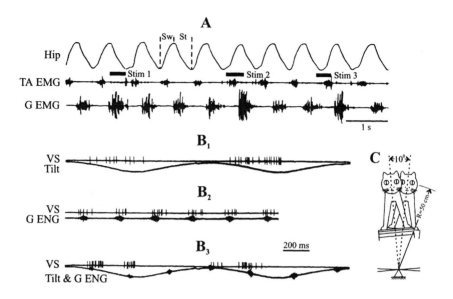

Fig. 13.10 Vestibular influences on the output motor pattern during stepping and scratching. A: Effects of stimulation of Deiters' nucleus on the muscle activity in the ipsilateral hind limb during locomotion. Stimuli (pulses 0.1 ms, 50 Hz, 150 μA) were applied during periods marked by bars. Movements of the hip (flexion up) and the EMGs of m. tibialis anterior and m. gastrocnemius were recorded. B_1–B_3: Vestibular reactions of a VS neuron during fictive scratching (the lateral tilts as shown in C). B_1: Reaction of the neuron to tilts at rest. B_2: Activity of the neuron during fictive scratching. B_3: Reactions of the neuron to tilts during fictive scratching. The lower trace is the tilt angle (ipsilateral tilt down) and the gastrocnemius ENG. A is from Orlovsky (1972*a*) and B_1–B_3 are from Arshavsky *et al.* (1978*d*).

neurons and related interneurons to different synaptic inputs, including those from the VS tract; this modulation is caused by the cycle-dependent influences from the rhythm generator (see Section 11.4).

Under the effect of the cerebellum, the VS neurons are also rhythmically modulated, with their peak of activity at the beginning of the stance phase (see Section 13.3.1 and Fig. 13.6J) (Orlovsky 1972*b*). This rhythmical activity in the VS tract, on the one hand, can be considered as phasic signals addressed specifically to the extensor motor neurons and promoting their excitation in the appropriate phase of the cycle. On the other hand, due to the rhythmical modulation of the VS neurons, a gating mechanism is also present at this level, affecting all inputs to these neurons. The effect of this mechanism on the transmission of signals from the vestibular organ is shown in Figs. 13.10B_1–B_3 (Arshavsky *et al.* 1978*d*). In the immobilized mesencephalic cat, a lateral tilt of the animal (Fig. 13.10C) resulted in activation of a VS neuron (Fig. 13.10B_1). Then fictive scratching was induced by pinna stimulation, and the rhythmical activity of the spinal CPG was monitored by periodical bursts in the G nerve (Fig. 13.10B_2). During fictive scratching, the cerebellum produces rhythmical modulation of VS neurons (see Section 13.3.1); under the effect of the cerebellum, the VS neuron (Fig. 13.10B_2) discharges in bursts in the extensor phase of the cycle. Interaction of the two inputs—from the vestibular organ and from the cerebellum—is shown in Fig. 13.10B$_3$: the VS neuron responds to tilt of the animal only during the extensor phase of the cycle.

The gating mechanism, operating at the level of the VS neurons, supplements the spinal gating mechanism. Their joint action secures that vestibular influences on the extensor activity can be efficiently transmitted only during a limited part of the cycle.

13.4.2   Rubro- and reticulospinal tracts

The RbS tract is functionally less homogeneous than the VS tract. Experiments with stimulation of the red nucleus in non-locomoting animals have shown that the main effect is an activation of the contralateral flexor muscles, but a smaller proportion of the RbS tract axons exert an excitatory action on extensors (see for example Hongo *et al.* 1969*a,b*; for a review, see Massion 1967). In the walking mesencephalic cat, the principal effect of red nucleus stimulation, that is excitation of the flexor motor neurons, persists but becomes strongly phase-dependent. The maximal effect occurs in the swing phase of the cycle, when the flexor motor neurons are activated by the spinal limb controller (Orlovsky 1972*a*). Thus, the main function of the RbS tract—enhancement of the flexor activity—persists during locomotion, but the efficiency of signal transmission by the tract is regulated by the spinal gating mechanism.

Under the effect of the cerebellum, the RbS neurons are rhythmically modulated, with the peak of activity in the swing phase (Fig. 13.6H) (Orlovsky 1972*e*) that is when the RbS influences on the spinal mechanisms are most efficient. This rhythmic modulation can be considered as phasic signals addressed to the swing controlling mechanism and affecting the level of flexor activity. In addition, the rhythmical modulation of the RbS neurons represents a gating mechanism at the brainstem level, similar to the gating at the VS neurons, and affecting all inputs to these neurons. One of the most powerful inputs to the red nucleus comes from the motor cortex (for a review, see Massion 1967). Transmission of cortical influences to the spinal cord via the RbS tract is thus phase-dependent. This gating mechanism, residing in the RbS neurons themselves, supplements the spinal gating mechanism.

The RS tract originates from a few different nuclei in the reticular formation (Brodal 1957), and is functionally even less homogeneous than the RbS tract (see for example Magoun and Rhines 1946; Sprague and Chambers 1953, 1954; Drew and Rossignol 1990*a,b*). Some RS neurons are responsible for activation of the spinal locomotor mechanisms (see Section 12.1). Experiments on the walking mesencephalic cat (Orlovsky 1972*a*), and intact cat (Drew 1991*b*; Drew and Rossignol 1984), have shown that stimulation of different sites in the reticular formation by brief trains of pulses primarily causes activation of the flexor muscles in the ipsilateral hind limb, but that stimulation also can affect the ipsilateral extensors, as well as some muscles of the contralateral hind limb. All these effects are strongly phase-dependent.

The pronounced rhythmical modulation of the RS neurons under the effect of the cerebellum (Fig. 13.6I) (Orlovsky 1970*b*) means that the RS system exerts a phasic action on the spinal networks. It also means that the RS neurons may gate inputs that they receive from different motor centres. In particular, the RS neurons receive powerful projections from the motor cortex and from the vestibular nuclei (see Brodal 1957). Due to the gating function of the RS neurons, the efficiency of the influences of these inputs on the spinal cord is phase-dependent. It seems likely that the high level of activity of RS neurons and their rhythmical modulation observed during locomotion of the intact cat (Drew *et al.* 1986) is caused by the summation of cerebellar and cortical inputs to these cells.

13.5 CONCLUSIONS: ROLE OF THE CEREBELLUM IN LOCOMOTOR COORDINATION

It is well established that the cerebellum is necessary for coordination of most motor acts, including locomotion. Damage to the cerebellum or to its parts, or their temporary functional inactivation, results in deviations of different movement parameters (amplitude, force, speed, acceleration) from their normal values, in abnormal phase relations between the activities of various muscle groups, etc. (Luciani 1915; Holmes 1939; Dow and Moruzzi 1958). These observations suggest that the cerebellum plays not a single but multiple roles in motor coordination. Experimental results obtained on the decerebrate cat performing stepping or scratching movements, while the input and output cerebellar signals were recorded (see Sections 13.1–13.4) allow a discussion of the different functions of the spino-cerebellum.

Figure 13.11A shows the principal functional units participating in the control of stepping (scratching) movements of the hind limb, and their interactions. The limb controller generates motor commands addressed to the limb muscles. An essential role in generating these commands is played by the central mechanisms (CPG) and by the feedback based on the afferent signals coming from the limb mechanoreceptors (see Chapter 11).

Some of these afferent signals are also delivered to the cerebellum by the DSCT (Input 1). During rhythmical limb movements, this input informs the cerebellum about different aspects of the movements—contraction of the flexor and extensor muscles, flexion and extension at joints, etc. (see Section 13.2.1). Another input to the cerebellum (Input 2) is formed by the VSCT and SRCP. This input delivers information about the activity of the rhythm generating network of the limb controller (the efference copy signals) (see Section 13.2.2).

The output cerebellar signals perform a modulation of the brainstem neurons giving rise to descending tracts (VS, RS, and RbS) (see Section 13.3.1). This modulation plays a double role: (1) it represents the commands sent by the cerebellum to the limb controller, and designated as Output 1 (direct cerebellar influences) in Fig. 13.11A; and (2) it is responsible for the regulation of signal transmission in the pathways from different brain motor centres to the limb controller, and designated as Output 2 (gating) in Fig. 13.11A.

From the diagram of Fig. 13.11A it is clear that the cerebellum may perform a number of principally different functions, depending on the relative significance of

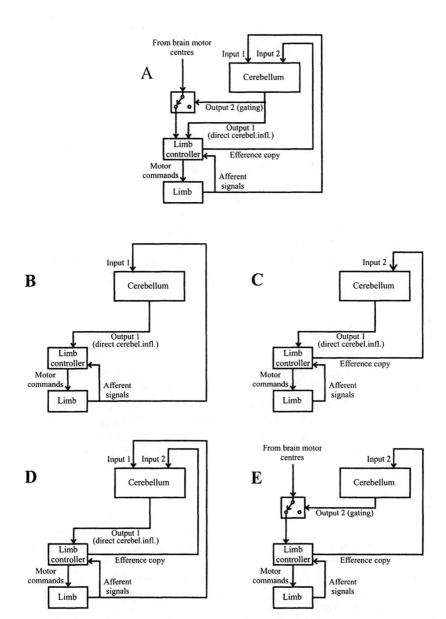

Fig. 13.11 Different functions of the cerebellum in locomotor coordination. A: Principal functional units participating in the control of stepping (scratching) movements of the hind limb, and their interactions. B–E: Four different cerebellar functions: B: Mediation of sensory feedback. C: Mediation of internal feedback. D: Optimization of the motor pattern. E: Organization of interactions between the spinal limb controllers and the supraspinal motor centres (see text for further explanation).

its two inputs, on their processing in the cerebellum, and on the relative significance of two cerebellar outputs. These functions are considered below:

1. *Mediation of sensory feedback*. A diagram for this cerebellar function is shown in Fig. 13.11B. The cerebellum receives information about limb movements (Input 1), then it processes this information, and generates commands (Output 1) addressed to the limb controller where they produce modification of the motor pattern.

2. *Mediation of internal feedback* (Fig. 13.11C). The cerebellum receives information about activity of the rhythm generating mechanisms of the limb controller (Input 2), processes this information, and generates commands (Output 1) for modifications of the efferent motor pattern.

3. *Optimization of the motor pattern* (Fig. 13.11D). The cerebellum compares Inputs 1 and 2, that is the efference copy ('intended movement') and sensory feedback ('executed movement'), and sends the relevant signals (Output 1) to the limb controller to compensate for the mismatch.

4. *Organization of interactions between the spinal limb controller and supraspinal motor centres* (Fig. 13.11E). The cerebellum receives information about activity of the limb controller (Input 1), processes this information, and via Output 2 regulates the signal transmission in the pathways from different supraspinal centres to the limb controller.

All these cerebellar functions play a role in motor coordination, and have received frequent and competent review along with other cerebellar functions (Ito 1984; Eccles *et al.* 1967; Bloedel and Bracha 1995; Bloedel 1992; Thach *et al.* 1992; Udo 1986; Brooks and Thach 1981; Arshavsky *et al.* 1986*b*). However, the experimental results obtained on the decerebrate cat strongly suggest that the main function of the cerebellum, when it takes part in the control of stepping limb movements, is the coordination of the spinal limb controllers, on the one hand, and the supraspinal motor centres, on the other. First, it has been found that Input 2 plays a predominant role in the generation of cerebellar output signals (see Section 13.3.2). Second, it has been found that the gating function of cerebellar Output 2 is very efficient (see Sections 13.4.1 and 13.4.2). Due to this function, any supraspinal command, addressed to the limb controllers, becomes locked to the appropriate phase of the cycle so that it will not disturb the basic locomotor pattern, but rather modify it to a permissible extent. In this sense, the spinal limb controllers dominate the supraspinal motor centres, and the motor cortex in particular during locomotion (see Chapter 14); they impose their rhythm upon the activity of these centres.

Gating is the simplest way to make supraspinal commands dependent on the phase of the locomotor cycle. In a general case, the generation and the final form of these commands themselves may be affected by the locomotor cycle-related signals that arrive from the spinal limb controllers, to a large extent, via the cerebellum (see Section 14.1).

14

Role of the motor cortex in locomotor coordination

The motor cortex does not play any significant role in the production of the basic locomotor pattern in the cat. This was demonstrated by the fact that the mesencephalic cat is capable of 'simple' locomotion, that is of walking and running in a straight line on a flat surface (see Section 10.3). The same conclusion was reached in experiments on cats and dogs with destruction or functional inactivation of the motor cortex (see for example Chambers and Liu 1957; Adkins *et al.* 1971; Dubrovsky *et al.* 1974; Beloozerova and Sirota 1988), or transection of the pyramidal tract (see for example Liddell and Phillips 1944). This situation strongly contrasts to that in man and other primates where even 'simple' locomotion is very severely disrupted by motor cortex lesions (see Section 15.2). In cats and dogs, however, elimination of cortical output dramatically affected their ability to locomote in more demanding circumstances ('skilled' locomotion), when considerable modifications of the basic locomotor pattern are needed, and especially when visuo-motor coordination is required. In this chapter, we will consider the signals transmitted from the motor cortex to the spinal cord, which are presumably responsible for different modifications of the basic locomotor pattern in the fore limb of the cat. The locomotion-related activity of the motor cortex has been reviewed by Armstrong (1986, 1988), Drew (1991*a,b*) and Kalaska and Drew (1993).

14.1 ACTIVITY OF CORTICAL NEURONS DURING LOCOMOTION ON A FLAT SURFACE

Neurons of the motor cortex giving rise to the pyramidal tract and projecting to the contralateral fore limb controller, can be found in area 4 of the cortex, in its forelimb zone (Fig. 14.1A). Most neurons in this zone exhibit rhythmic activity, related to the stepping movements of the contralateral limb, during 'simple' locomotion both on the ground and on a treadmill (Armstrong and Drew 1984*a,b*; Durelli *et al.* 1978; Palmer *et al.* 1985; Amos *et al.* 1989, 1990; Beloozerova and Sirota 1988, 1993*a,b*; Drew 1988, 1993). Figure 14.1B shows the activity of such a pyramidal tract neuron (PTN) recorded along with the elbow flexor (cleidobrachialis) and elbow extensor (triceps brachii, lateral head). Activity of this PTN

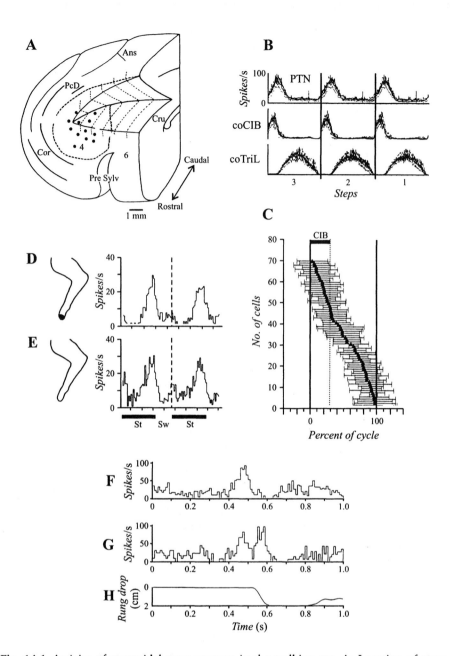

Fig. 14.1 Activity of pyramidal tract neurons in the walking cat. A: Location of some electrode trajectories (points of entrance to layer V) at which the pyramidal tract neurons (PTNs) related to the contralateral fore limb were encountered. (Abbreviations: Ans, ansate sulcus; Cor, coronal sulcus; Cru, cruciate sulcus; PcD, postcruciate dimple; Pre Sylv, presylvian sulcus; 4 and 6, cortical areas.) B: Averaged activity of a PTN during walking with no obstacles (thin lines) and in three steps (3, 2, 1) preceding the step over the obstacle (thick lines). The two curves practically coincide. Dotted lines indicate 0.01 confidence limits for the control walking. The PTN activity was recorded along with the EMGs of

was rhythmically modulated, with its peak in the swing phase of the contralateral limb. It was found that the phases of maximal activity in different PTNs are almost evenly distributed over the step cycle (Fig. 14.1C) (Drew 1993).

When tested in quiescent animals, PTNs can easily be activated by mechanical stimulation of different areas of skin of the contralateral limb. Afferent inputs from their receptive fields, however, do not play any significant role in the induction of rhythmic activity of the PTNs during walking. Two lines of evidence support this conclusion: (1) injection of local anesthetic into the receptive field resulted in a great reduction or abolishing of somatosensory responsiveness of PTNs, but their locomotion-related rhythmic discharges changed only slightly (Figs. 14.1D,E), and (2) considerable changes of the step-related afferent activity, resulting from a change of the speed of locomotion, only slightly affected the peak activity of PTNs and a position of the peak in the cycle. Also, the considerable increase of the muscular activity when running uphill, compared with locomotion on a horizontal surface, produced only minor changes in the rhythmical pattern of PTN activity (Armstrong and Drew 1984a; Beloozerova and Sirota 1988, 1993b).

Thus, it seems most likely that rhythmic modulation of the PTN activity during 'simple' locomotion is produced on the basis of signals coming from the rhythm generator of the spinal limb controller rather than on the basis of sensory feedback signals.

The spinal rhythm generators can exert their action on the motor cortex via different routes. One of them is through the cerebellum which receives input from the spinal rhythm generators (see Section 13.2) and, on the basis of this input, performs rhythmical modulation of different targets including the nucleus interpositus (see Section 13.3). In its turn, this nucleus has cortical projections mediated by the ventrolateral nucleus of thalamus (see Fig. 13.1C) (Eccles *et al.* 1967; Rispal-Padel 1979). Destruction of the ventrolateral nucleus markedly reduced the step-related modulation of PTNs (Beloozerova and Sirota 1988).

Evidently, the rhythmical modulation of PTNs during 'simple' locomotion (Fig. 14.1B) does not play any significant functional role since even a complete abolition of corticospinal influences (pyramidotomy, ablation of motor cortex) has a minor, if any, effect on the locomotor performance. Rather this modulation presents a basis for generation of corticospinal motor commands which must be coordinated with the activity of spinal limb controllers.

---

m. cleidobrachialis (ClB) and m. triceps brachii, lateral head (TriL). The data are aligned with the onset of ClB EMG. C: Mean phase of activity and angular deviation of 70 PTNs in the normalized step cycle during control walking. D,E: Effect of cutaneous anesthesia on the locomotor-related activity of a PTN. D: Receptive field and activity of the PTN in two successive steps before anesthesia. E: The same during local anesthesia. F–H: Activity of a PTN during walking on a horizontal ladder. F: Activity of a PTN during steps over stable rungs (averaged over 33 steps). G: Activity of the same PTN in the cycles when an unstable rung was encountered (averaged over 13 steps). The movement of the rung caused by the foot placement is shown in H. A–C are based on Drew (1993), D,E are based on Armstrong and Drew (1984b), and F–H are based on Marple-Horvat *et al.* (1993).

14.2   EFFECTS OF PERTURBATION OF THE LOCOMOTOR PATTERN

Considerable external perturbations of the basic pattern of stepping or abnormal afferent signals caused by peripheral stimulation, may evoke modification of the PTN discharges (Amos *et al.* 1989; Marple-Horvat *et al.* 1993; Palmer *et al.* 1985). Figure 14.1F shows the activity of a PTN recorded in a cat walking along a horizontal ladder. This PTN exhibited an increase of activity just before the onset of the stance phase. One of the rungs of the ladder was not fixed and could drop down when the cat stepped on it (Fig. 14.1H). This perturbation of the stepping movement evoked a short-latency response in the PTN (Fig. 14.1G). Such responses to perturbation were observed in relatively few PTNs, however (Amos *et al.* 1989; Marple-Horvat *et al.* 1993) suggesting that only some of the PTNs are involved in corrections of stepping movements based on sensory feedback. Similarly, some PTNs exhibited changes of their firing pattern when the fore limb was loaded by an additional weight during stepping, which resulted in a considerable modification of the motor pattern (Beloozerova and Sirota 1993*b*).

14.3   VISUALLY INDUCED MODIFICATIONS OF THE LOCOMOTOR PATTERN

Two major classes of visually-induced modifications of the step during locomotion have been investigated—stepping over an obstacle and placing the foot on a definite spot on the ground. In both cases, a dramatic change of the PTN activity was observed.

14.3.1   Stepping over obstacles

To step over an obstacle, the cat modifies the foot trajectory in the swing phase in accordance with the size and shape of the obstacle (Figs. 14.2A–C). In particular, to step over the obstacle of a larger height, the foot is lifted much more than in the case of a lower obstacle (compare B and C in Fig. 14.2). Almost all limb muscles modify their pattern of activity during the step over the obstacle. Figures 14.2D,E show that the elbow flexor m. brachialis dramatically increases its activity during a step over an obstacle as compared with the activity during ordinary steps. The modifications in kinematics and EMG patterns were different when the limb was the first stepping over the obstacle (the lead limb), and when it was second (the trailing limb).

The majority of the forelimb-related PTNs (80 per cent) changed their activity during a step over an obstacle as compared with ordinary steps (Drew 1988, 1993). The PTN shown in Fig. 14.2D increased its activity during the step over the obstacle. This increase was even larger during the step over a higher obstacle (Fig. 14.2E) when a larger modification of the limb trajectory was needed (Fig. 14.2C). An increase of activity during the step over an obstacle was observed in the majority of PTNs, as illustrated in the diagrams (Figs. 14.2F,G). The phase of activity within the step cycle was preserved in most PTNs, but in some of them

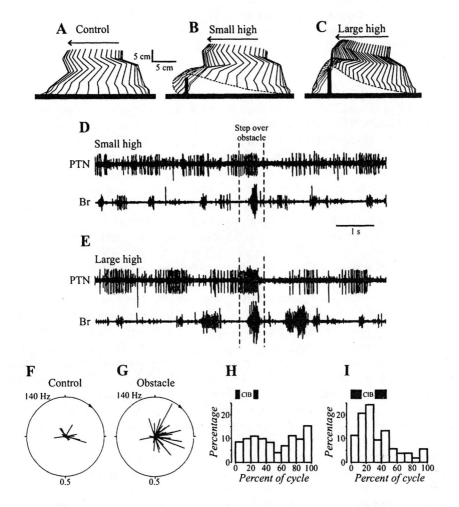

Fig. 14.2 Activity of pyramidal tract neurons when overstepping an obstacle. A–C: Stick figures showing the trajectory of the fore limb during the swing phase in the ordinary step (A) and in the steps over obstacles of different height (B,C). D,E: Activity of a pyramidal tract neuron (PTN) during ordinary steps and a step over obstacles of different height. The PTN was recorded along with the EMG of m. brachialis (Br). F,G: Vectoral representation of the activity of 53 PTNs in ordinary steps (F) and during steps over an obstacle (G). The length of each vector is proportional to the discharge frequency of a cell; the diameter of a circle represents a discharge of 140 Hz; the direction of each vector represents the phase of the PTN activity in the cycle. H,I: Histograms showing the percentage of cells discharging during different phases of the step cycle during control walking (H) and during steps over the obstacles (I). The cycle starts with activation of m. cleidobrachialis (ClB), whose phase of activity is shown by a bar. A–E are based on Drew (1991*a*) and F–I are based on Drew (1993).

(~25 per cent) a considerable displacement of the phase of activity was observed during the step over an obstacle. This most often occurred in the PTNs firing in the stance phase in ordinary steps: their peak activity moved to the swing phase when the animal stepped over an obstacle (Fig. 14.2H,I).

In many PTNs, which increased their activity during steps over obstacles, a strong correlation of the activity with the activity of a single muscle (or a small group of synergistic muscles acting around a single joint) was observed (Drew 1993), as in the PTN shown in Figs. 14.2D,E which appeared strongly linked to m. brachialis. These PTNs seem to precisely code specific aspects of the limb trajectory by affecting the activity of specific muscles (or of a few synergists). In many PTNs, however, a correlation of their activity with the activity of a particular muscle was not found. These latter PTNs seem to have wider projections in the spinal forelimb centre. Anatomical and electrophysiological studies have shown that there is a widespread branching of corticospinal axons in the spinal cord so that a single PTN can affect a number of motor neuron pools. A given pool is also affected by numerous PTNs, somewhat differing in their individual projection patterns (Futami *et al.* 1979; Shinoda *et al.* 1976, 1986).

The modifications of the pattern of stepping, that are necessary to overstep an obstacle, are incorporated into the locomotory rhythm so that the animal may continue its forward progression with minimal disruption and without loss of equilibrium. This is achieved, first of all, by a tight linkage of corticospinal commands to a particular phase of the ongoing step cycle. Although the cat sees the obstacle during a few steps preceding the modified step, most PTNs showed changes in their discharge pattern just prior to, or during, the step over the obstacle as illustrated in Figs. 14.2D,E (Drew 1993). This finding clearly shows (1) that the spinal rhythm generators impose temporal (phasic) constraints upon the processing of visual information (visuo-motor transformation), and (2) that this processing is fulfilled *before* formation of the corticospinal signals. The PTN activity thus represents pure motor commands.

The second mechanism promoting a preservation of the basic locomotor pattern during step modifications has already been considered (see Section 13.4). It is a phase-dependent modulation of the effect of any descending volleys, including the corticospinal ones, on the spinal locomotor networks, the modulation being performed by the spinal rhythm generators directly in the spinal cord. It was found that a weak stimulation of small loci in the motor cortex (or a weak stimulation of the pyramidal tract) during locomotion gave a very efficient activation of limb muscles when the stimulation was performed in that phase of the step in which the muscles have to be active according to the basic locomotor programme. With stronger or longer stimulation, however, the cortical influences may modify the basic locomotor pattern. For example, stimulation while the leg was in the air could prolong the swing phase, whereas stimulation while the leg was on the ground could curtail the stance and initiate a new phase of swing (Orlovsky 1972*a*; Armstrong and Drew 1985; Drew 1991*a*).

Modifications of the limb trajectory when overstepping an obstacle are accompanied by specific changes in the movement of the contralateral limb and, presumably, of the hind limbs and trunk. These changes can be considered as the postural support of the voluntary gait modifications. These postural reactions are presumably caused by the brainstem mechanisms. It was found that corticofugal neurons in area 4 not only send a command for overstepping an obstacle to the forelimb centre, but also a command addressed to the pontomedullary reticular formation. These signals can be used to trigger dynamic postural responses (Kably and Drew 1998*a*,*b*)

14.3.2   Accurate foot placement

In this locomotor task, the foot of the limb that moves forward in the swing-phase, has to be placed at a definite spot on the ground ('target') selected by means of vision (Fig. 14.3A). The location of this spot (black circle in Fig. 14.3A) may differ from the placing point determined by the spinal limb controller (empty circle in Fig. 14.3A) in any of its three spatial (x, y, or z) coordinates. If one considers only flat terrain, there are two possible strategies for solving the task of placing the foot on a definite spot: single step modification and mutual step modifications. These two strategies are illustrated in Figs. 14.3B,C for a simpler case in which corrections of the foot placement are needed only along the x-axis. While using a single step modification strategy, the cat is approaching the target with its normal (governed by the spinal controllers) steps, with the step length S_0 (1–3 in Fig. 14.3B), and only the very last step, aimed at placing the foot on the selected spot, is visually corrected (the value of correction is ΔS_b). This type of limb movement resembles reaching movements, i.e. the volitional movements aimed at reaching a certain target in space (Georgopoulos and Grillner 1989). There are, however, three major differences between these two types of movements. First, in reaching movements, the corticospinal system (and, to some degree, the rubrospinal one) are completely responsible for the initiation and performance of the movement. In contrast, their function during locomotion is only a correction of an ongoing movement generated by the spinal limb controller. Second, in ordinary reaching movements, the target has a stationary location in space, while during locomotion the target is continuously moving in relation to the animal at a speed equal to that of the walking animal. Third, ordinary reaching movements are usually under continuous visual feedback control. During locomotion, however, the cat does not see its limbs (Fig. 14.3A).

In a multiple step modification strategy (Fig. 14.3C), not only the very last step (4) but also a few preceding steps (1–3) are slightly modified in length (ΔS_i) as compared with ordinary steps (S_0), and these small changes of the step length are accumulated. This strategy has been analysed in detail for humans (Laurent and Thomson 1988).

A modification of the second strategy can be observed when the cat walks along a horizontal ladder with evenly spaced rungs (Fig. 14.3D). In this task, the stride length in each step differs from that determined by the spinal limb controller. The fact that one can continue walking on the stair for some time after shutting the eyes means that visual corrections of the step length are not performed in each step but rather that the spinal programme of stepping is modified to have a step length equal to the distance between the steps of the stair. It was found that the

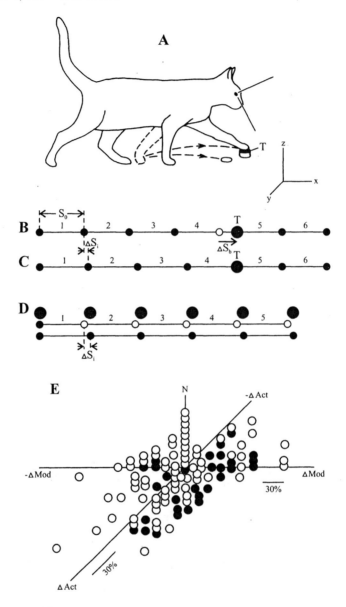

Fig. 14.3 Locomotion with accurate foot placement, and activity of neurons in motor cortex. A: A visually selected site for the foot placement (filled circle) may differ from the spinally pre-programmed site (empty circle) in any spatial coordinate. B,C: Two possible strategies for placing the foot at the 'target' spot (T)—single step modification (B) and multiple step modifications (C). Small filled circles show the real points of foot contact in successive step $(1, 2, \dots)$; an empty circle shows the point of foot contact in the fourth step as planned by the non-modified programme for stepping. S_0, the step length according to the non-modified programme; ΔS_b and ΔS_i, modifications of the step length with strategies shown in A and B, respectively. D: Walking on the rungs of the horizontal ladder (shown by large filled circles). Small empty circles show the pre-programmed points for foot placement,

step length modification is associated with a dramatic change in the activity of neurons of the forelimb area of the motor cortex, including PTNs (Beloozerova and Sirota 1988, 1993*b*). Figure 14.3E shows that 88 out 108 (81 per cent) of motor cortex neurons changed their activity during locomotion on a ladder as compared with overground locomotion. In most of them, the level of activity, as well as the degree of step-related rhythmical modulation increased considerably.

Thus, the majority of the fore limb-related PTNs considerably change their activity in two different tasks related to visually induced modifications of the step pattern: modifications of the step length (Figs. 14.3D,E) and modifications of foot trajectory (lifting the foot when overstepping an obstacle, Fig. 14.2). These findings correspond well to those obtained when studying reaching arm movements in the monkey: the majority of arm-related PTNs changed their activity during performance of a goal-directed movement in any part of the working space of the arm (Georgopoulos *et al.* 1993). There are two possible explanations for these results, differing mainly in the assumed content of the corticospinal commands. According to the first hypothesis, a corticospinal command is a rather general instruction addressed to the spinal cord in the form of activity of a large population of PTNs. The decoding of this command, i.e. the detailed specification of the activation patterns of different individual muscles, takes place in the spinal cord (Georgopoulos *et al.* 1983). Another explanation is that the corticospinal command is a rather detailed instruction, and the involvement of the majority of PTNs in the control of any reaching limb movement (or in any modification of the basic pattern in the case of stepping (Drew 1993)) simply reflects the fact that these very complicated movements involve numerous limb muscles, each of which needs supraspinal control. It does not seem unlikely that both hypotheses are partly true, and a corticospinal command contains both general instruction for movement modification and more specific details of muscle activation.

At the moment, information concerning the routes and processes by which the visuomotor transformation is performed is not readily available. Data from experiments in primates suggest that the visual signal passes from primary visual cortical areas to parietal and temporal cortex, from where it passes progressively to premotor cortex and finally to the primary motor cortex.

14.4 CONCLUSIONS

1. The motor cortex does not play any significant role in the control of 'simple' locomotion generated by the automatic control system. However, it plays a decisive role in the control of visually induced gait modifications. It also plays

---

small filled circles the real points after corrections (ΔS_i). E: Changes in the activity of the motor cortical neurons when walking on the ladder as compared with normal locomotion. Horizontal axis, changes in the average activity (ΔAct) and the depth of modulation (ΔMod) in individual neurons; vertical axis, number of neurons. Filled circles and empty circles, pyramidal and non-pyramidal neurons, respectively. E is from Beloozerova and Sirota (1988).

a role in compensation for unexpected, large perturbations of the locomotor pattern.

2. Spinal rhythm generators exert an influence on the motor cortex, causing a rhythmical bursting in the corticospinal and other cortical neurons. This rhythmic modulation of the motor cortex neurons and, presumably, also the neurons in other cortical areas processing visual information, is a basis for the generation of visually induced corticospinal motor commands strictly confined to a definite phase of the step cycle.

3. To step over an obstacle, the cat modifies its foot trajectory in the swing-phase in accordance with the size and shape of the obstacle. These modifications are caused, to a large extent, by the motor cortex. The majority of corticospinal neurons significantly change their firing pattern while overstepping an obstacle. In some of them, the activity is tightly linked with the activity of different limb muscles.

4. In the task of accurate foot placing—for example walking on a horizontal ladder—a modification of the step length is caused, to a large extent, by the motor cortex. This type of locomotion is also associated with a considerable modification of the activity in the corticospinal tract.

Part IV
Human locomotion

15

Walking and running in humans

15.1 MOTOR PATTERN IN WALKING AND RUNNING

The analysis of motor and EMG patterns of human locomotion has been performed in numerous studies (see for example Brandell 1973; Herman *et al.* 1976; Knutsson 1981; Milner *et al.* 1971; Elliot and Blanksby 1976; Nilsson *et al.* 1985; Grillner *et al.* 1979; Winter 1991). Several studies have also addressed the different modifications of the locomotor pattern that occur during training or in different visuo-locomotor tasks (see for example Thomson 1980; Laurent and Thomson 1988). In general, the locomotor activity in humans has been much more thoroughly studied than its neural control and in this matter we have to rely mainly on extrapolations from simpler animal models (Grillner and Orlovsky 1991).

Man is capable of locomotion with a very wide range of velocities, ranging from very slow speeds to extreme values of near $45\,\mathrm{km\,h^{-1}}$ toward the end of a $100\,\mathrm{m}$ race. The adaptation of the motor pattern to increasing speed is accomplished by increase in both frequency and amplitude of leg movement. In addition, man can change from one mode of progression, walking, to another mode, running.

The basic features of walking and running are the same (Fig 15.1): the legs perform alternating stepping movements, and the step cycle of each leg consists of a stance and a swing phase. At the same time, many differences exist between the motor patterns of walking and running, both with regard to the timing of various events within the step cycle and with regard to flexion–extension movements at different joints. These small but numerous distinctions indeed make walking and running two different forms of locomotion, and gradual transitions from one pattern to another have never been observed.

In walking, one or two legs are in contact with the ground throughout the step cycle, and the body weight is continuously supported either by the left leg, or by the right leg, or by both. In running, there are phases in the step cycle when the body has no support. Both in walking and in running, the knee and hip antigravitational muscles (extensors) are activated during and slightly before the stance phase, as illustrated in Fig. 15.1 for the hip extensor gluteus maximus (GM) and for the knee extensor vastus lateralis (VL). The main burst of activity in the ankle extensors is somewhat delayed in relation to the other extensors, as in the ankle extensor gastrocnemius lateralis (LG) in Fig. 15.1. The hip and knee extensors do not allow these joints to flex markedly under the action of the body weight. By the end of the stance phase, the extensor muscles provide force moving the body forward. An

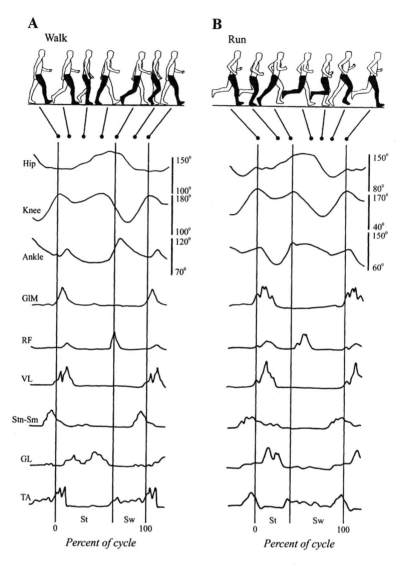

Fig. 15.1 Motor and EMG patterns of walking and running in man. A: Patterns for walking at the speed of 1.6 m s^{-1}. B: Patterns of running at the speed of 4 m s^{-1} in the same subject. There are shown the angular displacements in the hip, knee, and ankle joints of the right leg (flexion down) and integrated and rectified EMGs of some representative muscles of this leg. All values are averaged over several normalized cycles. Upper diagrams show the approximate body configuration in the corresponding phases of the step cycle. (Abbreviations: GlM, gluteus maximus; RF, rectus femoris; VL, vastus lateralis; Stn–Sm, semitendinosus and semimembranosus; GL, gastrocnemius lateralis; TA, tibialis anterior; St, stance phase; Sw, swing phase.) Based on Nilsson *et al.* (1985).

important source of this force development is a group of ankle extensors strongly contracting at the end of the support phase, which results in an ankle extension that pushes the body forward.

In the swing phase, the leg is transferred forward in relation to the body, and this work is done mainly by a group of hip flexors, including m. rectus femoris (RF in Fig. 15.1). In walking, the lower part of the leg is moderately elevated above ground during the transfer (Fig. 15.1A), whereas in fast running it is lifted much higher due to a stronger knee flexion (Fig. 15.1B). The biomechanical advantage of this strong flexion is that the centre of gravity of the leg gets closer to the hip, and less torque is needed to bring the leg forward during swing. At the end of the swing phase, the foot touches ground. In walking, this occurs with a 'heel strike', and at the moment of contact the foot points upward. Soon after this, the whole sole of the foot gets in contact with the ground because of an ankle extension. This extension is delayed to some extent by a group of ankle flexors, which become active shortly before the heel strike, as illustrated for m. tibialis anterior (TA) in Fig. 15.1A. The activated TA acts like a spring, softening the heel strike. In running, on the contrary, the front part of the entire sole of the foot touches ground initially, and all extensor muscles are coactivated. This contributes to a different force trajectory in walking and running, with one peak of the vertical component of the ground reaction force in running, and two peaks in walking (Nilsson and Thorstensson 1989).

These sequences of events in the step cycle are preserved at different speeds of progression. In contrast, the temporal characteristics of the cycle, and the amplitude of the movements, may change with speed. Figure 15.2 shows how these characteristics of the step cycle depend on the speed. In walking, the cycle duration decreases with speed, and this decrease is caused primarily by a reduction of the stance phase, whereas the swing phase changes only slightly (Fig. 15.2A). The amplitudes of hip and knee flexion at different speeds of walking are nearly constant (Fig. 15.2B). In this respect, kinematics of walking in humans is similar to that in cats (see Section 10.1), crustaceans (see Section 4.1), and insects (see Section 6.1), when they move in the lower range of their locomotor speeds. During running, the stance duration, and therefore the cycle duration, also decreases with speed, whereas the swing duration remains almost unchanged (Fig. 15.2A). The hip and knee amplitude increase almost twice in the speed range of 1 to $8\,\mathrm{m\,s^{-1}}$ (Fig. 15.2B). From Fig. 15.2 one can also see that man is able to chose between the gaits—walking or running—over a relatively wide range of velocities.

The main features that make walking and running motor patterns in humans different from those of other mammals are the following:

1. Due to the vertical body orientation, the hip excursions during the step cycle are between 90° and 180° in relation to the body axis. This contrasts with, for instance, quadrupeds such as the cat, the hind limbs of which are much more flexed during locomotion, and the hip angle varies between 70° and 110° (see Section 10.1).

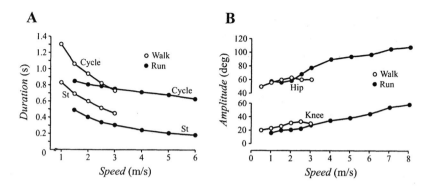

Fig. 15.2 Different characteristics of the step cycle as functions of speed. A: The cycle duration (Cycle) and the stance phase duration (St) plotted versus speed. B: The amplitude of movements at the hip and knee joints plotted versus speed. Curves with empty circles, walking; with filled circles, running. Based on Nilsson and Thorstensson (1989).

2. A coactivation of all extensors at the moment of foot contact is typical for quadrupeds (see Section 10.1). In humans a mixed muscle synergy (hip and knee extensors plus ankle flexors) becomes active at the moment of heel strike, while the ankle extensors come into action later, by the end of the stance phase.
3. Because of the upright, vertical body orientation during locomotion in humans, there are specific requirements for the maintenance of equilibrium different from the case of quadrupedal locomotion (see Section 15.4).

15.2   LEG CONTROLLERS AND THEIR ACTIVATION

The general scheme of the locomotor control system (Fig. 0.1) is also applicable to humans. The principal elements of the system are the controllers for the left and right legs, that can be activated by simple commands. Under special experimental conditions, these commands can be replaced by tonic afferent input (Gurfinkel *et al.* 1998). Figure 15.3G shows an experimental arrangement for reflexive elicitation of stepping movements in one of the legs. The leg was fastened to a double link suspension system that eliminated the effect of gravity on the leg. The subject was instructed to relax and not to intervene with movements that might be induced by peripheral stimuli. In response to sensory input—vibration (20–60 Hz) of one of the leg muscles—the leg performed stepping movements with alternating bursts in the flexor and extensor muscles, and coordinated flexion–extension movements in the hip and knee joints (Fig. 15.3A). The pattern of interjoint coordination in both flexor and extensor phases of the cycle (Figs. 15.3C,D) was similar to that in voluntary stepping (Figs. 15.3E,F). Occasionally, stimulation of a muscle evoked not 'forward' but 'backward' stepping (Fig. 15.3B). The stepping movements could be evoked by stimulation of various muscles of the leg. With a different experimental design, alternating stepping movements of both legs could be evoked by muscle vibration (Gurfinkel *et al.* 1998).

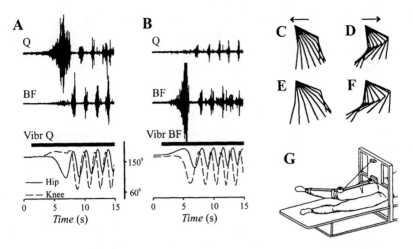

Fig. 15.3 Locomotor-like movements evoked by the leg muscle vibration in a normal subject. A: Rhythmic leg movements evoked by vibration (Vibr) of m. quadriceps (Q) are similar to forward stepping. B: Rhythmic movements evoked by vibration of m. biceps femoris (BF) are similar to backward stepping. There are shown the EMGs of Q and BF, as well as movements at the hip and knee joints. C–F: Stick diagrams showing leg configuration during voluntary stepping (C,D) and vibration-induced stepping (E,F). Successive leg configurations during its movement from the anterior to the posterior extreme position are shown in C,E; during the opposite movement, in D,F. G: Experimental arrangement for the horizontal leg suspension and for elicitation of 'air-stepping' by means of muscle vibration. From Gurfinkel *et al.* (1998).

These experiments have shown that:

1. Each of the legs in man has its own controller that can operate either alone or in coordination with the controller of the contralateral leg.
2. The controller can be subdivided into the nervous mechanisms controlling different joints. These mechanisms can operate with different phase lag in relation to each other, which determines the mode of locomotion, that is forward or backward stepping.
3. For activation of the leg controllers, a very simple command, that is a tonic drive, is sufficient.

A body of evidence indicates that, despite the cephalization of most motor functions in humans and other primates, the basic nervous mechanisms constituting the leg controller are located in the lumbosacral spinal cord, as in the cat and other quadrupeds (see Section 11.2). Observations on paraplegic patients, with a complete or almost complete rupture of the spinal cord, have shown that the lumbosacral spinal cord in these patients is not usually able to generate stepping movements spontaneously or in response to sensory stimulation (see Vilensky *et al.* 1992 for a review). A similar conclusion was reached on monkeys (Eidelberg *et al.* 1981). Stepping movements in spinal humans, however, could be induced, at least in some cases, when the patient was standing on a moving treadmill with weight support; these movements improved with daily training but still remained much weaker than in normal stepping. The improvement could be dramatic in patients with incomplete paraplegia, suggesting an important role of even weak supraspinal drive (Dietz *et al.* 1994). Similar results were obtained on monkeys with partial transection of the spinal cord (Vilensky *et al.* 1992).

The capacity of the lumbosacral spinal cord in paraplegic patients to generate stepping movements under the effect of a tonic drive was directly demonstrated in experiments with electrical stimulation of the spinal cord below the level of its rupture by means of implanted electrodes (Gerasimenko *et al.* 1996). Continuous stimulation (20–50 Hz) of the dorsal aspect of the spinal cord at the L2–L3 level elicited stepping-like movements of both legs.

In the decerebrated monkey, electrical stimulation of the posterior diencephalon and mesencephalon, that is the area corresponding to the mesencephalic loco-motor region in the cat (see Section 12.1) elicited stepping movements (Eidelberg *et al.* 1981). This finding suggests that the systems for initiation of locomotion in primates and other mammals are similar.

In the cat, a crucial role for the activation of the spinal locomotor mechanisms is played by the reticulospinal pathways (see Section 12.1). Experiments with partial transections of the spinal cord in the monkey (Eidelberg *et al.* 1981) have shown that recovery of locomotor function is faster and better if the ventrolateral quadrants of the spinal cord, that is the area where descending reticulo- and vestibulospinal tracts come, were left intact (Goldberger 1969). This area is not necessary for recovery to occur, however, and stepping movements could also be initiated via pathways—presumably corticospinal or propriospinal—descending in the dorsolateral quadrants (Mettler 1944; Mettler and Liss 1959; Goldberger 1965).

15.3 CENTRAL PATTERN GENERATOR AND SENSORY FEEDBACK

In the spinal cat, injection of DOPA can activate the locomotor network in the spinal cord (see Section 11.3). In spinal macaque monkeys, injection of DOPA did not induce the locomotor activity, however (Eidelberg *et al.* 1981). In a different species of monkey (*Callithrix jacchus*), a fictive locomotory rhythm could be induced by DOPA (Hultborn *et al.* 1993), though, indicating that a locomotor CPG exists also in primates. The role of this CPG in real locomotion is minor, however. It was found that patients suffering a loss of proprioception and touch usually are not able to walk, which indicates that sensory feedback is necessary for the generation of stepping (see for example Blouin *et al.* 1993). However, one case has been reported when the locomotor activity was restored in a patient without light touch and proprioception below the neck; the deficit was caused by a sensory neuropathy (Burnett *et al.* 1989; Lajoie *et al.* 1996). This deafferented subject managed to substitute the somatosensory feedback with visual feedback after long-lasting training. He was continuously looking at his legs when walking; with closed eyes, he was not able to walk.

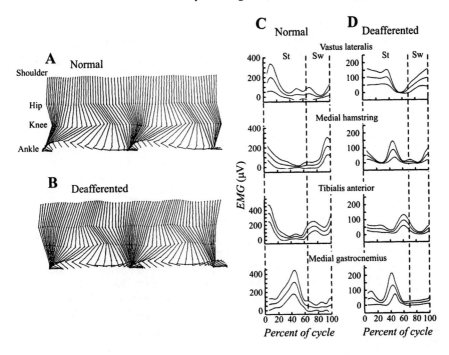

Fig. 15.4 Motor and EMG pattern of walking in the deafferented subject compared with normal subject. A,B: Stick diagrams of stepping movements in the normal (A) and deafferented (B) subjects. The cycle period in both cases was about 1 s. Two successive steps as viewed from the right side are shown. C,D: The EMG activity of some representative muscles during walking in the normal (C) and deafferented (D) subject. An averaged value of muscle activity ± SD is shown as a function of the phase in the normalized step cycle; the stance (St) and swing (Sw) phases are indicated. Based on Lajoie *et al.* (1996).

Figure 15.4 shows the kinematics and EMG patterns for the right leg in a normal subject (A,C) and in a deafferented subject (B,D). It is remarkable that the basic features of stepping can be generated without somatosensory feedback. Some differences between the subjects can be noticed, however, including a lower general level of the EMG activity, and abnormal phases of activity of some muscles in the step cycle of the deafferented subject. For example, m. tibialis anterior is normally active at the beginning of the stance phase (see also Section 15.1), whereas in the deafferented subject it is active at the end of this phase.

It seems highly unlikely that the deafferented subject is able to control and correct individually, via visual feedback, the contractions of each of about hundred muscles moving a leg. It seems more likely that visual information is used for updating the pre-existing central motor programmes for stepping, and for their adaptation to environmental conditions. This idea was first formulated by Ghez *et al.* (1995) when they investigated the effect of vision on the performance of reaching arm movements in deafferented patients. It was found that visual inspection of the limb during movement, and even before the onset of movement, considerably improved the motor performance. It was proposed that the improvements in performance produced after viewing the limb were mediated by visual updating of internal models of the limb. Vision of the limb at rest may provide configuration information, while vision of the limb in motion provides additional dynamic information. Both types of information make the central motor programme more adapted to reality.

15.4   MAINTENANCE OF EQUILIBRIUM DURING LOCOMOTION

In bipedal locomotion, the main aim of the stepping movements is to move the body forward. These movements, however, can also be considered as a means of preventing the body from falling in one direction or the other, since the equilibrium during bipedal locomotion is dynamic. The inherent instability of the vertical posture is also exploited to assist in propelling the body forward (Pedotti 1977; Gurfinkel and Shik 1973). The direction and amplitude of the leg movement in the swing phase are strictly linked to the motion of the body. On the other hand, the locomotor programme contains features that seem to maximize the stability during movement. For instance, in each step the body is moved toward the side of the supporting leg to ensure maximal lateral stability. The trunk and arm movements accompanying human locomotion also serve to provide stability (Thorstensson *et al.* 1982, 1984). Separate nervous mechanisms are responsible for stabilization of the head and eye positions during locomotion; they are driven by visual, vestibular, and somatosensory inputs (Berthoz and Pozzo 1988).

Various compensatory movements are aimed at maintaining the equilibrium during locomotion, despite different perturbations. The perturbations can be divided into two major categories, expected and unexpected ones. The corresponding postural correcting mechanisms operate in the feedforward or feedback mode. For many types of postural perturbations, both expected and unexpected, which a subject may encounter during locomotion, there are specific correcting programmes incorporated into the basic locomotor programme (Nashner 1980; Nashner and Forssberg 1986; Hirschfeld and Forssberg 1988, 1991).

15.4.1   Feedforward mode of postural control

Figure 15.5 illustrates postural adjustments associated with voluntary arm movements in a subject walking on a treadmill (Nashner and Forssberg 1986). The subject was instructed to pull or push a handle in response to tone stimuli which were presented in different phases of the step cycle. The EMGs of different muscles were recorded in ordinary steps and in disturbed steps. It was found that, depending on the motor task—pull or push—either the elbow flexor, m. biceps, or the elbow extensor, m. triceps were activated. This activity, however, was preceded by a 'postural response' in the leg muscles (the areas covered with a diagonal shading in Fig. 15.5). The anticipatory response depended on two factors: the direction of the force developed in the voluntary motor task, and the phase of the step cycle. Thus, several specific muscle synergies were formed depending on the combination of these factors, as shown in the stick diagrams (Fig. 15.5). In all

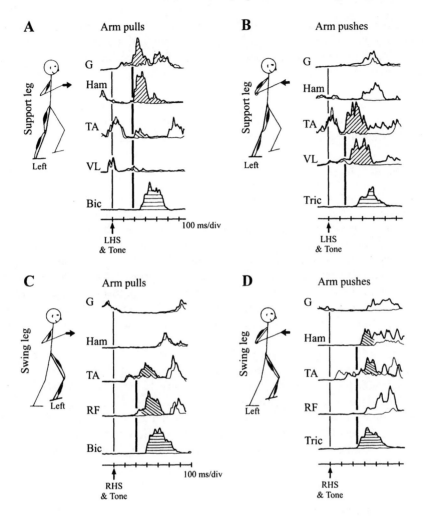

Fig. 15.5 Postural EMG responses during walking associated with voluntary arm movements. The subject walking on the treadmill at the speed of $1\,\mathrm{m\,s^{-1}}$ was instructed to pull (A,C) or push (B,D) the handle by its right arm in response to tone stimulus (Tone). The tone was presented at the moment of the left heel strike (LHS) in A,B, or the right heel strike (RHS) in C,D. There are shown the rectified and averaged EMGs of different muscles of the left leg recorded in normal cycles (thin lines) and disturbed cycles (thick lines). A difference between the EMGs in the disturbed and normal steps, that is a postural response, is shown as an area with diagonal shading. The EMG responses in the active arm muscles, that is biceps for pulling (A,C) and triceps for pushing (B,D) are also shown. Heavy vertical lines show the latency of postural responses. Stick figures illustrate muscle contractions and approximate orientation of the body. Arrows at the hands indicate the direction of force exerted on the subject. The EMGs were recorded from m. gastrocnemius (G), hamstring (Ham), tibialis anterior (TA), rectus femoris (RF), vastus lateralis (VL), biceps brachii (Bic), and triceps (Tric). Based on Nachner and Forssberg (1986).

cases, the response was aimed at counteracting the anticipated disturbance of the body orientation caused by interaction of the subject with the handle.

The strong dependence of the postural response on the phase of the step cycle indicates that the mechanisms responsible for postural corrections are under powerful influence of the limb controllers, so that corrections are always adjusted to the current state of the moving legs, as was also shown for the corrections of stepping movements in the cat (see for example 'stumbling reaction', Section 11.5) and in the stick insect (see Section 6.3).

15.4.2   Feedback mode of postural control

Nashner (1980) investigated EMG and motor responses to unexpected perturbations of stepping movements. The perturbations were caused by a sudden movement of the supporting surface in different directions. The corrective EMG responses occurred depending on two factors—the type of perturbation and the phase of the cycle, as was found for the postural feedforward adjustments (see Section 15.4.1). It was also found that the EMG responses closely resembled (in organization and latencies) those responses elicited by imposing the same movements of the substrate on the standing subjects (Nashner 1977; Nashner *et al.* 1979). These finding strongly suggest that the same postural control mechanisms are used in standing and walking subjects.

An important finding by Nashner (1980) was that, although the imposed perturbations were smaller in amplitude and rate than the normal walking movements, the EMG postural responses were significantly larger than the EMG activity in undisturbed step cycles. A question arises: how are the afferent signals from the leg mechanoreceptors processed in the CNS to reveal their small changes that occur in perturbed cycles? Comparison of 'anticipated sensation' with 'actual sensation' could be a possible solution of the problem of detecting postural disturbances (Nashner 1980).

15.5   CONCLUSIONS

1. The functional organization of the walking control system in humans is similar to that in cats and arthropods. Each of the legs is controlled by a semi-autonomous nervous mechanism—the leg controller. This mechanism is responsible for the generation of alternating activities in two groups of muscles that contract in the stance and swing phases of the step cycle, respectively. The controller can be activated by a simple command providing a tonic drive. It seems most likely that alternating stepping movements of the left and right legs are due to the interactions between their controllers. The leg controllers have two basic modes of operation—walking and running—somewhat differing in the timing and amplitude of contraction of different muscle groups in the step cycle.

2. The basic nervous mechanisms constituting the leg controller are located in the lumbosacral spinal cord. Afferent signals from the moving leg are very important for the generation of normal pattern of stepping. The neuronal

organization and the operation of the spinal networks generating stepping movements are not known.

3. It seems likely that the reticulospinal system plays an important role in activation of the spinal mechanisms for stepping. However, other descending system in primates may also activate these mechanisms. The real contribution of different descending systems in initiation of stepping is not known.

4. Complex postural mechanisms participate in the maintenance of a vertical body orientation during locomotion. They operate according to feedforward and feedback principles. The corrective postural responses, generated by these mechanisms, depend on the type of postural disturbance and on the phase of the step cycle. Very little is known about the localization of the postural mechanisms in the brain and about their neuronal organization.

16

General conclusions

In this book, we have considered neural mechanisms for the control of locomotion in 13 selected species belonging to very remote branches of the evolutionary tree, from molluscs to humans, and exhibiting very different forms of locomotion—crawling, swimming, walking, and flying. In the Preface we claimed that, despite the enormous diversity in the structure of the locomotor organs, in their motor pattern, and in the structure of the CNS in different species, the functional organization of the locomotor control system (Fig. 0.1) is similar. Indeed, as the reader can see in the book, all principal components of the system and their interactions, shown in Fig. 0.1, can be found in each of the investigated species. A remarkable diversity is observed, however, in the intrinsic structure of the functional components.

Controllers for locomotor organs. Each of the locomotor organs (leg, wing, trunk) has its own control nervous mechanism, the controller. A controller can be activated by a simple command (for example tonic excitatory drive), but it performs a very complex function—generation of the locomotory rhythm with the sequential activation of different muscle groups of the locomotor organ. In different species, the controllers differ in the role that is played by central mechanisms and sensory feedback. At one extreme we have the controllers that need minimal or no feedback for their function, that is they can operate as central pattern generators. Such mechanisms control wing flapping in *Clione*, and body undulations in *Aplysia*, *Tritonia*, leech, and tadpole. Close to this class of controllers are the controller for swimming body undulations in the lamprey, and the controller for wing beating in the locust.

At the other extreme we find the leg controller of the stick insect, which practically cannot operate under open-loop conditions. Finally, the leg controllers in the crayfish, lobster, locust, and cat occupy an intermediate position. Under open-loop conditions, they can generate rhythmic activity resembling, to some extent, a normal locomotor pattern. A closed feedback loop is necessary for their normal function, however.

These species differences confirm the intuitive notion that the control of movements in a homogeneous medium (swimming, flying) requires less sensory information than the control of walking on ground, where in each step the leg can be affected by irregularities of the substrate.

Another cause for differences between the design of controllers in different species is the varying degree of complexity of the locomotor organs. To control the wing beating in *Clione* or locust, or the body flexions in the swimming *Tritonia*, only simple alternating commands to the two antagonistic muscle groups are required. Correspondingly, the controller for locomotor organs in these species is relatively simple. The controller for a stepping limb is more complex and may consist of several subunits controlling the individual joints of the limb with definite phase-shifts in relation to each other (Fig. 0.1B). Finally, the controller for body undulations in the swimming leech or lamprey is most complex in the sense that it is composed of a great number of rhythmically active subunits, each of which affects the muscles in the corresponding body segments. Interactions between the subunits (segmental oscillators) determines their phase relations and gives rise to the propagating waves of body undulations.

For some of the controllers that can operate under open-loop conditions, an analysis of the central pattern generator network has been performed. A few principally different designs of the rhythm generator were found: (1) a biphasic generator, with inhibitory interactions between two antagonistic groups of interneurons (in *Clione*, lamprey, and tadpole); (2) a three-phasic generator, with excitatory and inhibitory interactions among three groups of interneurons (in *Tritonia*); (3) in the leech, the rhythm generator is more complex and is based primarily on interactions between numerous inhibitory neurons. One can thus see a number of different solutions for the same general problem—the generation of the locomotory rhythm.

A common feature of the controllers for locomotor organs in different species is that the rhythm generator produces a relatively simple temporal pattern, which is further processed and transformed into a more complicated pattern by the neuronal mechanisms constituting the output motor stage of the controller. The output motor stages in different species strongly differ in their neuronal organization, however. In *Clione*, it includes only the motor neurons, whereas in the cat it consists of different cell types—the alpha and gamma motor neurons, and Ia interneurons.

Initiation of locomotion. In all investigated species, locomotion is initiated by means of an excitatory drive to the locomotor organ controllers. The vigour of locomotion is proportional to the intensity of this drive. The drive is delivered by a command system. Experiments on simpler animals like *Clione* have shown that the command system consists of a number of subsystems that affect not only the locomotor controllers but also a number of non-locomotor mechanisms. Due to such a design, different gross motor synergies can be formed, and locomotion can be incorporated in different forms of behaviour. In vertebrates, different groups of reticulospinal neurons are an important component of the command system for initiation of locomotion. These neurons receive input from the mesencephalic locomotor region and other brain structures involved in the initiation of locomotion, and simultaneously activate all the spinal networks responsible for the generation of the locomotor pattern.

Postural control. A striking similarity can be found between the functional organization of postural mechanisms in swimming and flying animals belonging to phylogenetically remote groups—in *Clione*, locust, and lamprey. In all these animals a deviation from the normal body orientation affects two groups of antagonistic command neurons; the neurons are driven in a reciprocal way by orientation-dependent sensory inputs. The two groups elicit opposite postural corrective responses, and the body orientation at which they are equal will be stabilized. The postural mechanisms in these species differ, however, in that they are driven by sensory inputs of different modalities—by vestibular input in the lamprey and *Clione*, and by visual input in the locust. Also, the postural command systems evoke changes in the body orientation by affecting different motor systems—by tail bending in *Clione*, by modification of wing beating in the locust, and by modification of trunk undulations in the lamprey.

The nervous mechanisms for postural control in walking animals are very different from those in the swimming and flying ones. The postural control system in the walking animals rely, to a much larger extent, on somatosensory information which, due to the mechanical interaction of the animal with the ground, well reflects the current orientation of the body and its segments. Also, because of the complexity of the motor apparatus in the legged animals, very complex postural corrective programmes are required. These programmes are incorporated into the basic stepping programme.

Investigation of postural mechanisms in simpler animals like *Clione* and lamprey revealed an important principle of coding the spatial information: this information is presented as the activity of large populations of cells with wide angular zones of spatial sensitivity, rather than by the cells specifically tuned to narrow angular zones.

Are the conclusions reached on simple animal models applicable to mammals? Until the beginning of 1980s, the three authors of this book used cats as their main experimental model for studying the nervous control of locomotion. Between 1980 and 1985, however, S.G. switched to lampreys, whereas G.O. and T.D. moved to molluscs. One of the main reasons for this change was an increasing feeling of dissatisfaction caused by the fact that a number of principal questions concerning locomotor control could not be answered in the cat model. Above all we found it very difficult to describe the basic locomotor mechanisms in the cat (the leg controller, central pattern generator, command systems, etc.) in terms of activity of the corresponding neuronal networks. This difficulty was caused by the extreme complexity of the networks, with thousands of neurons involved in a coordinated activity.

As the reader can see from this book, the nervous mechanisms for locomotor control in invertebrates and lower vertebrates are much simpler, and some of them can be described in considerable detail, at the network and cellular level. The question arises, however, if these simple biological models can tell us anything substantial about nervous mechanisms for the corresponding functions in cats or humans. We believe they can. This belief is based on the numerous striking similarities between locomotor control mechanisms across the animal kingdom which we have tried to emphasize in this book.

References

Abraham, L. D. and Loeb, G. E. (1985). The distal hindlimb musculature of the cat. Patterns of normal use. *Experimental Brain Research*, 58, 580–93.

Acevedo, L. D., Hall, W. M., and Mulloney, B. (1994). Proctolin and excitation of the crayfish swimmeret system. *Journal of Comparative Neurology*, 345, 612–27.

Adkins, R. J., Cegnar, M. R., and Rafuse, D. D. (1971). Differential effects of lesions of the anterior and posterior sygmoid gyri in cats. *Brain Research*, 30, 411–14.

Advokat, C., Carew, T. J., and Kandel, E. R. (1976). Modification of a simple reflex in *Aplysia californica* by arousal with food stimuli. *Neuroscience Abstracts*, 2, 513.

Afelt, Z., Veber, N. B., and Maksimova, E. V. (1973). Reflex activity of chronically isolated spinal cord of the cat. (In Russian.) Nauka, Moscow.

Akazawa, K., Aldridge, J. W., Steeves, J. D., and Stein, R. B. (1982). Modulation of stretch reflexes during locomotion in the mesencephalic cat. *Journal of Physiology (London)*, 329, 553–67.

Alexander, R. M. N. (1969). Orientation of muscle fibres in the myomeres of fish. *Journal of mar. biol. Ass. U.K.*, 49, 263–90.

Alford, S. and Grillner, S. (1991). The involvement of $GABA_B$ receptors and coupled G-proteins in spinal GABAergic presynaptic inhibition. *Journal of Neuroscience*, 12, 3718–28.

Alford, S., Christenson, J., and Grillner, S. (1991). Presynaptic $GABA_A$ and $GABA_B$ receptor-mediated phasic modulation in axons of spinal motor interneurons. *European Journal of Neuroscience*, 3, 107–17.

Allen, G. I. and Tsukahara, N. (1974). Cerebrocerebellar communication systems. *Physiological Review*, 54, 957–1006.

Amos, A., Armstrong, D. M., and Marple-Horvat, D. E. (1989). Responses of motor cortical neurones in the cat to unexpected perturbations of locomotion. *Neuroscience Letters*, 104, 147–51.

Amos, A., Armstrong, D. M., and Marple-Horvat, D. E. (1990). Changes in the discharge patterns of motor cortical neurones associated with volitional changes in stepping in the cat. *Neuroscience Letters*, 109, 107–12.

Andersson, G. and Armstrong, D. M. (1985). Climbing fibre input to b zone Purkinje cells during locomotor perturbation in the cat. *Neuroscience Letters Supplement*, 22, S27.

Andersson, O. and Grillner, S. (1981). Peripheral control of the cat's step cycle. I. Phase dependent effects of ramp-movements of the hip during 'fictive locomotion'. *Acta Physiologica Scandinavica*, 113, 89–101.

Andersson, O. and Grillner, S. (1983). Peripheral control of the cat's step cycle. II. Entrainment of the central pattern generators for locomotion by sinusoidal hip movements during 'fictive locomotion'. *Acta Physiologica Scandinavica*, 118, 229–39.

Andersson, O., Forssberg, H., Grillner, S., and Lindquist, M. (1978). Phasic gain control of the transmission in cutaneous reflex pathways to motoneurons during 'fictive' locomotion. *Brain Research*, 149, 503–7.

Angstadt, J. D. and Friesen, W. O. (1993a). Modulation of swimming behavior in the medicinal leech. i. Effects of serotonin on the electrical properties of swim-gating cell 204. *Journal of Comparative Physiology A—Sensory Neurology and Behavioral Physiology*, 172, 223–34.

Angstadt, J. D. and Friesen, W. O. (1993*b*). Modulation of swimming behavior in the medicinal leech. ii. ionic conductances underlying serotonergic modulation of swim-gating cell 204. *Journal of Comparative Physiology A—Sensory Neural and Behavioral Physiology*, 172, 235–48.

Antziferova, L. I., Arshavsky, Y. I., Orlovsky, G. N., and Pavlova, G. A. (1980). Activity of neurons of cerebellar nuclei during fictitious scratch reflex in the cat. I. The fastigial nucleus. *Brain Research*, 200, 239–48.

Arbas, E. A. (1986). Control of hindlimb posture by wind-sensitive hairs and antennae during locust flight. *Journal of Comparative Physiology*, 159A, 849–57

Arkett, S. A. (1987). Ciliary arrest controlled by identified central neurons in a urochordate (Ascidiacea). *Journal of Comparative Physiology* 161, 837–47.

Arkett, S. A., Mackie, G. O., and Singla, C.L. (1987). Neuronal control of ciliary loco-motion in a gastropod veliger (*Calliostoma*). *Biological Bulletin of the Marine Biology Laboratory, Woods Hole*, 173, 513–26.

Armstrong, D. M. (1986). Supraspinal contributions to the initiation and control of loco-motion in the cat. *Progress in Neurobiology*, 26, 273–361.

Armstrong, D. M. (1988). The supraspinal control of mammalian locomotion. *Journal of Physiology*, 405, 1–37.

Armstrong, D. M. and Drew, T. (1984*a*). Discharges of pyramidal tract and other motor cortical neurones during locomotion in the cat. *Journal of Physiology*, 346, 471–95.

Armstrong, D. M. and Drew, T. (1984*b*). Locomotor-related neuronal discharges in cat motor cortex compared with peripheral receptive fields and evoked movements. *Journal of Physiology*, 346, 497–517.

Armstrong, D. M. and Drew, T. (1985). Forelimb electromyographic responses to motor cortex stimulation during locomotion in the cat. *Journal of Physiology*, 367, 327–51.

Armstrong, D. M. and Edgley, S. A. (1988). Discharges of interpositus and Purkinje cells of the cat cerebellum during locomotion under different conditions. *Journal of Physiology*, 400, 425–45.

Armstrong, D. M., Campbell, N. C., Edgley, S. A., Schild, R. F., and Trott, J. R. (1982). Investigations of the olivocerebellar and spinoolivary pathways. In *The cerebellum: new vistas* (eds. V. Chan-Palay and S. L. Palay), *Experimental Brain Research Supplement*, 6, pp. 195–232. Springer, New York.

Armstrong, D. M., Edgley, S. A., and Lidierth, M. (1988*a*). Complex spikes in Purkinje cells of the paravermal part of the anterior lobe of the cat cerebellum during locomotion. *Journal of Physiology*, 400, 405–14.

Arshavsky, Y. I., Kots, Y. M., Orlovsky, G. N., Rodionov, I. M., and Shik, M. L. (1965). Investigation of the biomechanics of running by the dog. *Biophysics*, 10, 737–46.

Arshavsky, Y. I., Berkinblit, M. B., Fukson, O. I., Gelfand, I. M., and Orlovsky, G. N. (1972*a*) Recordings of neurons of the dorsal spinocerebellar tract during evoked loco-motion. *Brain Research*, 43, 272–5.

Arshavsky, Y. I., Berkinblit, M. B., Fukson, O. I., Gelfand, I. M., and Orlovsky, G. N. (1972*b*). Origin of modulation in neurons of the ventral spinocerebellar tract during locomotion. *Brain Research*, 43, 276–9.

Arshavsky, Y. I., Berkinblit, M. B., Gelfand, I. M., Orlovsky, G. N., and Fukson, O. I. (1972*d*). Activity of the neurons of the dorsal spino-cerebellar tract during locomotion. *Biophysics*, 17, 506–14.

Arshavsky, Y. I., Berkinblit, M. B., Gelfand, I. M., Orlovsky, G. N., and Fukson, O. I. (1972*e*). Activity of the neurons of the ventral spino-cerebellar tract during locomotion. *Biophysics*, 17, 926–35.

Arshavsky, Y. I., Berkinblit, M. B., Gelfand, I. M., Orlovsky, G. N., and Fukson, O. I. (1972*f*). Activity of the neurons of the ventral spino-cerebellar tract during locomotion of cats with deafferented hindlimbs. *Biophysics*, 17, 1169–76.

Arshavsky, Y. I., Berkinblit, M. B., Gelfand, I. M., Orlovsky, G. N., and Fukson, O. I. (1974). Differences in the performans of spinocerebellar tract neurons during artificial stimulation and locomotion. In *Mechanisms of neuronal integration in nervous center* (ed. P. G. Kostyuk), pp. 99–105. Nauka, Leningrad. (In Russian.)

Arshavsky, Y. I., Gelfand, I. M., Orlovsky, G. N., and Pavlova, G. A. (1975*a*). Activity of neurons of the ventral spinocerebellar tract during 'fictive scratching'. *Biophysics*, 20, 748–9.

Arshavsky, Y. I., Gelfand, I. M., Orlovsky, G. N., and Pavlova, G. A. (1977). Activity of neurons of the lateral reticular nucleus during scratching. *Biophysics*, 22, 177–9.

Arshavsky, Y. I., Gelfand, I. M., Orlovsky, G. N., and Pavlova, G. A. (1978*a*). Messages conveyed by spinocerebellar pathways during scratching in the cat. I. Activity of neurons of the lateral reticular nucleus. *Brain Research*, 151, 479–91.

Arshavsky, Y. I., Gelfand, I. M., Orlovsky, G. N., and Pavlova, G. A. (1978*b*). Messages conveyed by spinocerebellar pathways during scratching in the cat. II. Activity of neurons of the ventral spinocerebellar tract. *Brain Research*, 151, 493–506.

Arshavsky, Y. I., Gelfand, I. M., Orlovsky, G. N., and Pavlova, G. A. (1978*c*). Messages conveyed by descending tracts during scratching in the cat. I. Activity of vestibulospinal neurons. *Brain Research*, 159, 99–110.

Arshavsky, Y. I., Orlovsky, G. N., and Panchin, Y. V. (1978*d*). Responses of Deiters' neurons to tilt during scratching. *Neirofiziologia*, 10, 316–18. (In Russian.)

Arshavsky, Y. I., Orlovsky, G. N., Pavlova, G. A., and Perret, C. (1978*e*). Messages conveyed by descending tracts during scratching in the cat. II. Activity of rubrospinal neurons. *Brain Research*, 159, 111–23.

Arshavsky, Y. I., Orlovsky, G. N., and Perret, C. (1980*b*). Activity of neurons of cerebellar nuclei during fictitious scratch reflex in the cat. II. The interpositus and lateral nuclei. *Brain Research*, 200, 249–58.

Arshavsky, Y. I., Gelfand, I. M. and Orlovsky, G. N. (1983). The cerebellum and control of rhythmical movements. *Trends in Neuroscience*, 6, 417–22.

Arshavsky, Y. I., Gelfand, I. M., Orlovsky, G. N., Pavlova, G. A., and Popova, L. B. (1984*a*). Origin of signals conveyed by the ventral spino-cerebellar tract and spino-reticulo-cerebellar pathway. *Experimental Brain Research*, 54, 426–31.

Arshavsky, Y. I., Orlovsky, G. N., and Popova, L. B. (1984*b*). Activity of cerebellar Purkinje cells during fictitious scratch reflex in the cat. *Brain Research*, 290, 33–41.

Arshavsky, Y. I., Beloozerova, I. N., Orlovsky, G. N., Panchin, Y. V., and Pavlova, G. A. (1985*a*). Control of locomotion in marine mollusc *Clione limacina*. I. Efferent activity during actual and fictitious swimming. *Experimental Brain Research*, 58, 255–62.

Arshavsky, Y. I., Beloozerova, I. N., Orlovsky, G. N., Panchin, Y. V., and Pavlova, G. A. (1985*b*). Control of locomotion in marine mollusc *Clione limacina*. II. Rhythmic neurons of pedal ganglia. *Experimental Brain Research*, 58, 263–72.

Arshavsky, Y. I., Beloozerova, I. N., Orlovsky, G. N., Panchin, Y. V., and Pavlova, G. A. (1985*c*). Control of locomotion in marine mollusc *Clione limacina*. III. On the origin of locomotory rhythm. *Experimental Brain Research*, 58, 273–84.

Arshavsky, Y. I., Beloozerova, I. N., Orlovsky, G. N., Panchin, Y. V., and Pavlova, G. A. (1985*d*). Control of locomotion in marine mollusc *Clione limacina*. IV. Role of type 12 interneurons. *Experimental Brain Research*, 58, 285–93.

Arshavsky, Y. I., Orlovsky, G. N., and Panchin, Y. V. (1985*e*). Control of locomotion in marine mollusc *Clione limacina*. V. Photoinactivation of efferent neurons. *Experimental Brain Research*, 59, 203–5.

Arshavsky, Y. I., Deliagina, T. G., Orlovsky, G. N., Panchin, Y. V., Pavlova, G. A., and Popova, L. B. (1986*a*). Control of locomotion in marine mollusc *Clione limacina*. VI. Activity of isolated neurons of pedal ganglia. *Experimental Brain Research*, 63, 106–12.

Arshavsky, Y. I., Gelfand, I. M., and Orlovsky, G. N. (1986*b*). *Cerebellum and rhythmical movements*. Springer, New York.

Arshavsky, Y. I., Orlovsky, G. N., Pavlova, G. A., and Popova, L. B. (1986*c*). Activity of C3-C4 propriospinal neurons during fictitious forelimb locomotion in the cat. *Brain Research*, 363, 354–7.

Arshavsky, Y. I., Deliagina, T. G., Orlovsky, G. N., and Panchin, Y. V. (1988*a*). Control of feeding movements in the freshwater snail *Planorbis corneus*. I. Rhythmical neurons of buccal ganglia. *Experimental Brain Research*, 70, 310–22.

Arshavsky, Y. I., Deliagina, T. G., Orlovsky, G. N., and Panchin, Y. V. (1988*b*). Control of feeding movements in the freshwater snail *Planorbis corneus*. II. Activity of isolated neurons of buccal ganglia. *Experimental Brain Research*, 70, 323–31.

Arshavsky, Y. I., Deliagina, T. G., Orlovsky, G. N., and Panchin, Y. V. (1988*c*). Control of feeding movements in the freshwater snail *Planorbis corneus*. III. Organization of the feeding rhythm generator. *Experimental Brain Research*, 70, 332–41.

Arshavsky, Y. I., Orlovsky, G. N., and Perret, C. (1988). Activity of rubrospinal neurons during locomotion and scratching in the cat. *Behavioural Brain Research*, 28, 193–9.

Arshavsky, Y. I., Deliagina, T. G., Orlovsky, G. N., and Panchin, Y. V. (1989*a*). Control of feeding movements in the pteropod mollusc, *Clione limacina*. *Experimental Brain Research*, 78, 387–97.

Arshavsky, Y. I., Orlovsky, G. N., Panchin, Y. V., and Pavlova, G. A. (1989*b*). Control of locomotion in marine mollusc *Clione limacina*. VII. Reexamination of type 12 interneurons. *Experimental Brain Research*, 78, 398–406.

Arshavsky, Y. I., Deliagina, T. G., Gelfand, I. M., Orlovsky, G. N., Panchin, Y. V., and Popova, L. B. (1990). Neural control of heart beat in the pteropod mollusc *Clione limacina*: coordination of circulatory and locomotor systems. *Journal of Experimental Biology*, 148, 461–75.

Arshavsky, Y. I., Deliagina, T. G., Orlovsky, G. N., Panchin, Y. V., Pavlova, G. A., and Popova, L. B. (1991). Locomotion in *Clione limacina* in relation to various types of behavior. In *Studies in neuroscience* (eds. D. A. Sakharov and W. Winlow), pp. 290–315. Manchester University Press.

Arshavsky, Y. I., Deliagina, T. G., Orlovsky, G. N., Panchin, Y. V., and Popova, L. B. (1992). Interneurons mediating the escape reaction of the marine mollusc *Clione limacina*. *Journal of Experimental Biology*, 164, 307–14.

Arshavsky, Y. I., Deliagina, T. G., Gamkrelidze, G. N., Orlovsky, G. N., Panchin, Y. V., Popova, L. B., and Shupliakov, O. V. (1993*a*). Pharmacologically induced elements of the hunting and feeding behaviour in the pteropod mollusc *Clione limacina*. I. Effects of GABA. *Journal of Neurophysiology*, 69, 512–21.

Arshavsky, Y. I., Deliagina, T. G., Gamkrelidze, G. N., Orlovsky, G. N., Panchin, Y. V., and Popova, L. B. (1993*b*). Pharmacologically induced elements of the hunting and feeding behavior in the pteropod mollusk *Clione limacina*. II. Effects of physostigmine. *Journal of Neurophysiology*, 69, 522–32.

Arshavsky, Y. I., Orlovsky, G. N., Panchin, Y. V., Roberts, A., and Soffe, S. R. (1993*c*). Neuronal control of swimming locomotion: analysis of the pteropod mollusc *Clione* and embryos of the amphibian *Xenopus*. *Trends in Neuroscience*, 16, 227–33.

Arshavsky, Y. I., Deliagina, T. G., Okshtein, I. L., Orlovsky, G. N., Panchin, Y. V., and Popova, L. B. (1994*a*). Defense reaction in the pond snail *Planorbis corneus*. 1. Activity of the shell-moving and respiratory systems. *Journal of Neurophysiology*, 71, 882–90.

Arshavsky, Y. I., Deliagina, T. G., Okshtein, I. L., Orlovsky, G. N., Panchin, Y. V., and Popova, L. B. (1994b). Defense reaction in the pond snail *Planorbis corneus*. 2. Central pattern generator. *Journal of Neurophysiology*, 71, 891–97.

Arshavsky, Y. I., Deliagina, T. G., Okshtein, I. L., Orlovsky, G. N., Panchin, Y. V., and Popova, L. B. (1994c). Defense reaction in the pond snail *Planorbis corneus*. 3. Response to input from statocysts. *Journal of Neurophysiology*, 71, 898–903.

Arshavsky, Y. I., Deliagina, T. G., Orlovsky, G. N., Panchin, Y. V., Popova, L. B., and Sadreyev, R. I. (1998). Analysis of the central pattern generator for swimming in the mollusk *Clione*. In *Neuronal mechanisms for generating locomotor activity* (eds. O. Keihn, R. M. Harris-Warrik, L. M. Jordan, H. Hultborn, and N. Kudo), Vol. 860, pp. 51–70. New York Academy of Sciences, New York.

Audesirk, G. J. (1977). Properties of central motor neurons exciting locomotory cilia in *Tritonia diomedea*. *Journal of Comparative Physiology*, 128, 259–67.

Audesirk, G. J. (1978). Central neuronal control of cilia in *Tritonia diomedea*. *Nature*, 272, 541–3.

Audesirk, G., McCaman, R. E., and Willows, A. O. (1979). The role of serotonin in the control of pedal ciliary activity by identified neurons in *Tritonia diomedea*. *Comparative Biochemistry and Physiology—C: Comparative Pharmacology*, 62C, 87–91.

Ayers, J. L. and Davis, W. J. (1977). Neuronal control of locomotion in the lobster, *Homarus americanus*. I. Motor programs for forward and backward walking. *Journal of Comparative Physiology*, 115, 1–27.

Bacon, J. and Möhl, B. (1983). The tritocerebral commissure gaint (TCG) wind-sensitive interneurone in the locust. I. Its activity in straight flight. *Journal of Comparative Physiology*, 150A, 439–52.

Bacon, J. and Tyrer, M. (1978). The tritocerebral commissure gaint (TCG): A bimodal interneurone in the locust, *Schistocerca gregaria*. *Journal of Comparative Physiology*, 126, 317–25.

Bacskai, B. J., Wallén, P., Lev-Ram, V., Grillner, S., and Tsien, R. Y. (1995). Activity-related calcium dynamics in lamprey motoneurons as revealed by video-rate confocal microscopy. *Neuron*, 14, 19–28.

Baev, K. V. (1978). Central locomotor program for the cat's hindlimb. *Neuroscience*, 3, 1081–92.

Baev, K. V. (1980). Polarization of primary afferent terminals in the lumbar spinal cord during fictitious locomotion. *Neurophysiology*, 12, 305–11.

Baev, K. V. and Kostyuk, P. G. (1981). Primary afferent depolarization evoked by the activity of spinal scratching generator. *Neuroscience*, 6, 205–15.

Baev, K. V. and Kostyuk, P. G. (1982). Polarization of primary afferent terminals of lumbosacral cord elicited by the activity of spinal locomotor generator. *Neuroscience*, 7, 1401–9.

Baev, K. V., Degtiarenko, A. M., Zavadskaia, T. V., and Kostiuk, P. G. (1979). Activity of interneurons of the lumbar region of the spinal cord during fictive locomotion of thalamic cats. *Neirofiziologiia*, 11, 329–38.

Baev, K. V., Degtyarenko, A. M., Zavadskaya, T. V., and Kostyuk, P. G. (1981). Activity of lumbosacral interneurons during fictitious scratching. *Neurophysiology*, 13, 45–52.

Baev, K. V., Beresovskii, V. K., Kebkalo, T. G., and Savoskina, L. A. (1988). Afferent and efferent connections of brainstem locomotor regions study by means of horseradish peroxidase transport technique. *Neuroscience*, 26, 871–92.

Baker, L. L., Chandler, S. H., and Goldberg, L. J. (1984). L-Dopa induced locomotor-like activity in ankle flexor and extensor nerves of chronic and acute spinal cats. *Experimental Neurology*, 86, 515–26.

Baker, P. S. (1979). The role of forewing muscles in the control of direction in flying locusts. *Journal of Comparative Physiology*, **131**, 59–66.

Baker, P. S. and Cooter, R. J. (1979). The natural flight of the migratory locust, *Locusta migratoria* L. I. Wing movements. *Journal of Comparative Physiology*, **131A**, 79–87.

Baker, P. S., Gewecke, M., and Cooter, R. J. (1981). The natural flight of the migratory locust *Locusta migratoria* L. III. Wing beat frequency, flight speed and altitude. *Journal of Comparative Physiology*, **141A**, 233–7.

Baldissera, F., Hultborn, H., and Illert, M. (1981). Integration in spinal neuronal systems. In *The nervous system. Handbook of physiology. Section 1* (eds. J. M. Brookhart and V. B. Mountcastle), Vol. 2, pp. 509–95. American Physiological Society, Bethesda, MD.

Ballantyne, D. and Rathmayer, W. (1981). On the function of the common inhibitory neuron in the walking legs of the crab *Eriphia spinifrons*. *Journal of Comparative Physiology*, **143**, 111–22.

Barajon, I., Gossard, J.-P., and Hultborn, H. (1992). Induction of *fos* expression by activity in the spinal rhythm generator for scratching. *Brain Research*, **588**, 168–72.

Barbeau, H. and Rossignol, S. (1987). Recovery of locomotion after chronic spinalization in the adult cat. *Brain Research*, **412**, 84–95.

Bard, P. and Macht, M. B. (1958). The behavior of chronically decerebrate cats. In *Neurological basis of behavior* (eds. G. E. W. Wolstenholme and C. M. O'Connor), pp. 55–71. Churchill, London.

Barnes, W. J. P. (1975). Leg coordination during walking in the crab, *Uca pugnas*. *Journal of Comparative Physiology*, **96**, 237–56.

Barnes, W. J. P., Spirito, C. P., and Evoy, W. H. (1972). Nervous control of walking in the crab *Cardisoma guanhumi*. II. Role of resistance reflexes in walking. *Zeitschrift für vergleichenden Physiology* **76**, 16–31.

Bässler, U. (1976). Reversal of a reflex to a single motoneuron in the stick insect *Carausius morosus*. *Biological Cybernetics*, **24**, 47–9.

Bässler, U. (1977). Sense organs in the femur of the stick insect and their relevance to the control of position of the femur-tibia-joint. *Journal of Comparative Physiology*, **121**, 99–113.

Bässler, U. (1983). *Neural basis of elementary behavior in stick insects*. Springer, Berlin.

Bässler, U. (1986). On the definition of central pattern generator and its sensory control. *Biological Cybernetics*, **54**, 65–9.

Bässler, U. (1987). Timing and shaping influences on the motor output for walking in stick insects. *Biological Cybernetics*, **55**, 397–401.

Bässler, U. (1988). Functional principles of pattern generation for walking movements of stick insect forelegs: the role of the femoral chordotonal organ afferents. *Journal of Experimental Biology*, **136**, 125–47.

Bässler, U. (1993). The walking- (and searching-) pattern generator of stick insects, a modular system composed of reflexes chains and endogenous oscillators. *Biological Cybernetics*, **69**, 305–17.

Bässler, U. and Büschges, A. (1998). Patter generation for stick insect walking movements. *Brain Research Reviews*, **27**, 65–88.

Bässler, U. and Nothof, U. (1994). Gain control in a proprioceptive feedback loop as a prerequisite for working close to instability. *Journal of Comparative Physiology A*, **175**, 23–33.

Bässler, U. and Wegner, U. (1983). Motor output of the denervated thoracic ventral nerve cord in the stick insect *Carausius morosus*. *Journal of Experimental Biology*, **105**, 127–45.

Bayev, K. V., Dekhtyarenko, A. M., Zavadskaya, T. V., and Kostyuk, P. G. (1979). Activity of lumbar interneurons during fictitious locomotion of thalamic cats. *Neurophysiology (Kiev)*, 11, 329–38.

Beloozerova, I. N. and Rossignol, S. (1994). Antidromic activity of dorsal root filaments during treadmill locomotion in thalamic cats. *Society of Neuroscience Abstracts*, 20, 1755 no. 716.6.

Beloozerova, I. N. and Sirota, M. G. (1988). Role of motor cortex in control of locomotion. In *Stance and motion: facts and concepts* (eds. V. S. Gurfinkel, M. E. Ioffe, J. Massion, and J. P. Roll), pp. 163–76. Plenum, New York.

Beloozerova, I. N. and Sirota, M. G. (1993a). The role of the motor cortex in the control of accuracy of locomotor movements in the cat. *Journal of Physiology*, 461, 1–25.

Beloozerova, I. N. and Sirota, M. G. (1993b). The role of the motor cortex in the control of vigour of locomotor movements in the cat. *Journal of Physiology*, 461, 27–46.

Benjamin, P. R. (1983). Gastropod feeding: Behavioural and neural analysis of a complex multicomponent system. In *Neural origin of rhythmic movements. Society for Experimental Biology Symposium 37* (eds. A. Roberts and B. L. Roberts), pp. 159–93. Cambridge University Press, Cambridge.

Beresovskii, V. K. and Baev, K. V. (1988). New locomotor regions of the brainstem revealed by means of electrical stimulation. *Neuroscience*, 26, 863–70.

Berkinblit, M. B., Deliagina, T. G., Orlovsky, G. N., and Feldman, A. G. (1977). Activity of propriospinal neurons during scratch reflex in the cat. *Nejrofiziologia*, 9, 504–11.

Berkinblit, M. B., Deliagina, T. G., Feldman, A. G., and Orlovsky, G. N. (1978a). Generation of scratching. 1. Activity of spinal interneurons during scratching. *Journal of Neurophysiology*, 41, 1040–57.

Berkinblit, M. B., Deliagina, T. G., Feldman, A. G., Gelfand, I. M., and Orlovsky, G. N. (1978b). Generation of scratching. II. Non-regular regimes of generation. *Journal of Neurophysiology*, 41, 1058–69.

Berkinblit, M. B., Deliagina, T. G., Orlovsky, G. N., and Feldman, A. G. (1980). Activity of motoneurons during fictitious scratch reflex in the cat. *Brain Research*, 193, 427–38.

Berthoz, A. and Pozzo, T. (1988). Intermittent head stabilization during postural and locomotory tasks in humans. In *Posture and gait: development, adaptation and modulation* (eds. B. Amblard, A. Bertoz, and F. Clarac), pp. 189–98. Elsevier, Amsterdam.

Bicker, G. and Pearson, K. G. (1983). Initiation of flight by an identified wind sensitive neuron (TCG) in the locust. *Journal of Experimental Biology*, 104, 289–94.

Blake, J. R. and Sleigh, M. A. (1974). Mechanics of ciliary locomotion. [review]. *Biological Reviews of the Cambridge Philosophical Society*, 49, 85–125.

Bloedel, J. R. (1992). Functional heterogenity with structural homogenity: how does the cerebellum operate? *Behavioural Brain Sciences*, 15, 666–78.

Bloedel, J. R. and Bracha, V. (1995). On the cerebellum, cutaneomuscular reflexes, movement control and the elusive engrams of memory. *Behavioural Brain Research*, 68, 1–44.

Blouin, J., Bard, C., Teasdale, N., Paillard, J., Fleury, M., Forget, R., and Lamarre, Y. (1993). Reference systems for coding spatial information in normal subjects and in a deafferented patient. *Experimental Brain Research*, 93, 324–31.

Boothby, K. M. and Roberts, A. (1992). The stopping response of *Xenopus laevis* embryos: pharmacology and intracellular physiology of rhythmic spinal neurons and hindbrain neurons. *Journal of Experimental Biology*, 169, 65–86.

Bowerman, R. F. and Larimer, J. L. (1974a). Command fibers in the circumesophageal connectives of crayfish. I. Tonic fibers. *Journal of Experimental Biology*, 60, 95–117.

Bowerman, R. F. and Larimer, J. L. (1974b). Command fibers in the circumesophageal connectives of crayfish. II. Phasic fibers. *Journal of Experimental Biology*, 60, 119–34.

Boylls, C. C. (1977). Olivary unit activity and effect of microstimulation during locomotion. *Neuroscience Abstracts*, **3**, 55.

Bradley, G. W., Euler, C. von, Martilla, I., and Roos, B. (1975). A model of the central and reflex inhibition of inspiration in the cat. *Biological Cybernetics*, **19**, 105–16.

Brandell, B. R. (1973). An analysis of muscle coordination in walking and running. In *Medicine and sport: biomechanics* (eds. S. Cerquiglini, A. Venerando, and J. Wartenweiler), Vol. 3, pp. 278–87. Karger, Basel.

Braun, G. and Mulloney, B. (1995). Coordination in the crayfish swimmeret system: differential excitation causes changes in intersegmental phase. *Journal of Neurophysiology*, **73**, 880–85.

Brodal, A. (1957). The reticular formation of the brain stem. Anatomical aspects and functional correlations. Oliver and Boyd, Edinburgh.

Brodal, A. (1958). *The reticular formation of the brain stem. Anatomical aspects and functional correlations.* Oliver and Boyd, London.

Brodal, A. (1974). Anatomy of vestibular nuclei and their connections. In *Handbook of sensory physiology, VI/I, Vestibular system, Part I: Basic mechanisms* (ed. H. H. Kornhuber), pp. 239–352. Springer, Berlin.

Brodal, A., Pompeiano, O., and Walberg, F. (1962). *The vestibular nuclei and their connections. Anatomy and functional correlations.* Oliver and Boyd, Edinburgh.

Brodfuehrer, P. D. and Burns, A. (1995). Neuronal factors influencing the decision to swim in the medicinal leech. *Neurobiology of Learning and Memory*, **63**, 192–9.

Brodfuehrer, P. D. and Cohen, A. H. (1990). Initiation of swimming activity in the medicinal leech by glutamate, quisqualate and kainate. *Journal of Experimental Biology*, **154**, 567–72.

Brodfuehrer, P. D. and Friesen, W. O. (1984). A sensory system initiating swimming activity in the medicinal leech. *Journal of Experimental Biology*, **108**, 341–55.

Brodfuehrer, P. D. and Friesen, W. O. (1986a). Initiation of swimming activity by trigger neurons in the leech subesophageal ganglion. I. Output pathways of Tr1 and Tr2. *Journal of Comparative Physiology A—Sensory Neural and Behavioral Physiology*, **159**, 489–502.

Brodfuehrer, P. D. and Friesen, W. O. (1986b). Initiation of swimming activity by trigger neurons in the leech subesophageal ganglion. II. Role of segmental swim-initiating interneurons. *Journal of Comparative Physiology A—Sensory Neural and Behavioral Physiology*, **159**, 503–10.

Brodfuehrer, P. D. and Friesen, W. O. (1986c). Initiation of swimming activity by trigger neurons in the leech subesophageal ganglion. III. Sensory inputs to Tr1 and Tr2. *Journal of Comparative Physiology A—Sensory Neural and Behavioral Physiology*, **159**, 511–19.

Brodfuehrer, P. D. and Friesen, W. O. (1986d). From simulation to undulation: a neuronal pathway for the control of swimming in the leech. *Science*, **234**, 1002–4.

Brodfuehrer, P. D., Debski, E. A., O'Gara, B. A., and Friesen, W. O. (1995a). Neuronal control of leech swimming. [review]. *Journal of Neurobiology*, **27**, 403–18.

Brodfuehrer, P. D., Parker, H. J., Burns, A., and Berg, M. (1995b). Regulation of the segmental swim-generating system by a pair of identified interneurons in the leech head ganglion. *Journal of Neurophysiology*, **73**, 983–92.

Brodin, L. and Grillner, S. (1985a). The role of putative excitatory amino acid neurotransmitters in the initiation of locomotion in the lamprey spinal cord. I. The effects of excitatory amino acid antagonists. *Brain Research*, **360**, 139–48.

Brodin, L. and Grillner, S. (1985b). The role of putative excitatory amino acid neurotransmitters in the initiation of locomotion in the lamprey spinal cord. II. The effects of amino acid uptake inhibitors. *Brain Research*, **360**, 149–58.

Brodin, L., Grillner, S., and Rovainen, C. M. (1985c). N-Methyl-D-aspartate (NMDA), kainate and quisqualate receptors and the generation of fictive locomotion in the lamprey spinal cord. *Brain Research*, **325**, 302–6.

Brodin, L., Buchanana, J., Hökfelt, T., Grillner, S., and Verhofstad, A. A. J. (1986b). A spinal projection of 5-hydroxytryptamine neurons in the lamprey brainstem; evidence from combined retrograde tracing and immunohistochemistry. *Neuroscience Letters*, **67**, 53–7.

Brodin, L., Ohta, Y., and Grillner, S. (1987). Retrograde transport of (3H)D-aspartate in lamprey reticulospinal neurons. *Acta Physiologica Scandinavia*, 633–4.

Brodin, L., Buchanan, J. T., Hökfelt, T., Grillner, S., Rehfeld, J. F., Frey, P., Verhofstad, A. A. J., Dockray, G. J., and Walsh, J. H. (1988a). Immuno-histochemical studies of cholecystokininlike peptides and their relation to 5-HT, CGRP, and bombesin immunoreactivities in the brainstem and spinal cord of lampreys. *Journal of Comparative Neurology*, **271**, 1–18.

Brodin, L., Grillner, S., Dubuc, R., Ohta, Y., Kasicki, S., and Hökfelt, T. (1988b). Reticulospinal neurons in lamprey: Transmitters, synaptic interactions and their role during locomotion. *Archives of Italian Biology*, **126**, 317–45.

Brooks, V. B. and Thach, W. T. (1981). Cerebellar control of posture and movement. In *Handbook of physiology. The nervous system* (ed. V. B. Brooks), Vol. II, pp. 877–946. American Physiological Society, Bethesda, MD.

Brown, G. D., Frost, W. N., and Getting, P. A. (1996). Habituation and iterative enhancement of multiple components of the *Tritonia* swim response. *Behavioral Neuroscience*, **110**, 478–85.

Brown, T. G. (1911). The intrinsic factors in the act of progression in the mammal. *Proceedings of the Royal Society of London Series B*, **84**, 309–19.

Brown, T. G. (1914). On the nature of the fundamental activity of the nervous centres; togerther with an analysis of the conditioning of rhythmic activity in progression and a theory of the evolution of function in the nervous system. *Journal of Physiology, London*, **48**, 18–46.

Brunn, D. E. and Dean, J. (1994). Intersegmental and local interneurons in the metathorax of the stick insect *Carausius morosus* that monitor middle leg position. *Journal of Neurophysiology*, **72**, 1208–19.

Buchanan, J. T. (1982). Identification of interneurons with contralateral, caudal axons in the lamprey spinal cord: synaptic interactions and morphology. *Journal of Neurophysiology*, **47**, 961–75.

Buchanan, J. T. and Cohen, A. H. (1982). Activities of identified interneurons, motoneurons, and muscle fibers during fictive swimming in the lamprey and effects of reticulospinal and dorsal cell stimulation. *Journal of Neurophysiology*, **47**, 948–60.

Buchanan, J. T. and Grillner, S. (1987). Newly identified 'glutamate interneurons' and their role in locomotion in the lamprey spinal cord. *Science*, **236**, 312–14.

Buchanan, J. and Grillner, S. (1991). 5-hydroxytryptamine depresses reticulospinal excitatory postsynaptic potentials in motoneurons of the lamprey. *Neuroscience Letters*, **112**, 71–4.

Buchanan, J. T., Brodin, L., Dale, N., and Grillner, S. (1987). Reticulospinal neurones activate excitatory amino acid receptors. *Brain Research*, **408**, 321–5.

Buchanan, J. T., Grillner, S., Cullheim, S., and Riesling, M. (1989). Identification of excitatory interneurons contributing to the generation of locomotion in lamprey: structure, pharmacology and function. *Journal of Neurophysiology*, **62**, 59–69.

Budakova, N. N. (1973). Stepping movements in a spinal cat due to DOPA administration. *Sechenov Physiological Journal of the USSR*, **59**, 1190–8. (In Russian).

Buford, J. A. and Smith, J. L. (1990). Adaptive control for backward quadrupedal walking. II. Hindlimb muscle synergies. *Journal of Neurophysiology*, 64, 756–66.

Buford, J. A., Zernicke, R. F., and Smith, J. L. (1990). Adaptive control for backward quadrupedal walking. I. Posture and hindlimb kinematics. *Journal of Neurophysiology*, 64, 745–55.

Burke, R. E. and Fleshman, J. W. (1986). Strategies to identify interneurons involved in locomotor pattern generation in the mammalian spinal cord. In *Neurobiology of vertebrate locomotion* (ed. S. Grillner, P. S. G. Stein, D. G. Stuart, H. Forssberg, and R. M. Herman), pp. 245–67. Macmillan, London.

Burke, R., Lundberg, A., and Weight, F. (1971). Spinal border cell origin of the ventral spinocerebellar tract. *Experimental Brain Research*, 12, 283–94.

Burnett, M. E., Cole, J. D., McLellan, D. L., and Sedgwick, E. M. (1989). Gait analysis in a man without proprioception below the neck. *Journal of Physiology*, 417, 102p.

Burns, M. D. (1973). The control of walking in Orthoptera. I. Leg movements in normal walking. *Journal of Experimental Biology*, 58, 45–58.

Burns, M. D. and Usherwood, P. N. R. (1979). The control of walking in Orthoptera. II. Motor neurone activity in normal free-walking animals. *Journal of Experimental Biology*, 79, 69–98.

Burrows, M. (1973). The morphology of an elevator and depressor motoneuron in the hindwing of a locust. *Journal of Comparative Physiology*, 83, 165–78.

Burrows, M. (1975). Monosynaptic connections between wing stretch receptors and flight motoneurons in the locust. *Journal of Experimental Biology*, 62, 189–219.

Burrows, M. (1987). Inhibitory interactions between spiking and nonspiking local interneurons in the locust. *Journal of Neuroscience*, 7, 3282–92.

Burrows, M. (1996). *The neurobiology of an insect brain.* Oxford University Press, Oxford.

Burrows, M. and Laurent, G. (1989). Reflex circuits and the control of movement. In *The computing neuron* (ed. R. Durbin, C. Miall, and G. Mitchison), pp. 244–61. Addison-Wesley, Wokingham.

Burrows, M. and Siegler, M. V. S. (1982). Spiking local interneurons mediate local reflexes. *Science*, 217, 650–2.

Burrows, M., Watson, A. H. D., and Brunn, D. E. (1989). Physiological and ultrastructural characterization of a central synaptic connection between identified motor neurons in the locust. *European Journal of Neuroscience*, 1, 111–26.

Büschges, A. (1990). Nonspiking pathways in a joint-control loop of the stick insect *Carausius morosus*. *Journal of Experimental Biology*, 151, 133–60.

Büschges, A. (1995). Role of local nonspiking interneurons in the generation of rhythmic motor activity in the stick insect. *Journal of Neurobiology*, 27, 488–512.

Büschges, A. (1998). Inhibitory synaptic drive patterns motoneuronal activity in rhythmic preparations of isolated thoracic ganglia in the stick insect. *Brain Research*, 783, 261–71.

Büschges, A. and Wolf, H. (1995). Nonspiking local interneurons in insect leg motor control. I. Common layout and species-specific response properties of femur-tibia joint control pathways in stick insect and locust. *Journal of Neurophysiology*, 73, 1843–60.

Büschges, A. and Wolf, H. (1996). Gain changes in sensorimotor pathways of the locust leg. *Journal of Experimental Biology*, 199, 2437–45.

Büschges, A., Kittmann, R., and Schmitz, J. (1994). Identified nonspiking interneurons in leg reflexes and during walking in the stick insect. *Journal of Comparative Physiology A*, 174, 685–700.

Büschges, A., Schmitz, J., and Bässler, U. (1995). Rhythmic patterns in the thoracic nerve cord of the stick insect induced by pilocarpine. *Journal of Experimental Biology*, 198, 435–56.

Bush, B. M. H. (1962). Proprioceptive reflexes in the legs of *Carcinus maenas* (L.). *Journal of Experimental Biology*, 39, 89–105.

Bush, B. M. H. (1965). Leg reflexes from chordotonal organs in the crab, *Carcinus maenas*. *Comparative Biochemical Physiology*, 15, 567–87.

Bush, B. M. H. (1976). Non-impulsive thoracic-coxal receptors in crustaceans. In *Structure and function of proprioceptors in the invertebrates*. (ed. P. J. Mill), pp. 115–51. Chapman and Hall, London.

Bussières, N. (1994). *Les systémes descendants chez la lamproie. Etude anatomique et fonctionnelle*. Ph.D. thesis, Faculté des études supérieures. Université de Montréal, Montréal.

Bussières, N. and Dubuc, R. (1992). Phasic modulation of vestibulospinal neurons during fictive locomotion in lampreys. *Brain Research*, 575, 174–9.

Bussières, N. and El Manira, A. E. (1997). GABA$_B$ receptor activation in lamprey sensory neurons modulates N- and P/Q-type calcium channels. *Society for Neuroscience Abstracts*, 23, p. 1182.

Cabelguen, J.-M. (1981). Static and dynamic fusimotor controls in various hindlimb muscles during locomotor activity in the decorticate cat. *Brain Research*, 213, 83–97.

Cabelguen, J.-M. (1986). Static and dymanic fusimotor controls during locomotion in the cat. In *Neurobiology of vertebrate locomotion* (eds. S. Grillner, P. S. G. Stein, D. G. Stuart, H. Forssberg, and R. M. Herman), pp. 577–92. Macmillan, London.

Cabelguen, J.-M., Orsal, D., and Perret, C. (1984). Discharges of forelimb spindle primary afferents during locomotor activity in the decorticate cat. *Brain Research*, 306, 359–64.

Camhi, J. (1969a). Locust wind receptors. I. Transducer mechanisms and sensory response. *Journal of Experimental Biology*, 50, 335–48.

Camhi, J. (1969b). Locust wind receptors. II. Contribution to flight initiation and lift control. *Journal of Experimental Biology*, 50, 363–73.

Camhi, J. M. (1970). Jaw-correcting postural changes in locusts. *Journal of Experimental Biology*, 52, 519–32.

Cannone, A. J. and Bush, B. M. H. (1980a). Reflexes mediated by non-impulsive afferent neurons of the thoracic-coxal muscle receptor organ in the crab, *Carcinus maenas*. I. Receptor potentials and promotor motoneuron responses. *Journal of Experimental Biology*, 86, 275–303.

Cannone, A. J. and Bush, B. M. H. (1980b). Reflexes mediated by non-impulsive afferent neurons of the thoracic-coxal muscle receptor organ in the crab, *Carcinus maenas*. II. Reflex discharge evoked by current injection. *Journal of Experimental Biology*, 86, 305–31.

Carlson, H., Halbertsma, J., and Zomlefer, M. (1979). Control of the trunk during walking in the cat. *Acta Physiologica Scandinavia*, 105, 251–3.

Carretta, M. (1988). The retzius cells in the leech: a review of their properties and synaptic connections. [review]. *Comparative Biochemistry and Physiology A—Comparative Physiology* 91, 405–13.

Carter, M. C. and Smith, J. L. (1986). Simultaneous control of two rhythmic behaviours. II. Hindlimb walking with paw-shake response in the spinal cat. *Journal of Neurophysiology*, 56, 184–95.

Cattaert, D., El Manira, A., Marchand, A., and Clarac, F. (1990). Central control of the sensory afferent terminals from a leg chordotonal organ in crayfish *in vitro* preparation. *Neuroscience Letters*, 108, 81–7.

Cattaert, D., El Manira, A., and Clarac, F. (1992). Direct evidence for presynaptic inhibitory mechanisms in crayfish sensory afferents. *Journal of Neurophysiology*, 67, 610–23.

Cazalets, J.-R., Borde, M., and Clarac, F. (1995). Localization and organization of the central pattern generator for hindlimb locomotion in newborn rat. *Journal of Neuroscience*, 15, 4943–51.

Chambers, W. W. and Liu, C. N. (1957). Corticospinal tract of the cat. An attempt to correlate the pattern of degeneration with deficits in reflex activity following neocortical lesions. *Journal of Comparative Neurology*, 108, 23–56.

Chambers, W. W. and Sprague, J. M. (1955a). Functional localization in the cerebellum. I. Organization in longitudinal corticonuclear zones and their contribution to the control of posture, both pyramidal and extrapyramidal. *Journal of Comparative Neurology*, 103, 105–30.

Chambers, W. W. and Sprague, J. M. (1955b). Functional localization in the cerebellum. II. Somatotopic organization of cortex and nuclei. *Archives of Neurology and Psychiatry*, 74, 653–80.

Chandler, S. H., Baker, L. L., and Goldberg, L. J. (1984). Characterization of synaptic potentials in hindlimb extensor motoneurons during L-Dopa-induced fictive locomotion in acute and chronic spinal cats. *Brain Research*, 303, 91–100.

Chrachri, A. and Clarac, F. (1987). Induction of rhythmic activity in motoneurons of crayfish thoracic ganglia by cholinergic agonists. *Neuroscience Letters*, 77, 49–54.

Chrachri, A. and Clarac, F. (1989). Synaptic connections between motor neurons and interneurons in the fourth thoracic ganglion of the crayfish *Procambarus clarkii. Journal of Neurophysiology*, 62, 1237–50.

Chrachri, A. and Clarac, F. (1990). Fictive locomotion in the fourth thoracic ganglion of the craysh, *Procambarus clarkii. Journal of Neuroscience*, 10, 707–19.

Chrachri, A. and Neil, D. M. (1993). Interaction and synchronization between two abdominal motor systems in crayfish. *Journal of Neurophysiology*, 69, 1373–83.

Chrachri, A., Neil, D., and Mulloney, B. (1994). State-dependent responses of two motor systems in the crayfish, *Pacifastacus leniusculus. Journal of Comparative Physiology A—Sensory Neural and Behavioral Physiology*, 175, 371–80.

Christenson, J. and Grillner, S. (1991). Primary afferents evoke excitatory amino acid receptor mediated EPSPs, that are modulated by presynaptic GABA$_B$ receptors in lamprey. *Journal of Neurophysiology*, 66, 2141–9.

Christenson, J., Franck, J., and Grillner, S. (1989). Increase in endogenous 5-hydroxytryptamine levels modulates the central network underlying locomotion in the lamprey spinal cord. *Neuroscience Letters*, 100, 188–92.

Clarac, F. (1976). Crustacean cuticular stress detectors. In *Structure and function of proprioceptors in the invertebrates* (ed. P. J. Mill), pp. 299–321. Chapman and Hall, London.

Clarac, F. (1977). Motor coordination in crustacean limbs. In *Identified neurons and behavior of arthropods* (ed. G. Hoyle), pp. 31–71. Plenum Press, New York and London.

Clarac, F. and Chasserat, C. (1979). Experimental modification of interlimb coordination during locomotion of a crustacean. *Neuroscience Letters*, 12, 217–26.

Clarac, F. and Chasserat, C. (1983a). Quantitative analysis of walking in a decapod crustacean, the rock lobster *Jasus lalaudii*. I. Comparative study of free and driven walking. *Journal of Experimental Biology*, 107, 189–217.

Clarac, F. and Chasserat, C. (1983b). Quantitative analysis of walking in a decapod crustacean, the rock lobster *Jasus lalaudii*. II. Spatial and temporal regulation of stepping in driven walking. *Journal of Experimental Biology*, 107, 219–43.

Clarac, F. and Chasserat, C. (1986). Basic processes of locomotor coordination in the rock lobster. I. Statistical analysis of walking parameters. *Biological Cybernetics*, 55, 159–70.

Clarac, F., Vedel, J. P., and Bush, B. M. H. (1978). Intersegmental reflex coordination by a single joint receptor organ (CB) in rock lobster walking legs. *Journal of Experimental Biology*, 73, 29–46.

Clarke, J. D. and Roberts, A. (1984). Interneurones in the *Xenopus* embryo spinal cord: sensory excitation and activity during swimming. *Journal of Physiology*, 354, 345–62.

Clarke, J. D. W., Hayes, B. P., Hunt, S. P., and Roberts, A. (1984). Sensory physiology and immunohistochemistry of Rohon–Beard neurons in embryos of *Xenopus laevis*. *Journal of Physiology*, 348, 511–25.

Clendenin, M., Ekerot, C.-F., Oscarsson, O., and Rosén, I. (1974a). The lateral reticular nucleus in the cat. I. Mossy fibre distribution in cerebellar cortex. *Experimental Brain Research*, 21, 473–86.

Clendenin, M., Ekerot, C.-F., Oscarsson, O., and Rosén, I. (1974b). The lateral reticular nucleus in the cat. II. Organization of component activated from bilateral ventral flexor reflex tract (bVFRT). *Experimental Brain Research*, 21, 487–500.

Clendenin, M., Ekerot, C.-F., Oscarsson, O., and Rosén, I. (1974c). The lateral reticular nucleus in the cat. III. Organization of component activated from ipsilateral forelimb tract. *Experimental Brain Research*, 21, 501–13.

Cohen, A. H. (1987). Effects of oscillators frequency on phase-locking in the lamprey central pattern generator. *Journal of Neuroscience Methods*, 21, 113–25.

Cohen, A. H. and Wallén, P. (1980). The neuronal correlate of locomotion in fish. 'Fictive swimming' induced in an *in vitro* preparation of the lamprey spinal cord. *Experimental Brain Research*, 41, 11–18.

Cohen, A. H., Holmes, P. J., and Rand, R. H. (1982). The nature of the coupling between segmental oscillators of the lamprey spinal generator for locomotion: a mathematical model. *Journal of Mathematical Biology*, 13, 345–69.

Cohen, M. I. (1979). Neurogenesis of respiratory rhythm in the mammal. *Physiological Review*, 59, 1105–73.

Cohen, M. I. and Feldman, J. L. (1977). Models of respiratory phase-switching. *Federation Proceedings*, 36, 2367–74.

Conway, B. A., Hultborn, H., and Kiehn, O. (1987). Proprioceptive input resets central locomotor rhythm in the spinal cat. *Experimental Brain Research*, 68, 643–56.

Crowe, A. and Matthews, P. B. C. (1964). Further studies of static and dynamic fusimotor fibres. *Journal of Physiology*, 174, 131–51.

Cruce, W. L. R. and Newman, D. B. (1984). Evolution of motor system: the reticulospinal pathways. *American Zoologist*, 24, 733–53.

Cruse, H. (1979). The control of the anterior extreme position of the hindleg of a walking insect. *Physiological Entomology*, 4, 121–4.

Cruse, H. (1980). A quantitative model of walking incorporating central and peripheral influences: II. The connections between the different legs. *Biological Cybernetics*, 37, 137–44.

Cruse, H. (1983). The influence of load and leg amputation upon coordination in walking crustaceans: a model calculation. *Biological Cybernetics*, 49, 1–7.

Cruse, H. (1985). Which parameters control the leg movement of a walking leg? II. The start of swing phase. *Journal of Experimental Biology*, 116, 357–62.

Cruse, H. (1990). What mechanisms coordinate leg movement in walking arthropods? *Trends in Neuroscience*, 13, 15–21.

Cruse, H. and Müller, U. (1986). Two coupling mechanisms which determine the coordination of ipsilateral legs in the walking crayfish. *Journal of Experimental Biology*, 121, 349–69.

Cruse, H., Dean, J., and Suilmann, M. (1984). The contributions of diverse sense organs to the control of leg movement by a walking insect. *Journal of Comparative Physiology A*, **154**, 695–705.

Dai, X., Douglas, J. I., Noga, B. R., and Jordan, L. M. (1990). Localization of spinal neurons activated during treadmill locomotion using the c-fos immunohistochemical method. *Society for Neuroscience Abstracts*, **16**, 889.

Dale, N. (1985). Reciprocal inhibitory interneurones in the *Xenopus* embryo spinal cord. *Journal of Physiology*, **363**, 61–70.

Dale, N. (1986). Excitatory synaptic drive for swimming mediated by excitatory amino acid receptors in the lamprey. *Journal of Neurophysiology*, **6**, 2662–75.

Dale, N. and Gilday, D. (1996). Regulation of rhythmic movements by purinergic neurotransmitters in frog embryos. *Nature*, **383**, 259–63.

Dale, N. and Grillner, S. (1986). Dual-component synaptic potentials in the lamprey mediated by excitatory amino acid receptors. *Journal of Neuroscience*, **69**, 2653–61.

Dale, N. and Kuenzi, E. M. (1997). Ion channels and the control of swimming in the *Xenopus* embryo. *Progresss in Neurobiology*, **53**, 729–56.

Dale, N. and Roberts, A. (1984) Excitatory amino acid receptors in *Xenopus* embryo spinal cord and their role in the activation of swimming. *Journal of Physiology*, **348**, 527–43.

Dale, N. and Roberts, A. (1985). Dual-component amino-acid-mediated synaptic potentials: excitatory drive for swimming in *Xenopus* embryos. *Journal of Physiology*, **363**, 35–59.

Davies, J., Evans, R. H., Jones, A. W., Smith, D. A. S., and Watkins, J. C. (1982). Differential activation and blockade of excitatory amino acid receptors in the mammalian and amphibian central nervous systems. *Comparative Biochemical Physiology*, **72C**, 211–24.

Davis, W. J. (1968a). The neuromuscular basis of lobster swimmeret beating. *Journal of Experimental Zoology*, **168**, 363–78.

Davis, W. J. (1968b). Lobster righting responses and their neural control. *Proceedings of the Royal Society of London B Biological Sciences*, **144**, 480–95.

Davis, W. J. (1968c). Quantitative analysis of swimmeret beating in the lobster. *Journal of Experimental Biology*, **48**, 643–62.

Davis, W. J. (1969). The neural control of swimmeret beating in the lobster. *Journal of Experimental Biology*, **50**, 99–117.

Davis, W. J. (1971). Functional significance of motorneuron size and soma position in swimmeret system of the lobster. *Journal of Neurophysiology*, **34**, 274–88.

Davis, W. J. and Kennedy, D. (1972a). Command interneurons controlling swimmeret movements in the lobster. I. Types of effects on motoneurons. *Journal of Neurophysiology*, **35**, 1–12.

Davis, W. J. and Kennedy, D. (1972b). Command interneurons controlling swimmeret movements in the lobster. II. Interaction of effects on motoneurons. *Journal of Neurophysiology*, **35**, 13–19.

Davis, W. J. and Kennedy, D. (1972c). Command interneurons controlling swimmeret movements in the lobster. III. Temporal relations among bursts in different motoneurons. *Journal of Neurophysiology*, **35**, 20–9.

de Burlet, H. M. and Versteegh, C. (1930). Uber Ban und Funktion des Petromyzonlabyrinthes. *Acta Oto-laringologica* (Suppl.), **13**, 5–58.

Dean, J. (1984). Control of leg protraction in the stick insect: a targeted movement showing compensation for externally applied forces. *Journal of Comparative Physiology A*, **155**, 771–81.

Dean, J. and Wendler, G. (1983). Stick insect locomotion on a walking wheel: interleg coordination of leg position. *Journal of Experimental Biology*, 103, 75–94.

Debski, E. A. and Friesen, W. O. (1987). Intracellular stimulation of sensory cells elicits swimming activity in the medicinal leech. *Journal of Comparative Physiology A— Sensory Neural and Behavioral Physiology*, 160, 447–57.

Delcomyn, F. (1985). Factors regulating insect walking. *Annual Review of Entomology*, 30, 239–56.

Delcomyn, F. (1991). Activity and directional sensitivity of leg campaniform sensilla in a stick insect. *Journal of Comparative Physiology A*, 168, 113–19.

Deliagina, T. G. (1977). The central pathway of the scratch reflex in the cat. *Nejrofiziologia*, 9, 619–21.

Deliagina, T. G. (1997a). Vestibular compensation in lamprey: impairment and recovery of equilibrium control during locomotion. *Journal of Experimental Biology*, 200, 1459–71.

Deliagina, T. G. (1997b). Vestibular compensation in lamprey: roll of vision at different stages of recovery of equilibrium control. *Journal of Experimental Biology*, 200, 2957–67.

Deliagina, T. G. (1997c). Responses of reticulospinal neurons in intact lamprey to vestibular and visual inputs. Effect of unilateral labyrinthectomy. *Society for Neuroscience Abstracts*, 23, Part 1, 765.

Deliagina, T. G. and Feldman, A. G. (1981). Activity of Renshaw cells during fictive scratch reflex in the cat. *Experimental Brain Research*, 42, 108–15.

Deliagina, T. G. and Orlovsky, G. N. (1980). Activity of Ia inhibitory interneurons during fictitious scratch reflex in the cat. *Brain Research*, 193, 439–47.

Deliagina, T. G. and Orlovsky, G. N. (1990a). Control of locomotion in the freshwater snail *Planorbis corneus*. 1. Locomotory repertoire of the snail. *Journal of Experimental Biology*, 152, 389–404.

Deliagina, T. G. and Orlovsky, G. N. (1990b). Control of locomotion in the freshwater snail *Planorbis corneus*. 2. Differential control of various zones of ciliated epithelium. *Journal of Experimental Biology*, 152, 405–23.

Deliagina, T. G., Feldman, A. G., Gelfand, I. M., and Orlovsky, G. N. (1975). On the role of central program and afferent inflow in the control of scratching movements in the cat. *Brain Research*, 100, 297–313.

Deliagina, T. G., Orlovsky, G. N., and Perret, C. (1981). Efferent activity during fictitious scratch reflex in the cat. *Journal of Neurophysiology*, 45, 595–604.

Deliagina, T. G., Orlovsky, G. N., and Pavlova, G. A. (1983). The capacity for generation of rhythmic oscillations is distributed in the lumbosacral spinal cord of the cat. *Experimental Brain Research*, 53, 81–90.

Deliagina, T. G., Orlovsky, G. N., Grillner, S., and Wallén, P. (1992a). Vestibular control of swimming in lamprey. II. Characteristics of spatial sensitivity of reticulospinal neurons. *Experimental Brain Research*, 90, 489–98.

Deliagina, T. G., Orlovsky, G. N., Grillner, S., and Wallén, P. (1992b). Vestibular control of swimming in lamprey. III. Activity of vestibular afferents. Convergens of vestibular inputs on reticulospinal neurons. *Experimental Brain Research*, 90, 499–507.

Deliagina, T. G., Grillner, S., Orlovsky, G. N., and Ullén, F. (1993). Visual inputs affects the response to roll in reticulospinal neurons of the lamprey. *Experimental Brain Research*, 95, 421–8.

Deliagina, T. G., Ullén, F., Gonzalez, M.-J., Ehrsson, H., Orlovsky, G. N., and Grillner, S. (1995). Initiation of locomotion by lateral line photoreceptors in lamprey: Behavioural and neurophysiological studies. *Journal of Experimental Biology*, 198, 2581–91.

Deliagina, T. G., Arshavsky, Y. I., and Orlovsky, G. N. (1998a). Control of spatial orientation in a mollusc. *Nature*, 393, 172–5.

Deliagina, T. G., Orlovsky, G. N., and Arshavsky, Y. I. (1998b). Control of body orientation in *Clione limacina*: spatial zones of activity of different neuron groups. *Society for Neuroscience Abstracts*, 24, Part 2, 2113.

DiCaprio, R. A. and Clarac, F. (1981). Reversal of a walking leg reflex elicited by a muscle receptor. *Journal of Experimental Biology*, 90, 197–203.

Dietz, V., Colombo, G., and Jensen, L. (1994). Locomotor activity in spinal man. *Lancet*, 334, 1260–2.

Douglas, J. R., Noga, B. R., Dai, X., and Jordan, L. M. (1993). The effects of intrathecal administration of excitatory amino acid agonists and antagonists on the initiation of locomotion in the adult cat. *Journal of Neuroscience*, 13, 990–1000.

Dow, R. S. and Moruzzi, G. (1958). *The physiology and pathology of the cerebellum*. University of Minnesota Press, Minneapolis.

Drew, T. (1988). Motor cortical cell discharge during voluntary gait modification. *Brain Research*, 457, 181–7.

Drew, T. (1991a). The role of the motor cortex in the control of gait modification in the cat. In *Neurobiological basis of human locomotion* (eds. M. Shimamura, S. Grillner, and V. R. Edgerton), pp. 201–12. Japan Scientific Societies Press, Tokyo.

Drew, T. (1991b). Functional organization within the medullary reticular formation of the intact unanesthetized cat. III. Microstimulation during locomotion. *Journal of Neurophysiology*, 66, 919–38.

Drew, T. (1991c). Visuomotor coordination in locomotion. *Current Opinions in Neurobiology*, 1, 652–7.

Drew, T. (1993). Motor cortical activity during voluntary gait modifications in the cat. I. Cells related to the forelimbs. *Journal of Neurophysiology*, 70, 179–99.

Drew, T. and Rossignol, S. (1984). Phase-dependent responses evoked in limb muscles by stimulation of medullary reticular formation during locomotion in thalamic cats. *Journal of Neurophysiology*, 52, 653–75.

Drew, T. and Rossignol, S. (1987). A kinematic and electromyographic study of cutaneous reflexes evoked from the forelimb of unrestrained walking cats. *Journal of Neurophysiology*, 57, 1160–84.

Drew, T. and Rossignol, S. (1990a). Functional organisation within the medullary reticular formation of the intact unanaesthetized cat. I. Movements evoked by microstimulation. *Journal of Neurophysiology*, 64, 767–81.

Drew, T. and Rossignol, S. (1990b). Functional organisation within the medullary reticular formation of the intact unanaesthetized cat. II. Electromyographic activity evoked by microstimulation. *Journal of Neurophysiology*, 64, 782–95.

Drew, T., Dubuc, R., and Rossignol, S. (1986). Discharge patterns of reticulospinal and other reticular neurons in chronic, unrestrained cats walking on a treadmill. *Journal of Neurophysiology*, 55, 375–401.

Driesang, R. B. and Büschges, A. (1993). The neuronal basis of catalepsy in the stick insect. IV. Properties of nonspiking interneurons. *Journal of Comparative Physiology A*, 173, 445–54.

Driesang, R. B. and Büschges, A. (1996). Physiological changes in central neuronal pathways contributing to the generation of a reflex reversal. *Journal of Comparative Physiology A*, 179, 45–57.

Dubrovsky, B., Garcia-Rill, E., and Surkes, M. A. (1974). Effects of discrete precruciate cortex lesions on motor behavior. *Brain Research*, 82, 328–33.

Dubuc, R. and Grillner, S. (1989). The role of spinal cord inputs in modulating the activity of reticulospinal neurons during fictive locomotion in the lamprey. *Brain Research*, 483, 196–200.

Dubuc, R., Cabelguen, J.-M., and Rossignol, S. (1988). Rhythmic fluctuations of dorsal root potentials and antidromic discharges of single primary afferents during fictive locomotion in the cat. *Journal of Neurophysiology*, 60, 2014–36.

Dubuc, R., Bongianni, F., Ohta, Y., and Grillner, S. (1993). Anatomical and physiological study of brainstem nuclei relaying dorsal column inputs in lampreys. *Journal of Comparative Neurology*, 327, 260–70.

Duch, C. and Pflüger, H.-J. (1995). Motor patterns for horizontal and upside-down walking and vertical climbing in the locust. *Journal of Experimental Biology*, 198, 1963–76.

Durelli, L., Schmidt, E. M., McIntosh, J. S., and Bak, M. J. (1978). Single unit chronic recordings from the sensorimotor cortex of unrestrained cats during locomotion. *Experimental Neurology*, 62, 580–94.

Duysens, J. and Pearson, K. G. (1980). Inhibition of flexor burst generation by loading ankle extensor muscles in walking cats. *Brain Research*, 187, 321–32.

Duysens, J., Trippel, M., Horstmann, G. A. (1990). Dietz V. Gating and reversal of reflexes in ankle muscles during human walking. *Experimental Brain Research*, 82, 351–8.

Eccles, J. C., Llinas, R., and Sasaki, K. (1966). The excitatory synaptic action of climbing fibres on the Purkinje cells of the cerebellum. *Journal of Physiology*, 182, 268–96.

Eccles, J. C., Ito, M., and Szentagothai, J. (1967). *The cerebellum as a neuronal machine.* Springer, New York.

Eccles, J. C., Provini, L., Strata, P., and Táboríková, H. (1968). Topographical investigations on the climbing fiber inputs from forelimb and hindlimb afferents to the cerebellar anterior lobe. *Experimental Brain Research*, 6, 195–215.

Eccles, J. C., Sabah, N. H., and Táboríková, H. (1974). The pathways responsible for excitation and inhibition of fastigial neurones. *Experimental Brain Research*, 19, 78–99.

Edgley, S. A. and Jankowska, E. (1987). Field potentials generated by group II muscle afferents in the middle lumbar segments of the cat spinal cord. *Journal of Physiology*, 385, 393–413.

Edgley, S. A., Jankowska, E., and Shefchyk, S. (1988). Evidence that mid-lumbar neurones in reflex pathways from group II afferents are involved in locomotion in the cat. *Journal of Physiology*, 403, 57–71.

Eidelberg, E. (1981). Consequences of spinal cord lesions upon motor function, with special reference to locomotor activity. *Progress in Neurobiology*, 17, 185–202.

Eidelberg, E., Walden, J. G., and Nguyen, L. H. (1981). Locomotor control in macaque monkeys. *Brain*, 104, 647–63.

Ekeberg, Ö., Wallén, P., Lansner, A., Tråvén, H., Brodin, L., and Grillner, S. (1991). A computer based model for realistic simulations of neural networks. *Biological Cybernetics*, 65, 81–90.

Ekeberg, Ö., Lansner, A., and Grillner, S. (1995). The neural control of fish swimming studied through numerical simulations. *Adaptive Behavior*, 3, 363–84.

Elliot, B. C. and Blanksby, B. A. (1976). Reliability of averaged integrated electromyograms during running. *Journal of Human Movement Studies*, 2, 28–35.

Elliott, C. J. H. and Benjamin, P. R. (1985). Interactions of pattern-generating interneurons controlling feeding in *Lymnaea stagnalis*. *Journal of Neurophysiology*, 54, 1396–411.

El Manira, A. and Bussières, N. (1997). Calcium channel subtypes in lamprey sensory and motor neurons. *Journal of Neurophysiology*, 78, 1334–40.

El Manira, A., DiCaprio, R. A., Cattaert, D., and Clarac, F. (1991). Monosynaptic interjoint reflexes and their central modulation during fictive locomotion in crayfish. *European Journal of Neuroscience*, 3, 1219–31.

El Manira, A., Tegnér, J., and Grillner, S. (1994). Calcium-dependent potassium channels play a critical role for burst termination in the locomotor network in lamprey. *Journal of Neurophysiology*, 72, 1852–61.

El Manira, A., Pombal, M. A., and Grillner, S. (1997a). Diencephalic projection to reticulospinal neurons involved in the initiation of locomotion in adult lampreys *Lampetra fluviatilis*. *Journal of Comparative Neurology*, 389, 603–16.

El Manira, A., Zhang, W., Svensson, E., and Bussières, N. (1997b). 5-HT inhibits calcium current and synaptic transmission from sensory neurons in lamprey. *Journal of Neuroscience*, 17, 1786–94.

El Manira, A., Parker, D., Kriger, P., Wikström, M., and Grillner, S. (1998). Presynaptic inhibition of sensory transmission from sensory interneuronal and supraspinal neurons to spinal target cells in lamprey. In *Presynaptic inhibition and neuronal control* (eds. P. Rudomin, R. Romo, and L. Mendell), pp. 329–48. Oxford University Press, Oxford.

Engberg, I. and Lundberg, A. (1969). An electromyographic analysis of muscular activity in the hindlimb of the cat during unrestrained locomotion. *Acta Physiologica Scandinavia*, 75, 614–30.

English, A. W. (1978a). An electromyographic analysis of forelimb muscles during overground stepping in the cat. *Journal of Experimental Biology*, 76, 105–22.

English, A. W. (1978b). Functional analysis of the shoulder girdle of cats during locomotion. *Journal of Morphology*, 156, 279–92.

English, A. W. (1980). Interlimb coordination during stepping in the cat: effects of dorsal column section. *Journal of Neurophysiology*, 44, 270–9.

English, A. W. (1984). An electromyographic analysis of compartments in cat lateral gastrocnemius muscle during unrestrained locomotion. *Journal of Neurophysiology*, 52, 114–25.

English, A. W. (1985). Interlimb coordination during stepping in the cat. The role of the dorsal spinocerebellar tract. *Experimental Neurology*, 87, 96–108.

Euler, C. von (1977). The functional organization of the respiratory phase switching mechanisms. *Federation Proceedings*, 36, 2375–80.

Euler, C. von (1983). On the origin and pattern control of breathing rhythmicity in mammals. In *Neural origin of rhythmic movements. Society for Experimental Biology Symposium 37* (eds. A. Roberts and B. L. Roberts), pp. 469–85. Cambridge University Press Cambridge.

Euler, C. von (1986). Brain stem mechanism for generation and control of breathing pattern. In *Handbook of physiology. The respiratory system* (eds. N. S. Cherniak and J. G. Widdicombe), Vol. 2, pp. 1–67. American Physiological Society, Bethesda, MD.

Evarts, E. V. and Thach, W. T. (1969). Motor mechanisms of the CNS: cerebrocerebellar interrelations. *Annual Review of Physiology*, 31, 451–98.

Evoy, W. H. and Kennedy, D. (1967). The central nervous organization underlying control of antagonist muscles in the crayfish. II. Types of command fibres. *Journal of Experimental Zoology*, 165, 223–38.

Fagerstedt, P., Wallén, P., and Grillner, S. (1995). Activity of interneurons during fictive swimming in the lamprey. *IBRO Congress of Neuroscience Abstracts*, 1, 346.

Fanardjan, V. V. and Gorodnov, V. L. (1983). Electrophysiological properties of cortical synaptic input of rubro-spinal neurons. *Neuroscience Letters*, 40, 269–73.

Feldberg, N. and Fleischhauer, K. (1960). Scratching movements evoked by drugs applied to the cervical cord. *Journal of Physiology*, 151, 502–17.

Feldman, A. G. and Orlovsky, G. N. (1975). Activity of interneurons mediating reciprocal Ia inhibition during locomotion. *Brain Research*, 84, 181–94.

Feldman, A. G., Orlovsky, G. N., and Perret, C. (1977). Activity of muscle spindle afferents during scratching in the cat. *Brain Research*, 129, 192–6.

Fenaux, F., Corio, M., Palisses, R., and Viala, D. (1991). Effects of NMDA-receptor antagonist, MK-801, on central locomotor programming in the rabbit. *Experimental Brain Research*, 86, 393–401.

Fleshman, J. W., Lev-Tov, A., and Burke, R. E. (1984). Peripheral and central control of flexor digitorium longus and flexor hallucis longus motoneurons: the synaptic basis of functional diversity. *Experimental Brain Research*, 54, 133–49.

Forssberg, H. and Grillner, S. (1973). The locomotion of the acute spinal cat injected with clonidine i.v. *Brain Research*, 50, 184–6.

Forssberg, H. and Hirschfeld, H. (1988). Phasic modulation of postural activation patterns during human walking. *Progress in Brain Research*, 76, 221–7.

Forssberg, H., Grillner, S., and Sjostrom, A. (1974). Tactile placing reactions in chronic spinal kittens. *Acta Physiologica Scandinavia*, 92, 114–20.

Forssberg, H. S., Grillner, S., and Rossignol, S. (1977). Phasic gain control of reflexes from the dorsum of the paw during spinal locomotion. *Brain Research*, 132, 121–39.

Forssberg, H., Grillner, S., and Halbertsma, J. (1980a). The locomotion of the low spinal cat. I. Coordination within a hindlimb. *Acta Physiologica Scandinavia*, 108, 269–81.

Forssberg, H., Grillner, S., Halbertsma, J., and Rossignol, S. (1980b). The locomotion of the low spinal cat: II. Interlimb coordination. *Acta Physiologica Scandinavia*, 108, 283–95.

Frank, K. and Fuortes, M. G. (1957). Presynaptic and postsynaptic inhibition of monosynaptic reflexes. *Federation Proceedings*, 16, 39–40.

Fredman, S. M. and Jahan-Parwar, B. (1980). Role of pedal ganglia motor neurons in pedal wave generation in *Aplysia*. *Brain Research Bulletin*, 5, 179–93.

Fredman, S. M. and Jahan-Parwar, B. (1983). Command neurons for locomotion in *Aplysia*. *Journal of Neurophysiology*, 49, 1092–117.

Freusberg, A. (1874). Reflexbewegungen beim Hunde. *Pfluegers Archives of Ges. Physiology*, 9, 358–91.

Friesen, W. O. (1985a). Neuronal control of leech swimming movements: interactions between cell 60 and previously described oscillator neurons. *Journal of Comparative Physiology*, 156, 231–42.

Friesen, W. O. (1985b). Inhibitory motor neurons are part of the network which generates leech (*Hirudo*) swimming activity. *Society for Neuroscience Abstracts*, 11 (Part 2), 1023.

Friesen, W. O. (1989a). Neuronal control of leech swimming movements. In *Neuronal and cellular oscillators* (ed. J. W. Jacklet), pp. 269–316. Marcel Dekker, New York.

Friesen, W. O. (1989b). Neuronal control of leech swimming movements. I. Inhibitory interactions between motor neurons. *Journal of Comparative Physiology A*, 166, 195–203.

Friesen, W. O. (1989c). Neuronal control of leech swimming movements. II. Motor neuron feedback to oscillator cells 115 and 28. *Journal of Comparative Physiology A*, 166, 205–15.

Friesen, W. O. (1994). Reciprocal inhibition: A mechanism underlying oscillatory animal movements. *Neuroscience and Biobehavior*, 18, 547–53.

Friesen, W. O. and Stent, G. S. (1977). Generation of locomotory rhythm by a neuronal network with recurrent cyclic inhibition. *Biological Cybernetics*, 28, 27–40.

Friesen, W. O. and Stein, G. (1978). Neuronal circuit for generating rhythmic movements. *Annual Review of Biophysics and Bioengineering*, 7, 37–61.

Friesen, W. O. and Wyman, R. J. (1979). Model circuit for the control of motor neuron activity pattern in *Drosophila*. *Society for Neuroscience Abstracts*, 5, 494.

Friesen, W. O., Poon, M., and Stent, G. S. (1976). An oscillatory neuronal circuit generating a locomotory rhythm. *Proceedings of the National Academy of Sciences of the United States of America*, 73, 3734–8.

Friesen, W. O., Poon, M., and Stent, G. S. (1978). Neuronal control of swimming in the medicinal leech. IV. Identification of a network of oscillatory interneurones. *Journal of Experimental Biology*, 75, 25–43.

Frost, W. N., Brown, G. D., and Getting, P. A. (1996). Parametric features of habituation of swim cycle number in the marine mollusc *Tritonia diomedea*. *Neurobiology of Learning and Memory*, 65, 125–34.

Futami, T., Shinoda, Y., and Yokota, J. (1979). Spinal axon collaterals of corticospinal neurons identified by intracellular injection of horseradish peroxide. *Brain Research*, 164, 279–84.

Gambarian, P. P., Orlovsky, G. N., Protopopova, F. V., Severin, F. V., and Shik, M. L. (1971). Muscular activity at different kinds of the cat locomotion, and adjusting changes of the organs of movements in the family *Felidae*. *Proceedings of the Zoological Institute of the USSR*, 48, 220–39. (In Russian).

Gamkrelidze, G. N., Laurienti, P. J., and Blankenship, J. E. (1995). Identification and characterization of cerebral ganglion neurons that induce swimming and modulate swim-related pedal ganglion neurons in *Aplysia brasiliana*. *Journal of Neurophysiology*, 74, 1444–62.

Garcia-Rill, E. (1986). The basal ganglia and the locomotor regions. *Brain Research Review*, 11, 47–63.

Garcia-Rill, E. and Skinner, R. D. (1986). The basal ganglia and the mesencephalic locomotor region. In *Neurobiology of vertebrate locomotion* (eds. S. Grillner, P. S. G. Stein, D. Stuart, H. Forssberg, and H. Herman), pp. 77–104. Macmillan, London.

Garcia-Rill, E. and Skinner, R. D. (1987a). The mesencephalic locomotor region i. Activation of a medullary projection site. *Brain Research*, 411, 1–12.

Garcia-Rill, E. and Skinner, R. D. (1987b). The mesencephalic locomotor region ii. Projections to reticulospinal neurons. *Brain Research*, 411, 13–20.

Garcia-Rill, E., Skinner, R. D., and Gilmore, S. A. (1981). Pallidal projections to the mesencephalic locomotor region (MLR) in the cat. *American Journal of Anatomy*, 161, 311–21.

Garcia-Rill, E., Skinner, R. D., Gilmore, S. A., and Owings, R. (1983a). Connections of the mesencephalic locomotor region (MLR). II Afferents and efferents. *Brain Research Bulletin*, 10, 63–71.

Garcia-Rill E., Skinner, R. D., and Fitzgerald, J. A. (1983b). Activity in the mesencephalic locomotor region during locomotion. *Experimental Neurology*, 82, 609–22.

Garcia-Rill, E., Skinner, R. D., and Fitzgerald, J. A. (1985). Chemical activation of the mesencephalic locomotor region. *Brain Research*, 330, 43–54.

Garcia-Rill, E., Skinner, R. D., Jackson, M. B., and Smith, M. M. (1983c). Connections of the mesencephalic locomotor region (MLR). I. Substantia nigra afferents. *Brain Research Bulletin*, 10 57–62.

Garcia-Rill, E., Kinjo, N., Atsuta, Y., Ishikawa, Y., Webber, M., and Skinner, R. D. (1990). Posterior midbrain-induced locomotion. *Brain Research Bulletin*, 24, 499–508.

Gelfand, I. M., Orlovsky, G. N., and Shik, M. L. (1988). Locomotion and scratching in tetrapods. In *Neural control of rhythmic movements in vertebrates* (eds. A. H. Cohen, S. Rossignol, and S. Grillner), pp. 167–99. Wiley, New York.

Georgopoulos, A. P. and Grillner, S. (1989). Visuomotor coordination in reaching and locomotion. *Science*, 245, 1209–10.

Georgopoulos, A. P., Caminiti, R., Kalaska, J. F., and Massey, J. T. (1983). Spatial coding of movement: a hypothesis corcerning the coding of movement direction by motor cortical populations. *Experimental Brain Research Supplement*, 7, 327–36.

Georgopoulos, A. P., Taira, M., and Lukashin, A. V. (1993). Cognitive neurophysiology of the motor cortex, *Science*, 260, 47–52.

Gerasimenko, Y., McKay, W. B., Pollo, F. E., and Dimitrijevic, M. R. (1996). Stepping movements in paraplegic patients induced by epidural spinal cord stimulation. *Society for Neuroscience Abstracts*, 22, 543–5.

Getting, P. A. (1976). Afferent neurons mediating escape swimming of the marine mollusc, *Tritonia*. *Journal of Comparative Physiology*, 110, 271–85.

Getting, P. A. (1977). Neuronal organization of escape swimming in *Tritonia*. *Journal of Comparative Physiology*, 121, 325–42.

Getting, P. A. (1981). Mechanisms of pattern generation underlying swimming in *Tritonia*. I. Neuronal network formed by monosynaptic connections. *Journal of Neurophysiology*, 46, 65–79.

Getting, P. A. (1983*a*). Mechanisms of pattern generation underlying swimming in *Tritonia*. II. Network reconstruction. *Journal of Neurophysiology*, 49, 1017–35.

Getting, P. A. (1983*b*). Mechanisms of pattern generation underlying swimming in *Tritonia*. III. Intrinsic and synaptic mechanisms for delayed excitation. *Journal of Neurophysiology*, 49, 1036–50.

Getting, P. A. and Dekin, M. S. (1985). Mechanisms of pattern generation underlying swimming in *Tritonia*. IV. Gating of central pattern generator. *Journal of Neurophysiology*, 53, 466–80.

Getting, P. A., Lennard, P. R., and Hume, R. I. (1980). Central pattern generator mediating swimming in *Tritonia*. I. Identification and synaptic interactions. *Journal of Neurophysiology*, 44, 151–64.

Gewecke, M. and Wendler, G. (eds.) (1985). *Insect locomotion*. Paul Parey, Berlin.

Ghez, C., Gordon, J., and Ghilardi, M. F. (1995). Impairments of reaching movements in patients without proprioception. II. Effects of visual information on accuracy. *Journal of Neurophysiology*, 73, 361–72.

Glover, J. C. and Kramer, A. P. (1982). Serotonin analog selectively ablates indentified neurons in the leech embryo. *Science*, 216, 317–19.

Goldberger, M. E. (1965). The extrapyramidal systems of the spinal cord: results of combined spinal and cortical lesions in the macaque. *Journal of Comparative Neurology*, 124, 161–74.

Goldberger, M. E. (1969). The extrapyramidal systems of the spinal cord. II. Results of combined pyramidal and extrapyramidal lesions in the macaque. *Journal of Comparative Neurology*, 135, 1–26.

Goslow, G. E., Reinking, R. M., and Stuart, D. G. (1973). The cat step cycle: hind limb joint angles and muscle lengths during unrestrained locomotion. *Journal of Morphology*, 141, 1–42.

Gossard, J. P. and Rossignol, S. (1990). Phase-dependent modulation of dorsal root potentials evoked by peripheral nerve stimulation during fictive locomotion in the cat. *Brain Research*, 537, 1–13.

Gossard, J.-P., Brownstone, R. M., Barajon, I., and Hultborn, H. (1994). Transmission in a locomotor-related group Ib pathway from hindlimb extensor muscles in the cat. *Experimental Brain Research*, 98, 213–28.

Gossard, J.-P., Cabelguen, J.-M., and Rossignol, S. (1991). An intracellular study of muscle primary afferents during fictive locomotion in the cat. *Journal of Neurophysiology*, 65, 914–26.

Graham, D. (1972). A behavioural analysis of the temporal organization of walking movements in the first instar and adult stick insect *Carausius morosus*. *Journal of Comparative Physiology*, 81A, 23–52.

Graham, D. (1978). Unusual step patterns in the free walking grasshopper *Neoconocephalus robustus*. I. General features of the step pattern. *Journal of Experimental Biology*, 73, 147–57.

Graham, D. (1985). Pattern and control of walking in insects. *Advances in Insect Physiology*, 18, 31–140.

Graham, D. and Wendler, G. (1981). Motor output to the protractor and retractor coxae muscles of Carausius morosus during walking on a tredwheel. *Physiological Entomology*, 6, 161–74.

Granit, R. (1950). Reflex self-regulation of muscle contraction and autogenetic inhibition. *Journal of Neurophysiology*, 13, 351–72.

Grant, G., Oscarsson, O., and Rosén, I. (1966). Functional organization of the spinoreticulo-cerebellar path with identification of its spinal component. *Experimental Brain Research*, 1, 306–19.

Granzow, B. and Kristan, W. B. (1986). Inhibitory connections between motor neurons modify a centrally generated motor pattern in the leech nervous system. *Brain Research*, 369, 321–5.

Gray, J. (1968). *Animal locomotion*. Weidenfeld & Nicolson, London.

Gray, J., Lissman, H. W., and Pumphrey, R. J. (1938). The mechanism of locomotion in the leech (*Hirudo medicinalis Ray*). *Journal of Experimental Biology*, 15, 408–30.

Grillner, S. (1972). The role of muscle stiffness in meeting the changing postural and locomotor requirements for force development by the ankle extensors. *Acta Physiologica Scandinavia*, 86, 92–108.

Grillner, S. (1973). Locomotion in the spinal cat. In *Control of posture and locomotion. Advances in Behavioral Biology 7* (eds. R. B. Stein, K. G. Pearson, R. S. Smith, and J. B. Redford), pp. 515–35. Plenum, New York.

Grillner, S. (1975). Locomotion in vertebrates: Central mechanisms and reflex interaction. *Physiological Review*, 55, 247–304.

Grillner, S. (1981). Control of locomotion in bipeds, tetrapods and fish. In *Handbook of physiology. The nervous system* (ed. V. Brooks), Vol. 2, pp. 1179–236. Waverly Press, Baltimore.

Grillner S. (1985). Neurobiological bases of rhythmic motor acts in vertebrates. *Science*, 228, 143–9.

Grillner, S. (1989). The segmental burst generating network used in lamprey locomotion: Experiments and simulations. In *The theoretical model for cell to cell signalling* (ed. A. Goldbeter), pp. 77–87. Academic, New York.

Grillner, S. (1997). Ion channels and locomotion. *Science*, 278, 1087–8.

Grillner, S. and Kashin, S. (1976). On the generation and performance of swimming in fish. In: *Neural control of locomotion* (eds. R. M. Herman, S. Grillner, P. S. G. Stein, and D. G. Stuart), Vol. 18, pp. 181–202. Plenum, New York.

Grillner, S. and Orlovsky, G. N. (1991). Locomotion, neural networks. In *Encyclopedia of Human Biology*, Vol. 4, pp. 769–81. Academic, New York.

Grillner, S. and Rossignol, S. (1978). On the initiation of the swing phase of locomotion in chronic spinal cats. *Brain Research*, 146, 269–77.

Grillner, S. and Wallén, P. (1980). Does the central pattern generation for locomotion in the lamprey depend on glycine inhibition? *Acta Physiologica Scandinavia*, **110**, 103–5.

Grillner, S. and Wallén, P. (1985). Central pattern generators for locomotion with special reference to vertebrates. *Annual Review of Neuroscience*, **8**, 233–61.

Grillner, S. and Zangger, P. (1974). Locomotor movements generated by the deafferented spinal cord. *Acta Physiologica Scandinavia*, **91**, 38A–39A.

Grillner, S. and Zangger, P. (1975). How detailed is the central pattern generator for locomotion? *Brain Research*, **88**, 367–71.

Grillner, S. and Zangger, P. (1979). On the central generation of locomotion in the low spinal cat. *Experimental Brain Research*, **34**, 241–61.

Grillner, S. and Zangger, P. (1984). The effect of dorsal root transection on the efferent motor pattern in the cat's hindlimb during locomotion. *Acta Physiologica Scandinavia*, **120**, 393–405.

Grillner, S., Hongo, T., and Lund, S. (1970). The vestibulospinal tract. Effects on alpha-motoneurons in the lumbosacral spinal cord in the cat. *Experimental Brain Research*, **10**, 94–120.

Grillner, S., Haltbertsma, J., Nilsson, J., and Thorstensson, A. (1979). The adaptation to speed in human locomotion. *Brain Research*, **165**, 177–82.

Grillner, S., McClellan, A., and Perret, C. (1981a). Entrainment of the spinal pattern generators for swimming by mechano-sensitive elements in the lamprey spinal cord *in vitro*. *Brain Research*, **217**, 380–6.

Grillner, S., McClellan, A., Sigvardt, K., Wallén, P., and Wilén, M. (1981b). Activation of NMDA-receptors elicits 'fictive locomotion' in lamprey spinal cord *in vitro*. *Acta Physiologica Scandinavia*, **113**, 549–51.

Grillner, S., McClellan, A., and Sigvardt, K. (1982). Mechano-sensitive neurons in the spinal cord of the lamprey. *Brain Research*, **235**, 169–73.

Grillner, S., Williams, T., and Lagerbäck, P.-Å. (1984a). The edge cell, a possible intraspinal mechanoreceptor. *Science*, **223**, 500–3.

Grillner, S., McClellan, A, Sigvardt, K., and Wallén, P. (1984b). On the spinal generation of locomotion with particular reference to a simple vertebrate: the lamprey. In *Nervous system regeneration* (eds. B. Haber and R. Perez-Polo), pp. 347–56. Alan Liss, New York.

Grillner, S., Brodin, L., Sigvardt, K., and Dale, N. (1986). On the spinal network generating locomotion in lamprey: transmitters, membrane properties and circuitry. In: *Neurobiology of vertebrate locomotion* (eds. S. Grillner, P. S. G. Stein, H. Forssberg, D. Stuart, and R. Herman), pp. 335–52. Macmillan, London.

Grillner, S., Buchanan, J. T., Wallén, P., and Brodin, L. (1988a). Neural control of locomotion in lower vertebrates—From behavior to ionic mechanisms. In *Neural control of rhythmic movements in vertebrates* (eds. A. H. Cohen, S. Rossignol, and S. Grillner), pp. 1–40. Wiley, New York.

Grillner, S., Wallén, P., and Viana di Prisco, G. (1990). Cellular network underlying locomotion as revealed in a lower vertebrate model: transmitters, membrane properties, circuitry, and simulation. *Cold Spring Harbor Symposia on Quantitative Biology*, **55**, 779–89.

Grillner, S., Matsushima, T., Wadden, T., Tegnér, J., El Manira, A., and Wallén, P. (1993). The neurophysiological bases of undulatory locomotion in vertebrates. *Seminars in Neuroscience*, **5**, 17–27.

Grillner, S., Deliagina, T., Ekeberg, Ö., El Manira, A., Hill, R., Lansner, A., Orlovsky, G., and Wallen, P. (1995). Neural networks controlling locomotion and body orientation in lamprey. *Trends in Neuroscience*, **18**, 270–9.

Grillner, S., Georgopoulos, A. P., and Jordan, L. M. (1997). Selection and initiation of motor behaviour. In *Neurons, networks and motor behavior* (eds. P. S. G. Stein, S. Grillner, A. Selverston, and D. G. Stuart), pp. 4–19. MIT Press, Cambridge, MA.

Grimm, K. and Sauer, A. E. (1995). The high number of neurons contributes to the robustness of the locust flight-CPG against parameter variation. *Biological Cybernetics*, 72, 329–35.

Grote, J. R. (1981). The effect of load on locomotion in crayfish. *Journal of Experimental Biology*, 92, 277–88.

Guertin, P., Angel, M., Perreault, M.-C., and McCrea, D. A. (1995). Ankle extensor group I afferents excite extensors throughout the hindlimb during MLR-evoked fictive locomotion in the cat. *Journal of Physiology*, 487, 197–209.

Gurfinkel, V. S. and Shik, M. L. (1973). The conrtol of posture and locomotion. In *Motor control* (eds. A. A. Gydikov, N. T. Tankov, and D. S. Kosarov), pp. 217–34. Plenum, New York.

Gurfinkel, V. S., Levik, Y. S., Kazennikov, O. V., and Selionov, V. A. (1998). Locomotor-like movements evoked by leg muscle vibration in humans. *European Journal of Neuroscience*, 10, 1608–12.

Halbertsma, J. M. (1983). The stride cycle of the cat: the modelling of locomotion by computerized analysis of automatic recordings. *Acta Physiologica Scandinavia*, Suppl., 521, 1–75.

Hamilton, P. V. and Ambrose, H. M. (1975). Swimming and orientation in *Aplysia brasiliana* (Mollusca: Gastropoda). *Marine Behavior and Physiology*, 3, 131–43.

Hamilton, P. V. and Russell, B. J. (1982). Field experiments on the sense organs and directional cues involved in offshore-oriented swimming by *Aplysia brasiliana* Rang (Mollusca: Gastropoda). *Journal of Experimental Marine Biology and Ecology*, 56, 123–43.

Hancox, J. C. and Pitman, R. M. (1991). Plateau potentials drive axonal impulse bursts in insect motoneurons. *Proceedings of the Royal Society of London B Biological Sciences*, 244, 33–8.

Harmon, L. D. (1964) Neuromimes: action of a reciprocally inhibitory pair. *Science*, 146, 1323–5.

Harmon, L. D. and Lewis, E. R. (1966). Neural modelling. *Physiological Review*, 46, 513–91.

Harris, J. E. (1936). The role of the fins in the equilibrium of the swimming fish. I. Wind-tunnel tests on a model of *Mustelus canis* (Mitchill). *Journal of Experimental Biology*, 13, 474–93.

Harris-Warrick, R. M. and Cohen, A. H. (1985). Serotonin modulates the central pattern generator for locomotion in the isolated lamprey spinal cord. *Journal of Experimental Biology*, 116, 27–46.

Harris-Warrick, R. M. and Marder, E. (1991). Modulation of neural networks for behaviour. *Annual Review of Neuroscience*, 14, 39–57.

Hashemzadeh-Gargari, H. and Friesen, W. O. (1989). Modulation of swimming activity in the medicinal leech by serotonin and octopamine. *Comparative Biochemistry and Physiology—C: Comparative Pharmacology and Toxicology*, 94, 295–302.

Hedwig, B. and Pearson, K. G. (1984). Pattern of synaptic input to identified flight motoneurons in the locust. *Journal of Comparative Physiology*, 154, 745–60.

Heitler, W. J. (1978). Coupled motoneurons are part of the crayfish swimmeret central oscillator. *Nature*, 275, 231–41.

Heitler, W. J. (1981). Neural mechanisms of central pattern generation in the crayfish swimmeret system. In *Neurobiology of invertebrates* (Advances in Physiological Science, Vol. 23) (ed. J. Salanki), pp. 369–83. Plenum, Oxford.

Heitler, W. J. (1985). Motor programme switching in the crayfish swimmeret system. *Journal of Experimental Biology*, 114, 521–49.

Heitler, W. J. (1986). Aspects of sensory integration in the crayfish swimmeret system. *Journal of Experimental Biology*, 120, 387–402.

Hellgren, J., Grillner, S., and Lansner, A. (1992). Computer simulation of the segmental neural network generating locomotion in lamprey by using populations of network interneurons. *Biological Cybernetics*, 68, 1–13.

Hening, W. A., Walters, E. T., Carew, T. J., and Kandel, E. R. (1979). Motorneuronal control of locomotion in *Aplysia*. *Brain Research*, 179, 231–53.

Hensbergen, E. and Kernell, D. (1992). Task-related differences in distribution of electromyographic activity within peroneus longus muscle of spontaneously moving cats. *Experimental Brain Research*, 89, 682–5.

Hensler, K. (1988). The pars intercerebralis neurone PI(2)5 of locusts: convergent processing of inputs reporting head movements and deviations from straight flight. *Journal of Experimental Biology*, 140, 511–33.

Hensler, K. (1989). Corrective flight steering in locusts: convergence of extero- and proprioceptive inputs in descending deviation detectors. In *Neurobiology of sensory systems* (eds. R. Naresh Singh and N. J. Strausfeld), pp. 531–54. Plenum, New York.

Hensler, K. and Rowell, C. H. F. (1990). Control of optomotor responses by descending deviation detector neurons in intact flying locust. *Journal of Experimental Biology*, 149, 191–205.

Herman, R., Wirta, A., Bampton, S., and Finley, F. R. (1976). Human solutions for locomotion: single limb analysis. In *Neural control of locomotion* (eds. R. Herman, S. Grillner, P. S. G. Stein, and D. G. Stuart), pp. 13–50. Plenum, New York.

Hinsey, J. C., Ranson, S. W., and McNattin R. F. (1930). The role of the hypothalamus and mesencephalon in locomotion. *Archives of Neurology and Psychiatry*, 23, 1–43.

Hirschfeld, H. and Forssberg, H. (1991). Phase-dependent modulations of anticipatory postural activity during human locomotion. *Journal of Neurophysiology*, 66, 12–19.

Ho, S. and O'Donovan, M. J. (1993). Regionalization and intersegmental coordination of rhythm-generating networks in the spinal cord of the chick embryo. *Journal of Neuroscience*, 13, 1354–71.

Hochman, S., Jordan, L. M., and Macdonald, J. F. (1994). N-methyl-D-aspartate receptor-mediated voltage oscillations in neurons surrounding the central canal in slices of rat spinal cord. *Journal of Neurophysiology*, 72, 565–77.

Hoffmann, P., Illert, M., and Wiedemann, E. (1985). EMG recordings from the cat forelimb during unrestrained locomotion. *Neuroscience Letters*, Suppl., 22, S126.

Hofmann, T. and Bässler, U. (1982). Anatomy and physiology of trochanteral campaniform sensilla in the stick insect, *Cuniculina impigra*. *Physiological Entomology*, 7, 413–26.

Holmes, G. (1939). The cerebellum of man. *Brain*, 62, 1–30.

Hongo, T., Jankowska, E., and Lundberg, A. (1969a). The rubrospinal tract. I. Effects on alpha-motoneurons innervating hindlimb muscles in cats. *Experimental Brain Research*, 7, 344–64.

Hongo, T., Jankowska, E., and Lundberg, A. (1969b). The rubrospinal tract. II. Facilitation of interneuronal transmission in reflex paths to motoneurons. *Experimental Brain Research*, 7, 365–91.

Horak, F. B. and Macpherson, J. M. (1995). Postural orientation and equilibrium. In *Integration of motor, circulatory, respiratory and metabolic control during excercise. Handbook of physiology, Section 12* (eds. J. Shepard and L. Rowell), pp. 1–39. Oxford University Press, New York.

Hounsgaard, J., Hultborn, H., Jespersen, J., and Kiehn, O. (1988). Bistability of alpha-motoneurones in the decerebrate cat and in the acute spinal cat after intravenous 5-hydroxytryptophan. *Journal of Physiology*, 405, 345–67.

Hoyle, G. (1964). Exploration of neural mechanisms underlying behaviour in insects. In *Neural theory and modelling* (ed. R. F. Reiss), pp. 346–76. Stanford University Press.

Huang, Z. and Satterlie, R. A. (1990) Neuronal mechanisms underlying behavioural switching in a pteropod mollusc. *Journal of Comparative Physiology A—Sensory Neural and Behavioural Physiology*, 166, 875–87.

Hubbard, J. I. and Oscarsson, O. (1962). Localization of the cell bodies of the ventral spinocerebellar tract in lumber segments of the cat. *Journal of Comparative Neurology*, 118, 199–204.

Hughes, G. and Wiersma, C. A. G. (1960). The co-ordination of swimmeret movements in the crayfish, *Procambarus clarkii* (Girard). *Journal of Experimental Biology*, 37, 657–70.

Hultborn, H. (1972). Convergence on interneurons in the reciprocal 1a inhibitory pathway to motoneurons. *Acta Physiologica Scandinavia*, Suppl. 375, 1–42.

Hultborn, H., Jankowska, E., and Lindström, S. (1971). Recurrent inhibition from motor axon collaterals of transmission in the 1a inhibitory pathway to motoneurons. *Journal of Physiology*, 215, 591–612.

Hultborn, H., Peterson, N., Brownstone, R., and Nielsen, J. (1993). Evidence of fictive spinal locomotion in the marmoset (*Callithrix jacchus*). *Society for Neuroscience Abstracts*, 19, 539.

Hume, R. I. and Getting, P. A. (1982a). Motor organization of *Tritonia* swimming. II. Synaptic drive to flexion neurons from premotor interneurons. *Journal of Neurophysiology*, 47, 75–90.

Hume, R. I. and Getting, P. A. (1982b). Motor organization of *Tritonia* swimming. III. Contribution of intrinsic membrane properties to flexion neuron burst formation. *Journal of Neurophysiology*, 47, 91–102.

Hume, R. I., Getting, P. A., and Del Beccaro, M. A. (1982). Motor organization of *Tritonia* swimming. I. Quantitative analysis of swim behavior and flexion neuron firing patterns. *Journal of Neurophysiology*, 47, 60–74.

Hunt, C. C. (1952). The effect of stretch receptors from muscle on the discharge of motoneurons. *Journal of Physiology*, 117, 359–79.

Ikeda, K. and Wiersma, C. A. G. (1964). Autogenic rhythmicity in the abdominal ganglia of the crayfish: the control of swimmeret movements. *Comparative Biochemistry and Physiology*, 12, 107–15.

Ito, M. (1984). *The cerebellum and neuronal control*. Raven Press, New York.

Ito, M. and Yoshida, M. (1964). The cerebellar-evoked monosynaptic inhibition of Deiters' neurons. *Experientia (Basel)*, 20, 515–16.

Jankowska, E. (1959). Instrumental scratch reflex of the deafferented limb in cats and rats. *Acta Biologica Experimentala Warszawa*, 19, 233–47.

Jankowska, E. and Edgley, S. (1993). Interaction between pathways controlling posture and gait at the level of spinal interneurones in the cat. *Progress in Brain Research*, 97, 161–71.

Jankowska, E. and Noga, B. R. (1990). Contralaterally projecting lamina VIII interneurones in middle lumbar segments in the cat. *Brain Research*, 535, 327–30.

Jankowska, E. and Roberts, W. (1971). Function of single interneurons established by their monosynaptic inhibitory effects on motoneurons. *Acta Physiologica Scandinavia*, 82, 24–25A.

Jankowska, E. and Roberts, W. J. (1972). Synaptic actions of single interneurons mediating reciprocal 1a inhibition of motoneurons. *Journal of Physiology*, 222, 623–42.

Jankowska, E., Jukes, M., Lund, S., and Lungberg, A. (1967a). The effect of DOPA on the spinal cord. 5. Reciprocal organization of pathways transmitting excitatory action to α-motoneurons of flexors and extensors. *Acta Physiologica Scandinavia*, 70, 369–88.

Jankowska, E., Jukes, M. G. M., Lund, S., and Lundberg, A. (1967b). The effect of DOPA on the spinal cord. 6. Half-centre organization of interneurons transmitting effects from the flexor reflex afferents. *Acta Physiologica Scandinavia*, 70, 389–402.

Jarre, F. and Büschges, A. (1995). Investigations on the structure of the flight generating system in the locust *Locusta migratoria*. *Verhalten Deutsche Zoologische Gesellschaft*, 88.1, 87.

Jones, H. D. (1975). Locomotion. In *Pulmonates* (eds. V. Fretter and J. Peake), Vol. 1, pp. 1–32. Academic, New York.

Jones, K. A. and Page, C. H. (1986a). Postural interneurons in the abdominal nervous system of lobsters. I. Organization, morphologies and motor programs for flexion, extension and inhibition. *Journal of Comparative Physiology A*, 158, 259–71.

Jones, K. A. and Page, C. H. (1986b). Postural interneurons in the abdominal nervous system of lobsters. II. Evidence for neurons having both command and driver role. *Journal of Comparative Physiology A*, 158, 273–80.

Jones, K. A. and Page, C. H. (1986c). Postural interneurons in the abdominal nervous system of lobsters. III. Pathways mediating intersegmental spread of excitation. *Journal of Comparative Physiology A*, 158, 281–90.

Jordan, L. M. (1983). Factors determining motoneuron rhythmicity during fictive locomotion. In *Neural origin of rhythmic movements, Society for Experimental Biology Symposium* 37 (eds. A. Roberts and B. L. Roberts), pp. 423–44. Cambridge University Press, Cambridge.

Jordan, L. M. (1986). Initiation of locomotion from the mammalian brainstem. In *Neurobiology of vertebrate locomotion* (eds. S. Grillner, P. S. G. Stein, D. G. Stuart, and H. Forssberg), pp. 21–37. Macmillan, London.

Jordan, L. M. (1991). Brainstem and spinal cord mechanisms for the initiation of locomotion. In *Neurobiological basis of human locomotion* (eds. M. Shimamura, S. Grillner, and V. R. Edgerton), pp. 3–20. Japan Scientific Societies Press, Tokyo.

Jordan, L. M., Pratt, C. A., and Menzies, J. E. (1979). Locomotion evoked by brain stem stimulation: occurrence without phasic segmental afferent input. *Brain Research*, 177, 204–7.

Jordan, L. M., Brownstone, R. M., and Noga, B. R. (1992). Control of functional systems in the brainstem and spinal cord. *Current Opinion in Neurobiology*, 2, 794–801.

Kably, B. and Drew, T. (1998a). Corticoreticular pathways in the cat. I. Projection patterns and collaterization. *Journal of Neurophysiology*, 80, 389–405.

Kably, B. and Drew, T. (1998b). Corticoreticular pathways in the cat. II. Discharge activity of neurons in area 4 during voluntary gait modifications. *Journal of Neurophysiology*, 80, 406–24.

Kahn, J. A. and Roberts, A. (1982). Experiments on the central pattern generator for swimming in amphibia embryos. *Philosophical Transactions of the Royal Society of London B*, 296, 229–43.

Kalaska, J. and Drew, T. (1993). Visuomotor coordination. *Exercise and Sports Science Review*, 21, 397–436.

Kandel, E. R. (1979). *Behavioural biology of Alysia: a contribution to the comparative study of Opisthobranch molluscs.* Freeman Press, San Francisco.

Kappers, A. C. U., Huber, G. C., and Crosby, E. (1936). *The comparative anatomy of the nervous system of vertebrates, including man.* Macmillan, New York.

Kasicki, S. and Grillner, S. (1986). Müller cells and other reticulospinal neurones are phasically active during fictive locomotion in the isolated nervous system of the lamprey. *Neuroscience Letters*, **69**, 239–43.

Kasicki, S., Grillner, S., Ohta, Y., Dubuc, R., and Brodin, L. (1989). Phasic modulation of reticulospinal neurones during fictive locomotion and other types of spinal motor activity in lamprey. *Brain Research*, **484**, 203–16.

Kato, M. (1988). Longitudinal myelotomy of lumbar spinal cord has little effect on coordinated locomotor activities of bilateral hindlimbs of the chronic cats. *Neuroscience Letters*, **93**, 259–263.

Kato, M. (1991). Chronically isolated lumbar half spinal cord and locomotor activities of the hindlimb. In *Neurobiological basis of human locomotion* (eds. M. Shimamura, S. Grillner, and V. R. Edgerton), pp. 407–10. Japan Scientific Societies Press, Tokyo.

Katz, P. S., Getting, P. A., and Frost, W. N. (1994). Dynamic neuromodulation of synaptic strength intrinsic to a central pattern generator circuit. *Nature*, **367**, 729–31.

Kawato, M. and Suzuki, R. (1980). Two coupled neural oscillators as a model of the circadian pacemaker. *Journal of Theoretical Biology*, **86**, 547–75.

Kazennikov, O. V., Shik, M. L., and Yakovleva, G. V. (1983). Stepping movements elicited by stimulation of the dorsal funiculus in the cat spinal cord. *Bulletin of Experimental Biology and Medicine (Moscow)*, **96**, 8–10.

Kazennikov, O. V., Selionov, V. A., and Shik, M. L. (1987). On the bulbospinal locomotor column in the cat. In *Stance and motion. Facts and concepts* (eds. V. S. Gurfinkel, M. E. Ioffe, J. Massion, and J. P. Roll), pp. 123–131. Plenum, New York.

Kennedy, D., Evoy, W. H., and Hanawalt, J. T. (1966). Release of coordinated behavior in crayfish by single central neurons. *Science*, **154**, 917–19.

Kennedy, D., Evoy, W. H., Dane, B., and Hanawalt, J. T. (1967). The central nervous organization underlying control of antagonistic muscles in the crayfish. II. Coding of position by command fibers. *Journal of Experimental Zoology*, **165**, 239–48.

Kien, J. (1990). Neuronal activity during spontaneous walking. I. Starting and stopping. *Comparative Biochemistry and Physiology A—Comparative Physiology*, **95**, 607–21.

Kittmann, R. (1991). Gain control in the femur-tibia feedback system of the stick insect. *Journal of Experimental Biology*, **157**, 503–22.

Kjaerulff, O. and Kiehn, O. (1996). Distribution of networks generating and coordinating locomotor activity in the neonatal rat spinal cord *in vitro*: a lesion atudy. *Journal of Neuroscience*, **16**, 5777–94.

Kjaerulff, O. and Kiehn, O. (1997). Crossed rhythmic synaptic input to motoneurons during selective activation of the contralateral spinal locomotor network. *Journal of Neuroscience*, **17**, 9433–47.

Klärner, D. and Barnes, W. J. P. (1986). The cuticular stress detector (CSD2) of the crayfish. II. Activity during walking and influences on leg coordination. *Journal of Experimental Biology*, **122**, 161–75.

Kleerekoper, H. (1963). Role of olfaction in the orientation of the petromyzon marinus in response to a single amine in prey's body odor. *Physiological Zoology*, **36**, 347–60.

Knox, P. and Neil, D. (1991). The coordinated action of abdominal postural and swimmeret motor systems in relation to body tilt in the pitch plane in the norway lobster *Nephrops norvegicus. Journal of Experimental Biology*, **155**, 605–27.

Knutsson, E. (1981). Gait control in hemiparesis. *Scandinavian Journal of Rehabilitation Medicine*, 13, 101–8.

Kopell, N. and Ermentrout, G. B. (1986). Symmetry and phaselocking in chains of weekly coupled oscillators. *Comments on Pure and Applied Mathematics*, 39, 623–60.

Kopell, N. and Ermentrout, G. B. (1988). Coupled oscillators and the design of central pattern generators. *Mathematical Bioscience*, 89, 14–23.

Koyama, H., Kishida, R., Goris, R. C., and Kusunoki, T. (1989). Afferent and efferent projections of the VIIIth cranial nerve in the lamprey *Lampetra Japonica*. *Journal of Comparative Neurology*, 280, 663–7.

Kretz, R., Shapiro, E., and Kandel E. R. (1986). Presynaptic inhibition produced by an identified presynaptic inhibitory neuron. I. Physiological mechanisms. *Journal of Neurophysiology*, 55, 113–46.

Krieger, P., El Manira, A., and Grillner, S. (1996). Activation of pharmacologically distinct metabotropic glutamate receptors depresses reticulospinal-evoked monosynaptic epsps in the lamprey spinal cord. *Journal of Neurophysiology*, 76, 3834–41.

Krieger, P., Grillner, S., and El Manira, A. (1998). Endogenous activation of metabotropic-glutamate receptors contributes to burst frequency regulation in the lamprey locomotor network. *European Journal of Neuroscience*, 10, 3333–42.

Kriellaars, D. J., Brownstone, R. M., Noga, B. R., and Jordan, L. M. (1994). Mechanical entrainment of fictive locomotion in the decerebrate cat. *Journal of Neurophysiology*, 71, 1–13.

Kristan, W. B. and Calabrese, R. L. (1976). Rhythmic swimming activity in neurones of the isolated nerve cord of the leech. *Journal of Experimental Biology*, 65, 643–68.

Kristan, W. B. and Weeks, J. C. (1983). Neurons controlling the initiation, generation and modulation of leech swimming. In *Neural origin of rhythmic movements. Society for Experimental Biology Symposium* 37 (eds. A. Roberts and B. L. Roberts), pp. 243–60. Cambridge University Press, Cambridge.

Kristan, W. B., Stent, G. S., and Ort, C. A. (1974a). Neuronal control of swimming in the medicinal leech. I. Dynamics of the swimming rhythm. *Journal of Comparative Physiology*, 94, 97–119.

Kristan, W. B., Stent, G. S., and Ort, C. A. (1974b). Neuronal control of swimming in the medicinal leech. II. Impulse patterns of the motor neurons. *Journal of Comparative Physiology*, 94, 155–70.

Kristan, W. B., Wittenberg, G., Nusbaum, M. P., and Stern-Tomlinson, W. (1988). Multifunctional interneurons in behavioral circuits of the medicinal leech. [review]. *Experientia*, 44, 383–9.

Kudo, N. and Yamada, T. (1987). N-Methyl-D,L-aspartate-induced locomotor activity in a spinal cord-hindlimb muscles preparation of the newborn rat studied in vitro. *Neuroscience Letters*, 75, 43–8.

Kuhta, P. C. and Smith, J. L. (1990). Scratch responses in normal cats: hindlimb kinematics and muscle synergies. *Journal of Neurophysiology*, 64, 1653–67.

Kulagin, A. S. and Shik, M. L. (1970). Interaction of symmetric extremities during controlled locomotion. *Biofizika*, 15, 164–70.

Kupfermann, I. (1974). Feeding behaviour in *Aplysia*: a simple system for study of motivation. *Behavioral Biology*, 10, 1–26.

Kupferman, I. and Weiss, K. R. (1978). The command neuron concept. *Behavioral Brain Sciences*, 1, 3–39.

Kuypers, H. G. J. M., Fleming, W. R., and Farinholt, J. W. (1962). Subcortical projections in the rhesus monkey. *Journal of Comparative Neurology*, 118, 107–37.

Lajoie, Y., Teasdale, N., Cole, J. D., Burnett, M., Bard, C., Fleury, M., Forget, R., Paillard, J., and Lamarre, Y. (1996). Gait of a deafferented subject without large myelinated sensory fibres below the neck. *Neurology*, 47, 109–15.

Larimer, J. (1976). Command interneurons and locomotor behavior in crustaceans. In *Neural control of locomotion* (eds. R. M. Herman, S. Grillner, P. S. G. Stein, and D. Stuart), pp. 293–326. Plenum, New York and London.

Larsell, O. (1953). The cerebellum of the cat and monkey. *Journal of Comparative Neurology*, 99, 135–200.

Laurent, G. (1987). The morphology of a population of thoracic intersegmental interneurons in the locust. *Journal of Comparative Neurology*, 256, 412–29.

Laurent, G. and Burrows, M. (1988). A population of ascending intersegmental interneurons in the locust with mechanosensory inputs from a hind leg. *Journal of Comparative Neurology*, 275, 1–12.

Laurent, G. and Burrows, M. (1989a). Intersegmental interneurons can control the gain of reflexes in adjacent segments by their action on nonspiking local interneurons. *Journal of Neuroscience*, 9, 3030–9.

Laurent, G. and Burrows, M. (1989b). Distribution of intersegmental inputs to nonspiking local interneurones and motor neurones in the locust. *Journal of Neuroscience*, 9, 3019–29.

Laurent, G. and Hustert, R. (1988). Motor neuronal receptive fields delimit patterns of motor activity during locomotion of the locust. *Journal of Neurophysiology*, 8, 4349–66.

Laurent, M. and Thomcon, J. A. (1988). The role of visual information in control of a constrained locomotor task. *Journal of Motor Behavior*, 20, 17–37.

Leibrock, C. S., Marchand, A. R., Barnes, W. J. P., and Clarac, F. (1996). Synaptic connections of the cuticular stress detectors in crayfish—mono- and polysynaptic reflexes and the entrainment of fictive locomotion in an *in vitro* preparation. *Journal of Comparative Physiology A—Sensory Neural and Behavioral Physiology*, 178, 711–25.

Lennard, P. R., Getting, P. A., and Hume, R. I. (1980). Central pattern generator mediating swimming in *Tritonia*. II. Initiation, maintenance, and termination. *Journal of Neurophysiology*, 44, 165–73.

Lent, C. M. and Dickinson, M. H. (1984). Serotonin integrates the feeding behavior of the medicinal leech. *Journal of Comparative Physiology A*, 154, 457–71.

Lent, C. M., Zundel, D., Freedman, E., and Groome, J. R. (1991). Serotonin in the leech central nervous system: anatomical correlates and behavioral effects. *Journal of Comparative Physiology A*, 168, 191–200.

Libersat, F., Zill, S., and Clarac, F. (1987). Single-unit responses and reflex effects of force-sensitive mechanoreceptors of the dactyl of the crab. *Journal of Neurophysiology*, 57, 1601–17.

Liddlell, E. G. T. and Phillips, C. G. (1944). Pyramidal section in the cat. *Brain*, 67, 1–9.

Litvinova, N. M. and Orlovsky, G. N. (1985). Feeding behaviour of *Clione limacina* (Pteropoda). *Proceedings of the Moscow Biological Society*, 90, 73–7.

Lliddell, E. G. T. and Sherrington, C. S. (1924). Reflexes in response to stretch. *Proceedings of the Royal Society of London Series B*, 96, 212–42.

Loeb, G. E. (1993). The distal hindlimb musculature of the cat: interanimal variability of locomotor activity and cutaneous reflexes. *Experimental Brain Research*, 96, 125–40.

Loeb, G. and Duysens, J. (1979). Activity patterns in individual hindlimb primary and secondary muscle spindle afferents during normal movements in unrestrained cats. *Journal of Neurophysiology*, 42, 420–40.

Loeb, G. and Hoffer, A. (1981). Muscle spindle function during normal and perturbed loco-motion in cats. In *Muscle receptors and movement* (eds. A. Taylor and A. Prochazka). Macmillan, London.

Lou, J.-S. and Bloedel, J. R. (1992). Responses of sagittally aligned Purkinje cells during perturbed locomotion: relation of climbing fibre activation to simple spike modulation. *Journal of Neurophysiology*, 68, 1820–33.

Lowenstein, O. (1970). The electrophysiological study of the responses of the isolated labyrinth of the lamprey (*Lampetra fluviatilis*) to angular acceleration, tilting and mechanical vibration. *Proceedings of the Royal Society of London*, B174, 419–34.

Lowenstein, O., Osborne, M. R., and Thornhill, R. A. (1968). The anatomy and ultrastruc-ture of the labyrinth of the lamprey (*Lampetra fluviatilis* L.). *Proceedings of the Royal Society of London*, B170, 113–34.

Luciani, L. (1915). Muscular and nervous system. In *Human physiology*, Vol. 3. Macmillan, London.

Lundberg, A. (1971). Function of the ventral spinocerebellar tract. A new hypothesis. *Experimental Brain Research*, 12, 317–30.

Lundberg, A. (1981). Half-centres revisited. In *Regulatory functions of the CNS. Principles of motion and organization* (eds. J. Szentagothai, M. Palkovits, and J. Hamori), *Adv. Physiol. Sci.* Vol. 1, pp. 155–67. Pergamon Press, Budapest.

Lundberg, A. and Oscarsson, O. (1956). Functional organization of the dorsal spino-cerebellar tract in the cat. IV. Synaptic connections of afferents from Golgi tendon organs and muscle spindles. *Acta Physiology Scand.*, 38, 53–75.

Lundberg, A. and Oscarsson, O. (1960). Functional organization of the dorsal spino-cerebellar tract in the cat. VII. Identification of units by antidromic activation from the cerebellar cortex with recognition of five functional subdivisions. *Acta Physiology Scand.*, 50, 356–74.

Lundberg, A. and Oscarsson, O. (1962a). Functional organization of the ventral spino-cerebellar tract in the cat. IV. Identification of units by antidromic activation from the cerebellar cortex. *Acta Physiology Scand.*, 54, 252–69.

Lundberg, A. and Oscarsson, O. (1962b). Two ascending spinal pathways in the ventral part of the cord. *Acta Physiology Scand.*, 54, 270–86.

Lundberg, A. and Weight, F. (1971). Functional organization of connections to the ventral spino-cerebellar tract. *Experimental Brain Res.*, 12, 295–316.

Lundberg, A. and Winsbury, G. (1960). Functional organization of the dorsal spino-cerebellar tract in the cat. VI. Further experiments on excitation from tendon organ and muscle spindle afferents. *Acta Physiologica Scandinavia*, 49, 165–70.

Macpherson, J. M., Deliagina, T. G., and Orlovsky, G. N. (1997). Control of body orien-tation and equilibrium in vertebrates. In *Neurons, networks and motor behavior* (eds. D. Stuart and P. Stein), pp. 257–67. MIT Press, Cambridge, MA.

Magni, F. and Willis, W. D. (1964). Subcortical and peripheral control of brain stem reticu-lar neurons. *Archives of Italian Biology*, 102, 434–48.

Magoun, H. W. and Rhines, R. (1946). An inhibitory mechanism in the bulbar reticular formation. *Journal of Neurophysiology*, 9, 165–71.

Mangan, P. S., Curran, G. A., Hurney, C. A., and Friesen, W. O. (1994a). Modulation of swimming behavior in the medicinal leech. III. Control of cellular properties in motor neurons by serotonin. *Journal of Comparative Physiology A—Sensory Neural and Behavioral Physiology*, 175, 709–22.

Mangan, P. S., Cometa, A. K., and Friesen, W. O. (1994b). Modulation of swimming behavior in the medicinal leech. IV. Serotonin-induced alteration of synaptic interactions between neurons of the swim circuit. *Journal of Comparative Physiology A—Sensory Neural and Behavioral Physiology*, **175**, 723–36.

Marchand, A. R., Leibrock, C. S., Auriac, M.-C., Barnes, W. J. P., and Clarac, F. (1995). Morphology, physiology and *in vivo* activity of cuticular stress detector afferents in crayfish. *Journal of Comparative Physiology A*, **176**, 409–24.

Marple-Horvat, D. E., Amos, A. J., Armstrong, D. M., and Criado, J. M. (1993). Changes in the discharge patterns of cat motor cortex neurones during unexpected perturbations of on-going locomotion. *Journal of Physiology*, **462**, 87–113.

Massion, J. (1967). The mammalian red nucleus. *Physiological Review*, **47**, 383–436.

Massion, J. and Sasaki, K. (1979). Cerebro-cerebellar interaction: solved and unsolved problems. In *Developments in neurosciences. Cerebro-cerebellar interactions* (eds. J. Massion and K. Sasaki), Vol. 6, pp. 261–87. Elsevier, Amsterdam.

Matsukawa, K. and Udo, M. (1985). Responses of cerebellar Purkinje cells to mechanical perturbations during locomotion of decerebrate cats. *Neuroscience Research*, **2**, 393–8.

Matsukawa, K., Kamei, H., Minoda, K., and Udo, M. (1982). Interlimb coordination in cat locomotion investigated with perturbation. I. Behavioural and electromyographic study on symmetric limbs of decerebrate and awake walking cats. *Experimental Brain Research*, **46**, 425–37.

Matsushima, T. and Grillner, S. (1990). Intersegmental co-ordination of undulatory movements—a 'trailing oscillator' hypothesis. *NeuroReport*, **1**, 97–100.

Matsushima, T. and Grillner, S. (1992). Neural mechanisms of intersegmental coordination in lamprey: local excitability changes modify the phase coupling along the spinal cord. *Journal of Neurophysiology*, **67**, 373–88.

Matsushima, T., TegnJr, J., Hill, R., and Grillner, S. (1993). GABA$_B$ receptor activation causes a depression of low- and high-voltage-activated Ca^{2+} currents, postinhibitory rebound, and postspike afterhyperpolarisation in lamprey neurons. *Journal of Neurophysiology*, **70**, 2606–19.

Matsuyama, K., Takakusaki, K., Nakajima, K., and Mori, S. (1997). Multi-segmental innervation of single pontine reticulospinal axons in the cervico-thoracic region of the cat: anterograde PHA-L tracing study. *Journal of Comparative Neurology*, **377**, 234–50.

Matthews, P. B. S. (1972). *Mammalian muscle receptors and their central actions*. Arnold, London.

McClellan, A. D. (1984). Descending control and sensory gating of 'fictive' swimming and turning responses elicited in an *in vitro* preparation of the lamprey brainstem/spinal cord. *Brain Research*, **302**, 151–62.

McClellan, A. (1986). Command systems for initiating locomotion in mammals. In *Neurobiology of vertebrate locomotion* (eds. S. Grillner, P. Stein, D. Stuart, H. Forsberg, and R. Herman), pp. 3–20. Macmillan, London.

McClellan, A. D. and Grillner, S. (1983). Initiation and sensory gating of 'fictive' swimming and withdrawal responses in an in vitro preparation of the lamprey spinal cord. *Brain Research*, **269**, 237–50.

McClellan, A. D., and Grillner, S. (1984). Activation of 'fictive swimming' by electrical micro-stimulation of brainstem locomotor regions in an in vitro preparation of the lamprey central nervous system. *Brain Research*, **300**, 357–61.

McClellan, A. D. and Hagevik, A. (1997). Descending control of turning locomotor activity in larval lamprey: neurophysiology and computer modeling. *Journal of Neurophysiology*, **78**, 214–28.

McCrea, D., Pratt, C. A., and Jordan, L. M. (1980). Renshaw cell activity and recurrent effects on motoneurons during fictive locomotion. *Journal of Neurophysiology*, **44**, 475–88.

McPherson, D. R. and Blankenship, J. E. (1991a). Neural control of swimming in *Aplysia brasiliana*. I. Innervation of parapodial muscle by pedal ganglion motoneurons. *Journal of Neurophysiology*, 66, 1338–51.

McPherson, D. R. and Blankenship, J. E. (1991b). Neural control of swimming in *Aplysia brasiliana*. II. Organization of pedal motoneurons and parapodial motor fields. *Journal of Neurophysiology*, 66, 1352–65.

McPherson, D. R. and Blankenship, J. E. (1991c). Neural control of swimming in *Aplysia brasiliana*. III. Serotonergic modulatory neurons. *Journal of Neurophysiology*, 66, 1366–79.

McPherson, D. R. and Blankenship, J. E. (1992). Neuronal modulation of foot and body-wall contractions in *Aplysia californica*. *Journal of Neurophysiology*, 67, 23–8.

Mettler, F. A. (1944). Observations on the consequences of large, subtotal lesions of the simian spinal cord. *Journal of Comparative Neurology*, 81, 339–60.

Mettler, F. A. and Liss, H. (1959). Functional recovery in primates after large subtotal spinal cord lesions. *Journal of Neuropathology and Experimental Neurology*, 18, 509–16.

Mill, P. J. (1976). Chordotonal organs of crustacean appendages. In *Structure and function of proprioceptors in the invertebrates* (ed. P. J. Mill), pp. 243–97. Chapman and Hall, London.

Miller, J. P. and Selverston, A. I. (1982). Mechanisms underlying pattern generation in lobster stomatogastric ganglion as determined by selective inactivation of identified neurons. IV. Network properties of pyloric system. *Journal of Neurophysiology*, 48, 1416–32.

Miller, S. L. (1974). Adaptive design of locomotion and foot form in prosobranch gastropods. *Journal of Experimental Marine Biology and Ecology*, 14, 99–156.

Milner, M., Basmajian, J. V., and Quanburg, A. O. (1971). Multifactorial analysis of walking by electromyography and computer. *American Journal of Physiological Medicine*, 50, 235–58.

Miyan, J. and Neil, D. (1986). Swimmeret proprioceptors in the lobsters *Nephrops norvegicus* L. and *Homarus gammarus* L. *Journal of Experimental Biology*, 126, 181–204.

Mogeston, G. J. (1991). The role of mesolimbic dopamine projections to the ventral striatum in response initiation. In *Neurobiological basis of human locomotion* (eds. M. Shimamura, S. Grillner, and V. R. Edgerton), pp. 33–44. Japan Scientific Societies Press, Tokyo.

Möhl, B. (1985). The role of proprioception in locust flight control. II. Information signalled by forewing stretch receptors during flight. *Journal of Comparative Physiology*, A156, 103–16.

Möhl, B. (1989). Sense organs and control of flight. In *Insect flight* (eds. G. J. Goldsworthy and C. H. Wheeler), pp. 75–97. CRC Press, Boca Raton, FL.

Möhl, B. and Bacon, J. (1983). The tritocerebral commissure gaint (TCG) wind-sensitive interneurone in the locust. II. Directional sensitivity and role in flight stabilization. *Journal of Comparative Physiology*, 150, 453–65.

Möhl, B. and Zarnack, W. (1977). Flight steering by means of time shifts in the activity of the direct downstroke muscles in the locust. *Fortschreitende Zoologie*, 24, 333–9.

Mori, S. (1987). Integration of posture and locomotion in acute decerebrate cats and in awake, freely moving cats. *Progress in Neurobiology*, 28, 161–95.

Mori, S., Shik, M. L., and Yagodnitsyn, A. S. (1977). Role of pontine tegmentum for locomotor control in mesencephalic cat. *Journal of Neurophysiology*, 40, 284–95.

Mori, S., Kawahara, K., Sakamoto, T., Aoki, M., and Tomiyama, T. (1982). Setting and resetting of postural muscle tone in the decerebrate cat by stimulation of the brain stem. *Journal of Neurophysiology* 48, 737–48.

Mori, S., Sakamoto, T., Ohta, Y., Takakusaki, K., and Matsuyama, K. (1989). Site-specific postural and locomotor changes evoked in awake, freely moving cats by stimulating the brainstem. *Brain Research*, 505, 66–74.

Mori, S., Matsuyama, K., Kohyama, J., Kobayashi, Y., and Takakusaki, K. (1992). Neuronal constituents of postural and locomotor control systems and their interactions in cats. *Brain Development*, 14, S109–S120.

Mori, S., Sakamoto, T., and Takakusaki, K. (1991). Interaction of posture and locomotion in cats: its automatic and volitional control aspects. In *Neurobiological basis of human locomotion* (eds. M. Shimamura, S. Grillner, and V. R. Edgerton), pp. 21–32. Japan Scientific Societies Press, Tokyo.

Mori, S., Matsuyama, K., Asanome, M., Nakajima, K., Matsui, T., and Kuze, B. (1997). Cerebellar control of locomotor movements in the cat. In *Brain and movement, International Symposium* p. 136. Institute for Information Transmission Problems RAS, Moscow.

Morin, F., Kennedy, D. T., and Gardner, E. (1966). Spinal afferents to the lateral reticular nucleus. I. An histological study. *Journal of Comparative Neurology*, 126, 511–22.

Mortin, L. I. and Stein, P. S. G. (1989). Spinal cord segments containing key elements of the central pattern generators for three forms of scratch reflex in the turtle. *Journal of Neuroscience*, 9, 2285–96.

Muller, K. J., Nicholls, J. G., and Stent, G. S. (1981). *Neurobiology of the leech*. Cold Spring Harbor Press, New York.

Mulloney, B. (1997). A test of the excitability-gradient hypothesis in the swimmeret system of cryfish. *Journal of Neuroscience*, 17, 1860–8.

Mulloney, B., Acevedo, L. D., and Bradbury, A. G. (1987). Modulation of the crayfish swimmeret rhythm by octopamine and the neuropeptide proctolin. *Journal of Neurophysiology*, 58, 584–97.

Murayama, M. and Takahata, M. (1996). Sensory control mechanisms of the uropod equilibrium reflexes during walking in the crayfish *Procambarus clarkii*. *Journal of Experimental Biology*, 199, 521–8.

Murchison, D., Chrachri, A., and Mulloney, B. (1993). A separate local pattern-generating circuit controls the movements of each swimmeret in crayfish. *Journal of Neurophysiology*, 70, 2620–31.

Murphy, P. R., Stein, R. B., and Taylor, J. (1984). Phasic and tonic modulation of impulse rates in gamma-motoneurones during locomotion in premammillary cats. *Journal of Neurophysiology*, 52, 228–43.

Nashner, L. M. (1977). Fixed patterns of rapid postural responses among leg muscles during stance. *Experimental Brain Research*, 30, 13–24.

Nashner, L. M. (1980). Balance adjustments of humans perturbed while walking. *Journal of Neurophysiology*, 44, 650–64.

Nashner, L. M. and Forssberg, H. (1986). Phase-dependent organization of postural adjustments associated with arm movements while walking. *Journal of Neurophysiology*, 55, 1382–94.

Nashner, L. M., Woollacott, M., and Tuma, G. (1974). Organization of rapid responses to postural and locomotor-like perturbations of standing man. *Experimental Brain Research*, 36, 463–76.

Nashner, L. M., Woollacott, M., and Tuma, G. (1979). Organization of rapid responses to postural and locomotor-like perturbations of standing man. *Experimental Brain Research*, 36, 463–76.

Neil, D. M. (1985). Multisensory interactions in the crustacean equilibrium system. In *Feedback and motor control in invertebrates and vertebrates* (eds. W. J. P. Barnes and M. Bladden), pp. 277–98. Croom Helm, London.

Neil, D. M. and Miyan, J. A. (1986). Phase-dependent modulation of auxiliary swimmeret muscle activity in the equilibrium reactions of the Norway lobster, *Nephrops norvegicus* L. *Journal of Experimental Biology*, 126, 157–79.

Neumann, L. (1985). Experiments on tegula function for flight coordination in the locust. In *Insect locomotion* (eds. M. Gewecke and G. Wendler), pp. 149–56. Paul Parey Verlag, Hamburg.

Newland, P. L. and Neil, D. M. (1987). Statocyst control of uropod righting reactions in different planes of body tilt in the Norway lobster, *Nephrops norvegicus*. *Journal of Experimental Biology*, 131, 301–21.

Nicholls, J. G. and Baylor, D. A. (1968). Specific modalities and receptive fields of sensory neurons in CNS of the leech. *Journal of Neurophysiology*, 31, 740–56.

Nieuwenhuys, R. (1972). Topological analysis of the brainstem of the lamprey *Lamperta fluviatilis*. *Journal of Comparative Neurology*, 145, 165–78.

Nieuwenhuys, R., Donkelaarten, H. J., and Nicholson, C. (1998). *The central nervous system of vertebrates*, Vol. 1. Springer, Berlin.

Nilsson, J. and Thorstensson, A. (1989). Ground reaction forces at different speeds of human walking and running. *Acta Physiologica Scandinavia*, 136, 217–27.

Nilsson, J., Thorstensson, A., and Hultbertsma, J. (1985). Changes in leg movements and muscle activity with speed of locomotion and mode of progression in humans. *Acta Physiologica Scandinavia*, 123, 457–75.

Noga, B. R., Kettler, J., and Jordan, L. M. (1988). Locomotion produced in mesencephalic cats by injections of putative transmitter substances and antagonists into the medial reticular formation and the pontomedullary locomotor strip. *Journal of Neuroscience*, 8, 2074–86.

Noga, B. R., Fortier, P. A., Kriellaars, D. J., Dai, X., Detillieux, G. R., and Jordan, L. M. (1995). Field potential mapping of neurons in the lumbar spinal cord activated following stimulation of the mesencephalic locomotor region. *Journal of Neuroscience*, 15, 2203–17.

Norekian, T. P. (1995). Prey capture phase of feeding behaviour in the pteropod mollusc, *Clione limacina*: neuronal mechanisms. *Journal of Comparative Physiology A*, 177, 41–53.

Norekian, T. P. (1997). Coordination of startle and swimming neural systems in the pteropod mollusk *Clione limacina*: role of the cerebral cholinergic interneuron. *Journal of Neurophysiology*, 78, 308–20.

Norekian, T. P. and Satterlie, R. A. (1993). Cerebral neurons underlying prey capture movements in the pteropod mollusc, *Clione limacina*. I. Physiology, morphology. *Journal of Comparative Physiology A—Sensory Neural and Behavioral Physiology*, 172, 153–69.

Norekian, T. P. and Satterlie, R. A. (1995). An identified cerebral interneuron initiates different elements of prey capture behaviour in the pteropod mollusc, *Clione limacina*. *Invertebrate Neuroscience*, 1, 235–48.

Norekian, T. P. and Satterlie, R. A. (1996a). Whole body withdrawal circuit and its involvement in the behavioral hierarchy of the mollusk *Clione limacina*. *Journal of Neurophysiology*, 75, 529–37.

Norekian, T. P. and Satterlie, R. A. (1996b). Cerebral serotonergic neurons reciprocally modulate swim and withdrawal neural networks in the mollusk *Clione limacina*. *Journal of Neurophysiology*, 75, 538–46.

Nusbaum, M. P. (1986). Synaptic basis of swim initiation in the leech. III. Synaptic effects of serotonin-containing interneurones (cells 21 and 61) on swim cpg neurones (cells 18 and 208). *Journal of Experimental Biology* 122, 303–21.

Nusbaum, M. P. and Kristan, W. B. (1986). Swim initiation in the leech by serotonin-containing interneurones, cells 21 and 61. *Journal of Experimental Biology*, **122**, 277–302.

Nusbaum, M. P., Friesen, W. O., Kristan, W. B., Jr., and Pearce, R. A. (1987). Neural mechanisms generating the leech swimming rhythm: swim-initiator neurons excite the network of swim oscillator neurons. *Journal of Comparative Physiology A—Sensory Neural and Behavioral Physiology*, **161**, 355–66.

O'Donovan, M. J., Pinter, M. J., Dum, R. P., and Burke, R. E. (1982). Actions of FDL and FHL muscles in intact cats: functional dissociation between anatomical synergists. *Journal of Neurophysiology*, **47**, 1126–43.

O'Gara, B. A. and Friesen, W. O. (1995). Termination of leech swimming activity by a previously identified swim trigger neuron. *Journal of Comparative Physiology A—Sensory Neural and Behavioral Physiology*, **177**, 627–36.

O'Gara, B. A., Chae, H., Latham, L. B., and Friesen, W. O. (1991). Modification of leech behavior patterns by reserpine-induced amine depletion. *Journal of Neuroscience*, **11**, 96–110.

Ohta, Y. and Grillner, S. (1989). Monosynaptic excitatory amino acid transmission from the posterior rhombencephalic reticular nucleus to spinal neurons involved in the control of locomotion in lamprey. *Journal of Neurophysiology*, **62**, 1079–89.

Ohta, Y., Dubuc, R., and Grillner, S. (1991). A new population of neurons with crossed axons in the lamprey spinal cord. *Brain Research*, **564**, 143–8.

Orlovsky, G. N. (1969). Spontaneous and induced locomotion of the thalamic cat. *Biophysics*, **14**, 1154–62.

Orlovsky, G. N. (1970a). Connexions of the reticulo-spinal neurons with the 'locomotor regions' of the brain stem. *Biophysics*, **15**, 178–86.

Orlovsky, G. N. (1970b). Work of the reticulo-spinal neurons during locomotion. *Biophysics*, **15**, 761–71.

Orlovsky, G. N. (1970c). Influence of the cerebellum on the reticulo-spinal neurons during locomotion. *Biophysics*, **15**, 928–36.

Orlovsky, G. N. (1972a). The effect of different descending systems on flexor and extensor activity during locomotion. *Brain Research*, **40**, 359–71.

Orlovsky, G. N. (1972b). Work of the Purkinje cells during locomotion. *Biophysics*, **17**, 935–41.

Orlovsky, G. N. (1972c). Work of the neurons of the cerebellar nuclei during locomotion. *Biophysics*, **17**, 1177–85.

Orlovsky, G. N. (1972d). Activity of vestibulospinal neurons during locomotion. *Brain Research*, **46**, 85–98.

Orlovsky, G. N. (1972e). Activity of rubrospinal neurons during locomotion. *Brain Research*, **46**, 99–112.

Orlovsky, G. N. (1991a). Cerebellum and locomotion. In: *Neurobiological basis of human locomotion* (eds. M. Shimamura, S. Grillner, and V. R. Edgerton), pp. 187–99. Japan Scientific Societies Press, Tokyo.

Orlovsky, G. N. (1991b). Gravistatic postural control in simpler systems. *Current Opinion in Neurobiology*, **1**, 621–7.

Orlovsky G. N. and Feldman, A. G. (1972a). On the role of afferent activity in generation of stepping movements. *Neurophysiology*, **4**, 401–9. (In Russian.)

Orlovsky G. N. and Feldman, A. G. (1972b). Classification of lumbosacral neurons according to their discharge patterns during evoked locomotion. *Neurophysiology*, **4**, 410–17. (In Russian.)

Orlovsky, G. N. and Shik, M. L. (1965). On standard elements of cyclic movements. *Biofizika*, 10, 847–56.

Orlovsky, G. N. and Shik, M. L. (1976). Control of locomotion: a neurophysiological analysis of the cat locomotor system. *International Review of Physiology, Neurophysiology*, 10, 281–317.

Orlovsky, G. N., Severin, F. V., and Shik, M. L. (1966a). Locomotion evoked by stimulation of the midbrain. *Proceedings of the Academy of Sciences of the USSR*, 169, 1223–6. (In Russian.)

Orlovsky, G. N., Severin, F. V., and Shik, M. L. (1966b). Effect of damage to the cerebellum on the coordination of movement in the dog on running. *Biophysics*, 11, 578–88.

Orlovsky, G. N., Deliagina, T. G., and Wallén, P. (1992). Vestibular control of swimming in lamprey. I. Responses of reticulospinal neurons to roll and pitch. *Experimental Brain Research*, 90, 479–88.

Orlovsky, G. N., Deliagina, T. G., and Grillner, S. (1997). Activity of reticulospinal neurons in freely behaving lamprey. *Society for Neuroscience Abstracts*, 23, Part 1, 765.

Orsal, D., Perret, C., and Cabelguen, J.-M. (1986). Evidence of rhythmic inhibitory synaptic influences in hindlimb motoneurons during fictive locomotion in the thalamic cat. *Experimental Brain Research*, 64, 217–24.

Ort, C. A., Kristan, W. B., and Stent, G. S. (1974). Neuronal control of swimming in the medicinal leech. II. Identification and connections of motor neurons. *Journal of Comparative Physiology*, 94, 121–54.

Oscarsson, O. (1957). Functional organization of the ventral spino-cerebellar tract in the cat. II. Connections with muscle, joint and skin nerve afferents and effects of adequate stimulation of various receptors. *Acta Physiologica Scandinavia*, 42, Suppl., 1–107.

Oscarsson, O. (1965). Functional organization of the spino- and cuneocerebellar tracts. *Physiological Review*, 45, 495–522.

Oscarsson, O. (1973). Functional organization of spinocerebellar paths. In *Handbook of sensory physiology* (ed. A. Iggo), Vol. II, pp. 339–80. Springer, Berlin.

Oscarsson, O. and Sjölund, B. (1977a). The ventral spino-olivocerebellar system in the cat. I. Identification of five paths and their termination in the cerebellar anterior lobe. *Experimental Brain Research*, 28, 469–86.

Oscarsson, O. and Sjölund, B. (1977b). The ventral spino-olivocerebellar system in the cat. II. Termination zones in the cerebellar posterior lobe. *Experimental Brain Research*, 28, 487–503.

Oscarsson, O. and Sjölund, B. (1977c). The ventral spino-olivocerebellar system in the cat. III. Functional characteristics of the five paths. *Experimental Brain Research*, 28, 505–20.

Palkovits, M., Magyar, P., and Szentágothai, J. (1971a). Quantitative histological analysis of the cerebellar cortex in the cat. I. Number and arrangement in space of the Purkinje cells. *Brain Research*, 32, 1–13.

Palkovits, M., Magyar, P., and Szentágothai, J. (1971b). Quantitative histological analysis of the cerebellar cortex in the cat. II. Cell number and densities in the granular layer. *Brain Research*, 32, 15–30.

Palkovits, M., Magyar, P., and Szentágothai, J. (1971c). Quantitative histological analysis of the cerebellar cortex in the cat. III. Structural organization of the molecular layer. *Brain Research*, 34, 1–18.

Palkovits, M., Magyar, P., and Szentágothai, J. (1972). Quantitative histological analysis of the cerebellar cortex in the cat. IV. Mossy fiber-Purkinje cell numerical transfer. *Brain Research*, 45, 15–29.

Palkovits, M., Mezey, E., Hamori, J., and Szentágothai, J. (1977). Quantitative histological analysis of the cerebellar nuclei in the cat. I. Numerical data on cells and on synapses. *Experimental Brain Research*, 28, 189–209.

Palmer, C. I., Marks, W. B., and Bak, M. J. (1985). The responses of cat motor cortical units to electrical cutaneous stimulation during locomotion and during lifting falling and landing. *Experimental Brain Research*, 58, 102–16.

Panchin, Y. V. (1984). [synchronization of the work of pedal ganglia of pteropod mollusks during locomotion]. [Russian]. *Neirofiziologiia*, 16, 540–3.

Panchin, Y. V., Popova, L. B., Deliagina, T. G., Orlovsky, G. N., and Arshavsky, Y. I. (1995a). Control of locomotion in marine mollusk *Clione limacina*. VIII. Cerebropedal neurons. *Journal of Neurophysiology*, 73, 1912–23.

Panchin, Y. V., Arshavsky, Y. I., Deliagina, T. G., Popova, L. B., and Orlovsky, G. N. (1995b). Control of locomotion in marine mollusk *Clione limacina*. IX. Neuronal mechanisms of spatial orientation. *Journal of Neurophysiology*, 73, 1924–37.

Panchin, Y. V., Sadreev, R. I., and Arshavsky, Y. I. (1995c). Control of locomotion in marine mollusc *Clione limacina*. X. Effects of acetylcholine antagonists. *Experimental Brain Research*, 106, 135–44.

Panchin, Y. V., Arshavsky, Y. I., Deliagina, T. G., Orlovsky, G. N., Popova, L. B., and Selverston, A. I. (1996). Control of locomotion in the marine mollusc *Clione limacina*. XI. Effects of serotonin. *Experimental Brain Research*, 109, 361–5.

Parker, D. and Grillner, S. (1996). Tachykinin-mediated modulation of sensory neurons, interneurons, and synaptic transmission in the lamprey spinal cord. *Journal of Neurophysiology*, 76, 4031–9.

Parker, D., Söderberg, C., Zotova, E., Shupliakov, O., Langel, U., Bartfai, T., Larhammar D., Brodin, L., and Grillner, S. (1997a). Co-localized neuropeptide Y and GABA have complementary actions in modulating spinal sensory inputs. *European Journal of Neuroscience*, 10, 2856–70.

Parker, D., Svensson, E., and Grillner, S. (1997b). Substance p modulates sensory action potentials in the lamprey via a protein kinase c-mediated reduction of a 4-aminopyridine-sensitive potassium conductance. *European Journal of Neuroscience*, 9, 2064–76.

Parker, D., Zang, W., and Grillner, S. (1998). Substance P modulates NMDA responses and causes long-term protein synthesis-dependent modulation of the lamprey locomotor network. *Journal of Neuroscience*, 18, 4800–13.

Parker, G. H. (1917). The pedal locomotion of the seahare *Aplysia*. *Journal of Experimental Zoology*, 24, 139–45.

Parsons, D. W. and Pinsker, H. M. (1988). Swimming in *Aplysia brasiliana*: identification of parapodial opener-phase and closer-phase neurons. *Journal of Neurophysiology*, 59, 717–39.

Paul, D. H. and Mulloney, B. (1985). Nonspiking local interneuron in the motor pattern generator for the crayfish swimmeret. *Journal of Neurophysiology*, 54, 28–39.

Paul, D. H. and Mulloney, B. (1986). Intersegmental coordination of swimmeret rhythms in isolated nerve cords of crayfish. *Journal of Comparative Physiology A*, 158, 215–24.

Pavlidis, T. (1973). *Biological oscillators: their mathematical analysis*. Academic, New York.

Pavlova, G. A. (1977). Activity of reticulospinal neurons during scratch reflex. *Biofizika*, 22, 740–2.

Pearce, R. A. and Friesen, W. O. (1985a). Intersegmental coordination of the leech swimming rhythm. I. Roles of cycle period gradient and coupling strength. *Journal of Neurophysiology*, 54, 1444–59.

Pearce, R. A. and Friesen, W. O. (1985b). Intersegmental coordination of the leech swimming rhythm. II. Comparison of long and short chains of ganglia. *Journal of Neurophysiology*, 54, 1460–72.

Pearce, R. A. and Friesen, W. O. (1988). A model for intersegmental coordination in the leech nerve cord. *Biological Cybernetics*, 58, 301–11.

Pearson, K. G. (1972). Central programming and reflex control of walking in the cockroach. *Journal of Experimental Biology*, 56, 173–93.

Pearson, K. G. (1993). Common principles of motor control in vertebrates and invertebrates. *Annual Review of Neuroscience*, 16, 265–97.

Pearson, K. G. and Collins, D. F. (1993). Reversal of the influence of group Ib afferents from plantaris on activity in medial gastrocnemius muscle during locomotor activity. *Journal of Neurophysiology*, 70, 1009–17.

Pearson, K. G. and Duysens, J. (1976). Function of segmental reflexes in the control of stepping in cockroaches and cats. In *Neural control of locomotion* (eds. R. M. Herman, S. Grillner, P. S. G. Stein, and D. G. Stuart), pp. 519–37. Plenum Press, New York.

Pearson, K. G. and Fourtner, C. R. (1975). Nonspiking interneurons in walking system of the cockroach. *Journal of Neurophysiology*, 38, 33–52.

Pearson, K. G. and Iles, J. F. (1970). Discharge patterns of coxal levator and depressor motoneurons of the cockroach, *Periplaneta americana*. *Journal of Experimental Biology*, 52, 139–65.

Pearson, K. G. and Ramirez, J. M. (1990). Influence of input from the forewing stretch receptors on motoneurons in flying locusts. *Journal of Experimental Biology*, 151, 317–40.

Pearson, K. G. and Robertson, R. M. (1987). Structure predicts synaptic function of two classes of interneurons in the thoracic ganglia of *Locusta migratoria*. *Cell and Tissue Research*, 250, 105–14.

Pearson, K. G. and Rossignol, S. (1991). Fictive motor patterns in chronic spinal cats. *Journal of Neurophysiology*, 66, 1874–87.

Pearson, K. G. and Wolf, H. (1988). Connections of hindwing tegulae with flight neurons in the locust, *Locusta migratoria*. *Journal of Experimental Biology*, 135, 381–409.

Pearson, K. G., Wong, R. K. S., and Fourtner, C. R. (1976). Connections between hair-plate afferents and motoneurons in the cockroach leg. *Journal of Experimental Biology*, 64, 251–66.

Pearson, K. G., Reye, D. N., Parsons, D. W., and Bicker, G. (1985). Flight-initiating interneurons in the locust. *Journal of Neurophysiology*, 53, 910–25.

Pedotti, A. (1977). A study of motor coordination and neuromuscular activities in human locomotion. *Biological Cybernetics*, 26, 53–62.

Perell, K. L., Gregor, R. J., Buford, J. A., and Smith, J. L. (1993). Adaptive control for backward quadrupedal walking. IV. Hindlimb kinetics during stance and swing. *Journal of Neurophysiology*, 70, 2226–40.

Perkel, D. H. and Mulloney, B. (1974). Motor pattern production in reciprocally inhibitory neurons exhibiting postinhibitory rebound. *Science*, 185, 181–3.

Perret, C. (1976). Neural control of locomotion in the decorticate cat. In *Neural control of locomotion, advances in behavioral biology* (eds. R. M. Herman, S. Grillner, P. G. Stein, and D. G. Stuart), pp. 587–615. Plenum, New York.

Perret, C. (1983). Centrally generated pattern of motoneuron activity during locomotion in the cat. In *Neural origin of rhythmic movements. Society for Experimental Biology Symposium* 37 (eds. A. Roberts and B. L. Roberts), pp. 405–22. Cambridge University Press, Cambridge.

Perret, C. and Buser, P. (1972). Static and dymanic fusimotor activity during locomotor movements in the cat. *Brain Research*, 40, 165–9.

Perret, C. and Cabelguen, J.-M. (1976). Central and reflex participation in the timing of locomotor activations of a bifunctional muscle, the semi-tendinosus, in the cat. *Brain Research*, 106, 390–5.

Perret, C. and Cabelguen, J.-M. (1980). Main characteristics of the hindlimb locomotor cycle in the decorticate cat with special reference to bifunctional muscles. *Brain Research*, **187**, 333–52.

Peterson, B. W. (1979). Reticulospinal projections to spinal motor nuclei. *Annual Review of Physiology*, **41**, 127–40.

Peterson, B. W., Maunz, R. A., Pitts, N. G., and Mackel, R. G. (1975). Patterns of projection and branching of reticulospinal neurons. *Experimental Brain Research*, **23**, 333–51.

Pflüger, M.-J., Brauning, P., and Hubbert, R. (1981). Distribution and specific central projections of mechanoreceptors in the thorax and proximal leg joints of locusts. II. The external mechanoreceptors: hair plates and tactile hairs. *Cell and Tissue Research*, **216**, 79–96.

Philippson, M. (1905). L'autonomie et la centralisation dans le système nerveux des animaux. *Travaux du Laboratoire de Physiologie Institut Solvay. (Bruxelles.)*, **7**, 1–208.

Pierotti, D. J., Roy, R. R., Gregor, R. J., and Edgerton, V. R. (1989). Electromyographic activity of cat hindlimb flexors and extensors during locomotion at varying speeds and inclines. *Brain Research*, **481**, 57–66.

Platt, C. (1983). The peripheral vestibular system of fishes. In *Fish neurobiology. Brainstem and sense organs*, Vol. 1 (eds. R. G. Northcutt and R. E. Davis), pp. 89–123. University of Michigan Press, Ann Arbor.

Pointis, D. and Borenstein, P. (1985). The mesencephalic locomotor region in cat: effects of local applications of diazepam and gamma-aminobutyric acid. *Neuroscience Letters*, **53**, 297–302.

Pombal, M., El Manira, A., and Grillner, S. (1997a). Afferents of the lamprey striatum with special reference to the dopaminergic system: A combined tracing and immunohistochemical study. *Journal of Comparative Neurology*, **386**, 71–91.

Pombal, M., El Manira, A., and Grillner, S. (1997b). Organization of the lamprey striatum—transmitters and projections. *Brain Research*, **766**, 249–54.

Pompeiano, O. (1973). Reticular formation. In *Handbook of sensory physiology*, Vol. II (ed. A. Iggo), pp. 381–8. Springer, Berlin.

Poon, M. L. T. (1980). Induction of swimming in lamprey by L-Dopa and amino acids. *Journal of Comparative Physiology*, **136**, 337–44.

Poon, M., Friesen, W. O., and Stent, G. S. (1978). Neuronal control of swimming in the medicinal leech. V. Connexions between the oscillatory interneurones and the motor neurones. *Journal of Experimental Biology*, **75**, 45–63.

Porten, K. von, Redmann, G., Rothman, B., and Pinsker, H. (1980). Neuroethological studies of freely swimming *Aplysia brasiliana*. *Journal of Experimental Biology*, **84**, 245–57.

Porten, K. von, Parsons, D. W., Rothman, B. S., and Pinsker, H. (1982). Swimming in *Aplysia brasiliana*: analysis of behaviour and neuronal pathways. In *Behavioral and neural biology*, Vol. 36, pp. 1–23. Academic Press.

Pratt, C. A. and Jordan, L. M. (1980). Recurrent inhibition of motoneurons in decerebrate cats during controlled treadmill locomotion. *Journal of Neurophysiology*, **44**, 489–500.

Pratt, C. A. and Jordan, L. M. (1987). Ia inhibitory interneurons and Renshaw cells as contributors to the spinal mechanisms of fictive locomotion. *Journal of Neurophysiology*, **57**, 56–71.

Pratt, C. A., and Loeb, G. E. (1991). Functionally complex muscles of the cat hindlimb. I. Patterns of activation across sartorius. *Experimental Brain Research*, **85**, 243–56.

Pratt, C. A., Chanaud, C. M., and Loeb, G. E. (1991). Functionally complex muscles of the cat hindlimb. IV. Intramuscular distribution of movement command signals and cutaneous reflexes in broad, bifunctional thigh muscles. *Experimental Brain Research*, 85, 281–99.

Preston, R. J. and Lee, R. M. (1973). Feeding behaviour in *Aplysia californica*: role of chemocal and tactile stimulation. *Journal of Comparative Physiology and Psychology*, 82, 368–81.

Prochazka, A. and Gorassini, M. (1998*a*). Models of ensemble firing of muscle spindle afferents recorded during normal locomotion in cats. *Journal of Physiology*, 507, 277–91.

Prochazka, A. and Gorassini, M. (1998*b*). Ensemble firing of muscle afferents recorded during normal locomotion in cats. *Journal of Physiology*, 507, 293–304.

Prochazka, A., Westerman, R. A., and Ziccone, S. P. (1976). Discharges of single hindlimb afferents in the freely moving cat. *Journal of Neurophysiology*, 39, 1090–104.

Ramirez, J. M. and Pearson, K. G. (1988). Generation of motor patterns for walking and flight in motoneurons supplying bifunctional muscles in the locust. *Journal of Neurobiology*, 19, 257–82.

Ramirez, J. M. and Pearson, K. G. (1991*a*). Octopamine induces bursting and plateau potentials in insect neurons. *Brain Research*, 549, 332–7.

Ramirez, J. M. and Pearson, K. G. (1991*b*). Octopaminergic modulation in the flight system of the locust. *Journal of Neurophysiology*, 66, 1522–37.

Ramirez, J. M. and Pearson, K. G. (1993). Alteration of bursting properties in interneurons during locust flight. *Journal of Neurophysiology*, 70, 2148–60.

Rand, R. H., Cohen, A. H., and Holmes, P. J. (1988). Systems of coupled oscillators as models of central pattern generators. In *Neural control of rhythmic movements in vertebrates* (eds. A. H. Cohen, S. Rossignol, and S. Grillner), pp. 333–67. Wiley, New York.

Rasmussen, S., Chan, A. K., and Goslow, G. E. J. (1978). The cat step cycle: electromyographic patterns for hindlimb muscles during posture and unrestrained locomotion. *Journal of Morphology*, 155, 253–70.

Reichert, H. and Rowell, C. H. F. (1989). Invariance of oscillator interneurone activity during variable motor output by locusts. *Journal of Experimental Biology*, 141, 231–9.

Renshaw, B. (1941). Influence of the discharge of motoneurons upon excitation of neighboring motoneurons. *Journal of Neurophysiology*, 4, 167–83.

Rexed, B. (1954). A cytoarchitectonic atlas of the spinal cord in the cat. *Journal of Comparative Neurology*, 100, 297–379.

Rispal-Padel, L. (1979). Functional characteristics of the cerebello-thalamo-cortical pathway in the cat. In *Cerebro-cerebellar interactions* (eds. J. Massion and K. Sasaki), pp. 67–103. Elsevier/North-Holland, Amsterdam.

Ritter, D. (1992). Lateral bending during lizard locomotion. *Journal of Experimental Biology*, 173, 1–10.

Roberts, A. (1978). Pineal eye and behaviour in *Xenopus* tadpoles. *Nature*, 273, 774–5.

Roberts, A. (1989) A mechanism for swimming in the nervous system: turning on swimming in a frog tadpole. In *The computing neuron* (eds. R. Durbin, C. Mial, and G. Mitchson), pp. 229–43. Addison Wesley, Wokingham.

Roberts, A. (1990). How does a neurons system produce behaviour? A case study in neurobiology. *Science Progress*, 74, 31–51.

Roberts, A. and Clarke, J. D. W. (1982). The neuroanatomy of an amphibian embryo spinal cord. *Philosophical Transactions of the Royal Society. Series B*, 296, 195–212.

Roberts, A. and Sillar, K. T. (1990). Characterization and function of spinal excitatory interneurons with commissural projections in *Xenopus laevis* embryos. *European Journal of Neuroscience*, 2, 1051–62.

Roberts, A. and Tunstall, M. J. (1990). Mutual re-excitation with post-inhibitory rebound: a simulation study on the mechanisms for locomotor rhythm generation in the spinal cord of *Xenopus* embryos. *European Journal of Neuroscience*, 2, 11–23.

Roberts, A. and Tunstall, M. J. (1994). Longitudinal gradients in the spinal cord of *Xenopus* embryos and their possible role in coordination of swimming. *European Journal of Morphology*, 32, 176–84.

Roberts, A., Kahn, J. A., Soffe, S. R., and Clarke, J. D. W. (1981). Neuronal control of swimming in a vertebrate. *Science*, 213, 1032–4.

Roberts, A., Soffe, S. R., Clarke, J. D. W., and Dale, N. (1983). Initiation and control of swimming in amphibian embryos. In *Neuronal origin of rhythmic movements* (eds. A. Roberts and B. L. Roberts), pp. 261–84. Cambridge University Press, Cambridge.

Roberts, A., Dale, N., and Soffe, S. R. (1984). Sustained responses to brief stimuli: swimming in *Xenopus* embryos. *Journal of Experimental Biology*, 112, 321–35.

Roberts, A., Dale, N., Evoy, W. H., and Soffe, S. R. (1985). Synaptic potentials in motoneurons during fictive swimming in spinal *Xenopus* embryos. *Journal of Neurophysiology*, 54, 1–10.

Roberts, A., Soffe, S. R., and Dale, N. (1986). Spinal interneurons and swimming in frog embryos. In *Neurobiology of vertebrate locomotion* (eds. S. Grillner, P. S. G. Stein, D. G. Stuart, H. Forssberg, and R. M. Herman), pp. 279–306. Macmillan, London.

Robertson, R. M. and Pearson, K. G. (1982). A preparation for the intracellular analysis of neuronal activity during flight in the locust. *Journal of Comparative Physiology*, 146, 311–20.

Robertson, R. M. and Pearson, K. G. (1983). Interneurons in the flight system of the locust: distribution, connections, and resetting properties. *Journal of Comparative Neurology*, 215, 33–50.

Robertson, R. M. and Pearson, K. G. (1985*a*). Neural circuits in the flight system of the locust. *Journal of Neurophysiology*, 53, 110–28.

Robertson, R. M. and Pearson, K. G. (1985*b*). Neural networks controlling locomotion in locust. In *Model neural networks and behavior* (ed. A. I. Selverston), pp. 21–35. Plenum, New York.

Romanes, G. J. (1964). The motor pools of the spinal cord. In *Organization of the spinal cord. Progress in Brain Research*, Vol. II (eds. J.C. Eccles and J.P. Shade), pp. 93–119. Elsevier, Amsterdam.

Ronacher, B., Wolf, H., and Reichert, H. (1988). Locust flight behaviour after hemisection of individual thoracic ganglia: evidence for hemiganglionic premotor centers. *Journal of Comparative Physiology*, 161A, 749–59.

Rose, R. M. and Benjamin, P. R. (1981). Interneuronal control of feeding in the pond snail *Lymnaea stagnalis*. II. The interneuronal mechanism generating feeding cycles. *Journal of Experimental Biology*, 22, 203–28.

Rossignol, S. (1996). Neural control of stereotypic limb movements. In *Handbook of physiology* (eds. L. B. Rowell and J. T. Sheperd), pp. 173–216. Oxford University Press, New York.

Rossignol, S. and Drew, T. (1986). Phasic modulation of reflexes during rhythmic activity. In *Neurobiology of vertebrate locomotion* (eds. S. Grillner, P. S. G. Stein, D. G. Stuart, H. Forssberg, and R. M. Herman), pp. 517–34. Macmillan, London.

Rossignol, S. and Dubuc, R. (1994). Spinal pattern generation. *Current Opinion in Neurobiology*, 4, 894–902.

Rossignol, S. and Gauthier, L. (1980). An analysis of mechanisms controlling the reversal of crossed spinal reflexes. *Brain Research*, 182, 31–45.

Rossignol, S., Julien, C., Gauthier, L., and Lund, J. P. (1981). State-dependent responses during locomotion. In *Muscle receptors and movement* (eds. A. Taylor and A. Prochazka), pp. 389–402. Macmillan, London.

Rossignol, S., Barbeau, H., and Julien, C. (1986). Locomotion of the adult chronic spinal cat and its modification by monoaminergic agonists and antagonists. In *Development and plasticity of the mammalian spinal cord* (Fidia Research Series III) (eds. M. Goldberger, A. Gorio, and M. Murray), pp. 323–45. Liviana Press, Padova.

Rossignol, S., Lund, J. P., and Drew, T. (1988). The role of sensory inputs in regulating patterns of rhythmical movements in higher vertebrates. A comparison between locomotion, respiration and mastication. In *Neural control of rhythmic movements in vertebrates* (eds. A. Cohen, S. Rossignol, and S. Grillner), pp. 201–83. Wiley, New York.

Rossignol, S., Belanger, M., Barbeau, H., and Drew, T. (1989). Assessment of locomotor functions in the adult chronic spinal cat. In *Conference proceedings: 'Criteria for assessing recovery of function: behavioral methods'* (eds. M. Brown and M. E. Goldberger), pp. 62–5. A.P.A, Springfield, NJ.

Rossignol, S., Saltiel, P., Perreault, M.-C., Drew, T., Pearson, K., and Belanger, M. (1993). Intralimb and interlimb coordination in the cat during real and fictive rhythmic motor programs. *Seminars in the Neurosciences*, 5, 67–75.

Rovainen, C. M. (1967). Physiological and anatomical studies on large neurons of central nervous system of the sea lamprey (*Petromyzon marinus*). I. Müller and Mauthner cells. *Journal of Neurophysiology*, 30, 1000–23.

Rovainen, C. M. (1974). Synaptic interactions of reticulospinal neurons and nerve cells in the spinal cord of the sea lamprey. *Journal of Comparative Neurology*, 154, 207–23.

Rovainen, C. M. (1978). Müller cells, 'Mauthner' cells, and other identified reticulospinal neurons in the lamprey. In *Neurobiology of the Mauthner cell* (eds. D. S. Faber and H. Korn), pp. 245–69. Raven Press, New York.

Rovainen, C. M. (1979a). Electrophysiology of vestibulospinal and vestibuloreticulospinal systems in lampreys. *Journal of Neurophysiology*, 42, 745–66.

Rovainen, C. M. (1979b). Neurobiology of lampreys. *Physiological Review*, 59, 1007–77.

Rovainen, C. M. (1982). Neurophysiology. In *Biology of lampreys* (eds. M. W. Hardisty and I. C. Potter), pp. 1–136. Academic, London.

Rovainen, C. M. (1986). The contribution of multisegmental interneurons to the longitudinal coordination of fictive swimming in the lamprey. In *Neurobiology of vertebrate locomotion* (eds. S. Grillner, P. S. G. Stein, D. G. Stuart, H. Forssberg, and R. M. Herman), pp. 353–70. Macmillan, London.

Rowell, C. H. F. (1988). Mechanisms of flight steering in locusts. *Experientia*, 44, 389–95.

Rowell, C. H. F. (1989). Descending interneurons of the locust reporting deviation from flight course: what is their role in steering? *Journal of Experimental Biology*, 146, 177–94.

Rowell, C. H. F. and Pearson, K. G. (1983). Ocellar input to the flight motor system of the locust: structure and function. *Journal of Experimental Biology*, 103, 265–88.

Rowell, C. H. F. and Reichert, H. (1986). Three descending interneurons reporting deviation from course in the locust. II. Physiology. *Journal of Comparative Physiology*, 158A, 775–94.

Rubinson, K. (1974). The central distribution of VIII nerve afferents in larval *Petromyzon marinus*. *Brain and Behavioral Evolution*, 10, 121–9.

Rudomin, P., Romo, R., and Mendell, L. (1998). Presynaptic inhibition and neural control. Oxford University Press, New York.

Russel, D. F. and Wallén, P. (1983). The control of myotomal motoneurons during 'fictive swimming' in the lamprey spinal cord *in vitro*. *Acta Physiologica Scandinavia*, 117, 161–70.

Ryckebusch, S. and Laurent, G. (1993). Rhythmic patterns evoked in locust leg motor neurons by the muscarinic agonist pilocarpine. *Journal of Neurophysiology*, **69**, 1583–95.

Satterlie, R. A. (1989). Reciprocal inhibition and rhythmicity: swimming in a pteropod mollusc. In *Neuronal and cellular oscillators* (Cellular Clock Series, Vol. 2), (ed. J. Jacklet), pp. 151–72. Marcel Dekker, New York.

Satterlie, R. A. (1993). Neuromuscular organization in the swimming system of the pteropod mollusc *Clione limacina*. *Journal of Experimental Biology*, **181**, 119–40.

Satterlie, R. A. (1995). Serotonergic modulation of swimming speed in the pteropod mollusc *Clione limacina*. *Journal of Experimental Biology*, **198**, 905–16.

Satterlie, R. A. and Norekian, T. P. (1995). Serotonergic modulation of swimming speed in the pteropod mollusc *Clione limacina*. III. Cerebral neurons. *Journal of Experimental Biology*, **198**, 917–30.

Satterlie, R. A. and Spencer, A. N. (1985). Swimming in the pteropod mollusc *Clione limacina*. II. Physiology. *Journal of Experimental Biology*, **116**, 205–22.

Satterlie, R. A., LaBarbera, M., and Spencer, A. N. (1985). Swimming in the pteropod mollusc *Clione limacina*. I. Behaviour and morphology. *Journal of Experimental Biology*, **116**, 189–204.

Satterlie, R. A., Norekian, T. P., and Robertson, K. J. (1997). Startle phase of escape swimming is controlled by pedal motoneurons in the pteropod mollusk *Clione limacina*. *Journal of Neurophysiology*, **77**, 272–80.

Sauer, A. E., Driesang, R. B., Büschges, A., and Bässler, U. (1995). Information processing in the femur-tibia control loop of stick insects. I. The response characteristics of two nonspiking interneurons result from parallel excitatory and inhibitory inputs. *Journal of Comparative Physiology A*, **177**, 145–58.

Sauer, A. E., Büschges, A., and Stein, W. (1997). The role of presynaptic afferent inhibition in tuning sensorimotor pathways in an insect joint-control network. *Journal of Neurobiology*, **32**, 359–76.

Sawyer, R. Y. (1981). Leech biology and behaviour. In *Neurobiology of the leech* (eds. K. Muller, J. Nicholls, and G. Stent), pp. 7–26. Cold Spring Harbor Laboratory Press, New York.

Schomburg, E. D. (1990). Spinal sensorimotor systems and their supraspinal control. *Neuroscience Research*, **7**, 265–340.

Schotland, J., Shupliakov, O., Wikström, M., Brodin, L., Srinivasan, M., You, Z., Herrera-Marshitz, M., Zhang, W., Hökfelt, T., and Grillner, S. (1995). Control of lamprey locomotor neurons by colocalized monoamine transmitters. *Nature*, **374**, 266–8.

Schotland, J. L., Shupliakov, O., Grillner, S., and Brodin, L. (1996). Synaptic and nonsynaptic monoaminergic neuron systems in the lamprey spinal cord. *Journal of Comparative Neurology*, **372**, 229–44.

Selverston, A. I. (1985). Oscillatory neural networks. *Annual Review of Physiology*, **47**, 29–48.

Selverston, A. I. and Miller, J. P. (1980). Mechanisms underlying pattern generation in lobster stomatogastric ganglion as determined by selective inactivation of identified neurons. I. Pyloric system. *Journal of Neurophysiology*, **44**, 1102–21.

Selverston, A. I. and Moulins, M. (1985). Oscillatory neural networks. [review]. *Annual Review of Physiology*, **47**, 29–48.

Selverston, A. I. and Moulins, M. (ed.) (1987). *The crustacean stomatogastric system*. Springer, Berlin.

Severin, F. V. (1970). On the role of γ-motor system for extensor α-motoneuron activation during controlled locomotion. *Biophysics*, **15**, 1138–45.

Severin, F. V., Orlovsky, G. N., and Shik, M. L. (1967). Work of the muscle receptors during controlled locomotion. *Biophysics*, 12, 575–86.

Shadmehr, R. (1989). A neural model for generation of some behaviors in the fictive scratch reflex. *Neural Computation*, 1, 242–52.

Shefchyk, S. J. and Jordan, L. M. (1985). Excitatory and inhibitory post-synaptic potentials in alpha-motoneurons produced during fictive locomotion by stimulation of the mesencephalic locomotor region. *Journal of Neurophysiology*, 53, 1345–55.

Shefchyk, S. J., Jell, R. M., and Jordan, L. M. (1984). Reversible cooling of the brainstem reveals areas required for mesencephalic locomotor region evoked treadmill locomotion. *Experimental Brain Research*, 56, 257–62.

Shefchyk, S., McCrea, D., Kriellaars, D., Fortier, P., and Jordan, L. (1990). Activity of interneurons within the L4 spinal segment of the cat during brainstem-evoked fictive locomotion. *Experimental Brain Research*, 80, 290–5.

Sherff, C. M. and Mulloney, B. (1996). Tests of the motor neuron model of the local pattern-generating circuits in the swimmeret system. *Journal of Neuroscience*, 16, 2839–59.

Sherrington, C. S. (1906a). *The intergrative action of the nervous system*. Yale University Press, New Haven, CT.

Sherrington, C. S. (1906b). Observations on scratch-reflex in the spinal dog. *Journal of Physiology (London)*, 34, 1–50.

Sherrington, C. S. (1910). Notes on the scratch-reflex of the cat. *Quarterly Journal of Experimental Physiology*, 3, 210–13.

Shik, M. L. (1983). Action of the brainstem locomotor region on spinal stepping generators via propriospinal pathways. In *Spinal cord reconstruction* (eds. C. C. Kao, R. P. Bunge, and P. J. Reier), pp. 421–34. Raven Press, New York.

Shik, M. L. and Orlovsky, G. N. (1965) Coordination of the limbs during running of the dog. *Biophysics*, 10, 1048–59.

Shik, M. L. and Orlovsky, G. N. (1976). Neurophysiology of locomotor automatism. *Physiological Review*, 56, 465–501.

Shik, M. L. and Yagodnitsyn, A. S. (1977). The pontobulbar 'locomotor strip'. *Neurophysiology (Kiev)*, 9, 95–7.

Shik, M. L., Severin, F. V., and Orlovsky, G. N. (1966a). Control of walking and running by means of electrical stimulation of the mid-brain. *Biophysics*, 11, 756–65.

Shik, M. L., Orlovsky, G. N., and Severin, F. V. (1966b). Organization of locomotor synergism *Biophysics*, 11, 1011–19.

Shik, M. L., Severin, F. V., and Orlovsky, G. N. (1967). Structures of the brain stem responsible for evoked locomotion. *Sechenov Physiological Journal of the USSR*, 53, 1125–32.

Shik, M. L., Orlovsky, G. N., and Severin, F. V. (1968). Locomotion of the mesencephalic cat elicited by stimulation of the pyramids. *Biophysics*, 13, 143–52.

Shimamura, M., Tanaka, I., and Fuwa, T. (1991). Supraspinal control mechanisms of coordinated movements among four limbs in cat during stepping. In *Neurobiological basis of human locomotion* (eds. M. Shimamura, S. Grillner, and V. R. Edgerton), pp. 57–74. Japan Scientific Societies Press, Tokyo.

Shinoda, Y., Arnold, A. P., and Asanuma, H. (1976). Spinal branching of corticospinal axons in the cat. *Experimental Brain Research*, 26, 215–34.

Shinoda, Y., Yamaguchi, T., and Futami, T. (1986). Multiple axon collaterals of single corticospinal axons in the cat spinal cord. *Journal of Neurophysiology*, 55, 425–48.

Sillar, K. T. and Roberts, A. (1993). Control of frequency during swimming in *Xenopus* embryos: a study on interneuronal recruitment in a spinal rhythm generator. *Journal of Physiology*, 472, 557–72.

Sillar, K. T. and Skorupski, P. (1986). Central input to primary afferent neurons in crayfish, *Pacifastacus leniusculus*, is correlated with rhythmic motor output of thoracic ganglia. *Journal of Neurophysiology*, **55**, 678–88.

Sillar, K. T., Skorupski, P., Elson, R. C., and Bush, B. M. H. (1986). Two identified afferent neurons entrain a central locomotor rhythm generator. *Nature*, **323**, 440–3.

Sillar, K. T., Wedderburn, J. F. S., and Simmers, J. A. (1991). The development of swimming rhythmicity in post-embryonic *Xenopus laevis*. *Proceedings of the Royal Society of London*, B**246**, 147–53.

Sillar, K. T., Simmers, J. A., and Wedderburn, J. F. S. (1992). The post-embryonic development of cell properties and synaptic drive underlying locomotor rhythm generation in *Xenopus laevis*. *Proceedings of the Royal Society of London*, B**249**, 65–70.

Simmons, P. (1980). A locust wind and ocellar neurone. *Journal of Experimental Biology*, **85**, 281–94.

Sirota, M. G. and Shik, M. L. (1973). The cat locomotion elicited through the electrode implanted in the mid-brain. *Sechenov Physiological Journal of the USSR*, **59**, 1314–21. (In Russian.)

Sirota, M., Viana Di Prosco, G., and Dubuc, R. (1994). Activation of swimming by electrical microstimulation of brainstem locomotor regions in semi-intact lampreys. *Physiology Canada*, **25**, 142.

Sjöström, A. and Zangger, P. (1976). Muscle spindle control during locomotor movements generated by the deafferented spinal cord. *Acta Physiologica Scandinavia*, **97**, 281–91.

Skorupski, P. (1992). Synaptic connections between nonspiking afferent neurons and motoneurons underlying phase-dependent reflexes in crayfish. *Journal of Neurophysiology*, **67**, 664–79.

Skorupski, P. and Sillar, K.T. (1986). Phase-dependent reversal of reflexes mediated by the thoracocoxal muscle receptor organ in the crayfish, *Pacifastacus leniusculus*. *Journal of Neurophysiology*, **55**, 689–95.

Skorupski, P., Rawat, B. M., and Bush, B. M. H. (1992). Heterogeneity and central modification of feedback reflexes in crayfish motor pool. *Journal of Neurophysiology*, **67**, 648–63.

Smith, J. L., Betts, B., Edgerton, V. R., and Zernicke, R. F. (1980). Rapid ankle extension during paw shakes: Selective recruitment of fast ankle extensors. *Journal of Neurophysiology*, **43**, 612–20.

Smith, J. L., Smith, L. A., Zernicke, R. F., and Hoy, M. (1982). Locomotion in exercised and non-exercised cats cordotomized at two or twelve weeks of age. *Experimental Neurology*, **76**, 393–413.

Smith, J. L., Hoy, M. G., Koshland, G. F., Phillips, D. M., and Zernicke, R. F. (1985). Intralimb coordination of the paw-shake response: a novel mixed synergy. *Journal of Neurophysiology*, **54**, 1271–81.

Smith, J. L., Buford, J. A., and Zernicke, R. F. (1988). Constraints during backward walking in the quadruped. In *Posture and gait: development, adaptation and modulation* (eds. B. Amblard, A. Berthoz, and F. Clarac), pp. 391–400. Elsevier, Amsterdam.

Smith, J. L., Chung, S. H., and Zernicke, R. F. (1993). Gait-related motor pattern and hindlimb kinetics for the cat trot and gallop. *Experimental Brain Research*, **94**, 308–22.

Soffe, S. R. (1989). Roles of glicinergic inhibition and N-methyl-D-aspartate receptor-mediated excitation in the locomotor rhythmicity of one half of the *Xenopus* embryo CNS. *European Journal of Neuroscience*, **1**, 561–71.

Soffe, S. R. (1990). Active and passive membrane properties of spinal cord neurons that are rhythmically active during swimming in *Xenopus* embryos. *European Journal of Neuroscience*, **2**, 1–10.

Soffe, S. R., Clarke, J. D. W., and Roberts, A. (1984). Activity of commissural inter-neurons in the spinal cord of *Xenopus* embryos. *Journal of Neurophysiology*, 51, 1257–67.

Söderberg, C. (1996). Molecular evolution of the neuropeptide Y family of peptides. PhD Dissertation, Uppsala.

Sprague, J. M. and Chambers, W. W. (1953). Regulation of posture in intact and decere-brate cat. I. Cerebellum, reticular formation, vestibular nuclei. *Journal of Neurophysiology*, 16, 451–63.

Sprague, J. M. and Chambers, W. W. (1954). Control of posture by reticular formation and cerebellum in the intact, anesthetized and unanesthetized and in the decerebtared cat. *American Journal of Physiology*, 176, 52–64.

Steeves, J. D. and Jordan, L. M. (1980). Localization of a descending pathway in the spinal cord which is necessary for controlled treadmill locomotion. *Neuroscience Letters*, 20, 283–8.

Steeves, J. D. and Jordan, L. M. (1984). Autoradiographic demonstration of the projections from the mesencephalic locomotor region. *Brain Research*, 307, 263–76.

Steeves, J. D., Schmidt, B. J., Skovgaard, B. J., and Jordan, L. M. (1980). Effect of noradrenaline and 5-hydroxytryptamine depletion on locomotion in the cat. *Brain Research*, 185, 349–62.

Stein, P. S. G. (1971). Intersegmental coordination of swimmeret motoneurone activity in crayfish. *Journal of Neurophysiology*, 34, 310–18.

Stein, P. S. G. (1974). Neural control of interappendage phase during locomotion. *American Zoologist*, 14, 1003–16.

Stein, P. S. G. (1976). Mechanisms of interlimb phase control. In *Neural control of loco-motion* (eds. R. M. Herman, S. Grillner, P. S. G. Stein, and D. G. Stuart), pp. 465–87. Plenum, New York.

Stein, P. S. G. (1977a). Application of the mathematics of coupled oscillator systems to the analysis of the neural control of locomotion. *Federation Proceedings*, 36, 2056–9.

Stein, P. S. G. (1977b). A comparative approach to the control of locomotion. In *Identified neurons and behaviour of arthropods* (ed. G. Hoyle), pp. 227–39. Plenum, New York.

Stein, P. S. G. (1978). Motor systems, with specific reference to the control of locomotion. *Annual Review of Neuroscience*, 1, 61–81.

Stein, P. S. (1983). The vertebrate scratch reflex. In *Neural origin of rhythmic movements. Society for Experimental Biology Symposium.* 37 (eds. A. Roberts and B. L. Roberts), pp. 383–403. Cambridge University Press, Cambridge.

Stevenson, P. A. and Kutsch, W. (1987). A reconsideration of the central pattern generator concept for locust flight. *Journal of Comparative Physiology*, 161A, 115–29.

Stoll, C. J., Goldschmeding, J. T., Janse, C., and de Vlieger, T. A. (1978). Observations on parapodial reflexes in *Aplysia fasciata*. *Proceedings of the Koninklijke Nederlandse Adademie van Wetenschappen*, 81, 115–25.

Stuart, A. E. (1970). Physiological and morphological properties of motoneurons in the central nervous system of the leech. *Journal of Physiology*, 209, 627–46.

Stuart, D. G., Withey, T. P., Wetzel, M. L., and Goslow G. E. (1973). Time constraints for interlimb coordination in the cat during unrestrained locomotion. In *Control of posture and locomotion* (eds. R. B. Stein, K. G. Pearson, R. S. Smith, and J. B. Redford), pp. 537–60. Plenum, New York.

Syed, N., Harrison, D., and Winlow, W. (1988). Locomotion in *Lymnaea*—role of sero-tonergic motoneurons controlling the pedal cilia. *Symposia Biologica Hungarica*, 36, 387–99.

Takahata, M. and Hisada, M. (1979). Functional polarization of statocyst receptors in the crayfish *Procambarus clarkii* Girard. *Journal of Comparative Physiology*, 130, 201–7.

Takahata, M. and Hisada, M. (1982a). Statocyst interneurons in the crayfish *Procambarus clarkii* Girard. I. Identification and response characteristics. *Journal of Comparative Physiology*, 149, 287–300.

Takahata, M. and Hisada, M. (1982b). Statocyst interneurons in the crayfish *Procambarus clarkii* Girard. II. Directional sensitivity and its mechanisms. *Journal of Comparative Physiology*, 149, 301–6.

Takahata, M. and Hisada, M. (1986a). Sustained membrane potential change of uropod motor neurons during the fictive abdominal posture movement in crayfish. *Journal of Neurophysiology*, 56, 702–17.

Takahata, M. and Hisada, M. (1986b). Local nonspiking interneurons involved in gating of the descending motor pathway in crayfish. *Journal of Neurophysiology*, 56, 718–31.

Takahata, M., Yoshino, M., and Hisada, M. (1985). Neuronal mechanisms underlying crayfish steering behaviour as an equilibrium respomse. *Journal of Experimental Biology*, 114, 599–617.

Takakusaki, K., Ohta, Y., and Mori, S. (1989). Single medullary reticular neurons exert postsynaptic inhibitory effects via inhibitory interneurons upon alpha-motoneurons innervating cat hindlimb muscles. *Experimental Brain Research*, 74, 11–23.

Taylor, C. P. (1981a). Contribution of compound eyes and ocelli to steering of locusts in flight. I. Behavioural analysis. *Journal of Experimental Biology*, 93, 1–18.

Taylor, C. P. (1981b). Contribution of compound eyes and ocelli to steering of locusts in flight. II. Timing changes in flight motor units. *Journal of Experimental Biology*, 93, 19–31.

Tegnér, J. (1997). Modulation of cellular mechanisms in a spinal locomotor network—an experimental and computational study in lamprey. PhD thesis, Nobel institute for Neurophysiology, Karolinska Institute.

Tegnér, J., Hellgren-Kotaleski, J., Lansner, A., and Grillner, S. (1997). Low voltage activated calcium channels in the lamprey locomotor network-simulation and experiment. *Journal of Neurophysiology*, 77, 1795–812.

Tegnér, J., Lansner, A., and Grillner, S. (1998). Modulation of burst frequency by calcium-dependent potassium channels in the lamprey locomotor system-dependence of the activity level. *Journal of Computational Neuroscience*, 5, 121–40.

Ten Donkelaar, H. J. (1982). Organisation of descending pathways to the spinal cord in amphibians and reptiles. In *Descending pathways to the spinal cord. Progress in Brain Research*, Vol. 57 (eds. H. G. J. M. Kuypers and G. F. Martin), pp. 25–67. Elsevier, Amsterdam.

Terakado, Y. and Yamaguchi, T. (1990). Last-order interneurons controlling activity of elbow flexor motoneurons during forelimb fictive locomotion in the cat. *Neuroscience Letters*, 111, 292–6.

Teräväinen, H. and Rovainen, C. M. (1971). Fast and slow motoneurons to body muscle of the sea lamprey. *Journal of Neurophysiology*, 34, 990–8.

Thach, W. T., Goodkin, H. P., and Keating, J. G. (1992). The cerebellum and the adaptive coordination of movement. *Annual Review of Neuroscience*, 15, 403–42.

Thomson, C. S. and Page, C. H. (1982). Command fibre activation of superficial flexor motoneurons in the lobster abdomen. *Journal of Comparative Physiology*, 148, 515–27.

Thomson, J. A. (1980). How do we use visual information to control locomotion? *Trends in Neuroscience*, 3, 247–50.

Thorstensson, A., Carlson, H., Zomlefer, M. R., and Nilsson, J. (1982). Lumbar back muscle activity in relation to trunk movements during locomotion in man. *Acta Physiologica Scandinavia*, 131, 211–14.

Thorstensson, A., Nilsson, J., Carlson, H., and Zomlefer, M. R. (1984). Trunk movements in human locomotion. *Acta Physiologica Scandinavia*, 121, 9–22.

Thüring, D. A. (1986). Variability of motor output during flight steering in locusts. *Journal of Comparative Physiology*, 158A, 653–64.

Timmerick, S. J. B., Paul, D. H., and Roberts, B. L. (1990). Dynamic characteristics of vestibular-driven compensatory fin movements in the dogfish. *Brain Research*, 516, 318–21.

Tråvén, H., Brodin, L., Lansner, A., Ekeberg, Ö., Wallén, P., and Grillner, S. (1993). Computer simulations of NMDA and non-NMDA receptor-mediated synaptic drive—sensory and supraspinal modulation of neurons and small networks. *Journal of Neurophysiology*, 70, 695–709.

Trueman, E. R. (1983). Locomotion in molluscs. In *The Mollusca. Physiology, Part 1*, Vol. 4, pp. 155–98. Academic, New York.

Tsirylis, T. P. (1974). The fine structure of the statocyst in the pteropod mollusk *Clione limacina*. *Journal of Evolutional Biochemistry and Physiology*, 10, 181–8.

Tsukahara, N., Bando, T., Murakami, F., and Oda, Y. (1983). Properties of cerebellar-precerebellar reverberating circuits. *Brain Research*, 274, 249–59.

Tunstall, M. J. and Roberts, A. (1990). NMDA applied to the spinal cord in *Xenopus* embryos reduces rostro-caudal delay during fictive swimming. *Journal of Physiology*, 425, 92p.

Tunstall, M. J. and Roberts, A. (1991). Longitudinal co-ordination of motor output during swimming in *Xenopus* embryos. *Proceedings of the Royal Society*, B244, 27–32.

Tunstall, M. J. and Roberts, A. (1994). A longitudinal gradient of synaptic drive in the spinal cord of *Xenopus* embryos and its role in co-ordination of swimming. *Journal of Physiology*, 474, 393–405.

Tyrer, N. M. and Altman, J. S. (1974) Motor and sensory flight neurons in a locust demonstrated using cobalt chloride. *Journal of Comparative Neurology*, 157, 117–38.

Udo, M. (1986). Role of selected lobules of the cerebellum in the control of locomotion. In *Neurobiology of vertebrate locomotion* (eds. S. Grillner, P. S. G. Stein, D. G. Stuart, H. Forssberg, and R. Herman), pp. 691–704. Macmillan, London.

Udo, M., Matsukawa, K., and Kamei, H. (1979a). Effects of partial cooling of cerebellar cortex at lobules V and IV of the intermediate part in the decerebrate walking cat under monitoring vertical floor reaction forces. *Brain Research*, 160, 559–64.

Udo, M., Matsukawa, K., and Kamei, H. (1979b). Hyperflexion and changes in interlimb coordination of locomotion induced by cooling of the cerebellar intermediate cortex in normal cats. *Brain Research*, 166, 405–8.

Udo, M., Matsukawa, K., Kamei, H., and Oda, Y. (1980). Cerebellar control of locomotion: effects of cooling cerebellar intermediate cortex in high decerebrate and awake walking cats. *Journal of Neurophysiology*, 44, 119–34.

Udo, M., Matsukawa, K., Kamei, H., Minoda, K. and Oda, Y. (1981). Simple and complex spike activities of Purkinje cells during locomotion in the cerebellar vermal zones of decerebrate cats. *Experimental Brain Research*, 41, 292–300.

Udo, M., Kamei, H., Matsukawa, K., and Tanaka, K. (1982). Interlimb coordination in cat locomotion investigated with perturbation. II. Correlations in neuronal activity of Deiters' cells of decerebrate walking cat. *Experimental Brain Research*, 46, 438–47.

Ullén, F., Orlovsky, G. N., Deliagina, T. G., and Grillner, S. (1993). Role of dermal photoreceptors and lateral eyes in initiation and orientiation of locomotion in lamprey. *Behavioral Brain Research*, 54, 107–10.

Ullén, F., Deliagina, T.G., Orlovsky, G. N., and Grillner, S. (1995a). Spatial orientation in the lamprey. I. Control of pitch and roll. *Journal of Experimental Biology*, **198**, 665–73.

Ullén, F., Deliagina, T. G., Orlovsky, G. N., and Grillner, S. (1995b). Spatial orientation in the lamprey. II. Visual influence on orientation during locomotion and in attached state. *Journal of Experimental Biology*, **198**, 675–81.

Ullén, F., Deliagina, T. G., Orlovsky, G. N., and Grillner, S. (1996). Visual potentiation of vestibular responses in lamprey reticulospinal neurons. *European Journal of Neuroscience*, **8**, 2298–307.

Ullén, F., Deliagina, T., Orlovsky, G., and Grillner, S. (1997). Visual pathways for postural control and negative phototaxis in lamprey. *Journal of Neurophysiology*, **78**, 960–76.

Van Dongen, P. A., Hokfelt, T., Grillner, S., Rehfeld, J. F., and Verhofstad, A. J. (1985). A cholecystokinin-like peptide is present in 5-hydroxytryptamine neurons in the spinal cord of the lamprey. *Acta Physiologica Scandinavica*, **125**, 557–60.

Van Dongen, P., Theodorsson-Norheim, E., Brodin, E., Hökfelt, T., Grillner, S., Peters, A., Cuello, A., Forssmann, W., Reinecke, M., Singer, E., and Lazarus, L. (1986). Immunohistochemical and chromatographic studies of peptides with tachykinin-like immunoreactivity in the central nervous system of the lamprey. *Peptides*, **7**, 297–313.

Viala, D., Buisseret-Delmas, C., and Portal, J. J. (1988). An attempt to localize the lumbar locomotor generator in the rabbit using 2-deoxy-[14C]glucose autoradiography. *Neuroscience Letters*, **86**, 139–43.

Viala, D. and Vidal, C. (1978). Evidence for distinct spinal locomotion generators supplying respectively fore- and hindlimbs in the rabbit. *Brain Research*, **155**, 182–6.

Viana di Prisco, G., Wallén, P., and Grillner, S. (1990). Synaptic effects of intraspinal stretch receptor neurons mediating movement-related feedback during locomotion. *Brain Research*, **530**, 161–6.

Viana Di Prisco, G., Ohta, Y., Bongiani, F., Grillner, S., and Dubuc, R. (1995). Trigeminal inputs to reticulospinal neurons in lamprey are mixed by excitatory and inhibitory amino acids. *Brain Research*, **695**, 76–80.

Viana Di Prisco, G., Pearlstein, E., Robitaille, R., and Dubuc, R. (1997). Role of sensory-evoked NMDA plateau potentials in the initiation of locomotion. *Science*, **278**, 1122–5.

Vilensky, J. A., Moore, A. M., Eidelberg, E., and Walden, J. G. (1992). Recovery of locomotion in monkeys with spinal cord lesions. *Journal of Motor Behaviour*, **24**, 288–96.

von Holst, E. (1935). Über den Lichtrückenreflex bei Fischen. *Pubblicazione Stazione Zoologica Napoli*, **15**, 143–58.

von Holst, E. (1938). Über relative Koordination bei Säugern und beim Menschen. *Pfluegers Archiv*, **240**, 44–9.

von Porten, K., Redmann, G., Rothman, B., and Pinsker, H. (1980). Neuroethological studies of freely swimming *Aplysia brasiliana*. *Journal of Experimental Biology*, **84**, 245–57.

von Porten, K., Parsons, D. W., Rothman, B. S., and Pinsker, H. (1982). Swimming in *Aplysia brasiliana*: analysis of behaviour and neuronal pathways. In *Behavioral and neural biology*, Vol. 36, pp. 1–23. Academic, New York.

Wadden, T., Hellgren-Kotaleski, J., Lansner, A., and Grillner, S. (1997). Intersegmental co-ordination in the lamprey—simulations using a continuous network model. *Biological Cybernetics*, **76**, 1–9.

Wagner, N. (1885). Die Wirbellosen des Weissen Meeres. Verlag von Wilhelm Engelmann, Leipzig.

Walberg, F., Pompeiano, O., Westrum, L. E., and Hauglie-Hanssen, E. (1962). Fastigo-reticular fibres in the cat. An experimental study with the silver method. *Journal of Comparative Neurology*, 119, 187–99.

Waldron, I. (1967). Mechanisms for the production of the motor output pattern in flying locust. *Journal of Experimental Biology*, 47, 201–12.

Wallén, P. and Williams, T. L. (1984). Fictive locomotion in the lamprey spinal cord *in vitro* compared with swimming in the intact and spinal animal. *Journal of Physiology*, 347, 225–39.

Wallén, P. and Grillner, S. (1987). N-Methyl-D-Aspartate receptor-induced, inherent oscillatory activity in neurons active during locomotion in the lamprey. *Journal of Neuroscience*, 7, 2745–55.

Wallén, P., Grillner, S., Feldman, L., and Bergelt, S. (1985). Dorsal and ventral myotome motoneurones and their input during fictive locomotion in lamprey. *Journal of Neuroscience*, 53, 654–61.

Wallén, P., Buchanan, J. T., Grillner, S., and H'kfelt, T. (1989). Effects of 5-hydroxytryptamine on the afterhyperpolarization, spike frequency regulation and oscillatory membrane properties in lamprey spinal cord neurons. *Journal of Neurophysiology*, 61, 759–68.

Wallén, P., Shupliakov, O., and Hill, R. H. (1993). Origin of phasic synaptic inhibition in myotomal motoneurons during fictive locomotion in the lamprey. *Experimental Brain Research*, 96, 194–202.

Waller, W. H. (1940). Progression movements elicited by subthalamic stimulation. *Journal of Neurophysiology*, 3, 300–7.

Walmsley, B., Hodgson, J. A., and Burke, R. E. (1978). Forces produced by medial gastrocnemius and soleus muscles during locomotion in freely moving cats. *Journal of Neurophysiology*, 41, 1203–16.

Walters, E. T., Carew, T. J., and Kandel, E. R. (1978). Conflict and response selection in the locomotor system of *Aplysia*. *Neuroscience Abstracts*, 4, 209.

Wannier, T., Orlovsky, G., and Grillner, S. (1995). Reticulospinal neurons provide monosynaptic glycinergic inhibition of spinal neurons in lamprey. *NeuroReport*, 6, 1597–600.

Wannier, T., Deliagina, T. G., Orlovsky, G. N., and Grillner, S. (1998). Differential effects of the reticulospinal system on locomotion in lamprey. *Journal of Neurophysiology*, 80, 103–13.

Watkins, J. C. and Evans, R. H. (1981). Excitatory amino acid neuro-transmitters. *Annual Review of Pharmacology and Toxicology*, 21, 165–206.

Weeks, J. C. (1981). Neuronal basis of leech swimming: separation of swim initiation, pattern generation, and intersegmental coordination by selective lesions. *Journal of Neurophysiology*, 45, 698–723.

Weeks, J. C. (1982a). Synaptic basis of swim initiation in the leech. I. Connections of a swim-initiating neuron (cell 204) with motor neurons and pattern-generating 'oscillator' neurons. *Journal of Comparative Physiology A*, 148, 253–63.

Weeks, J. C. (1982b). Synaptic basis of swim initiation in the leech. II. A pattern-generating neuron (cell 208) which mediates motor effects of swim-initiating neurons. *Journal of Comparative Physiology A*, 148, 265–79.

Weeks, J. C. (1982c). Segmental specialization of a leech swim-initiating interneuron, cell 205. *Journal of Neuroscience*, 2, 972–85.

Weeks, J. C. and Kristan, W. B. (1978). Initiation, maintenance and modulation of swimming in the medicinal leech by the activity of a single neuron. *Journal of Experimental Biology*, 77, 71–88.

Wehner, R. (1981) Spatial vision in arthropods. In *Handbook of sensory physiology* (ed. H. Autrum), vol. VII/6C, pp. 287–616. Springer, Berlin.

Weiland, G. and Koch, U. (1987). Sensory feedback during active movements of stick insects. *Journal of Experimental Biology*, 133, 137–56.

Weis-Fogh, T. (1949). An aerodynamic sense organ stimulating and regulating flight in locusts. *Nature*, 164, 873–4.

Weis-Fogh, T. (1956). Biological and physics of locust flight. II. Flight performance of the desert locust *Schistocerca gregaria*. *Philosophical Transactions of the Royal Society of London B*, 239, 459–510.

Weiss, K. R., Cohen, J. L., and Kupferman, I. (1978). Modulatory control of buccal musculature by a serotonergic neuron (metacerebral cell) in *Aplysia*. *Journal of Neurophysiology*, 41, 181–203.

Wendler, G. (1974). The influence of proprioceptive feedback on locust flight coordination. *Journal of Comparative Physiology*, A88, 173–200.

Wetzel, M. C. and Stuart, D. G. (1976). Ensemble characteristics of cat locomotion and its neural control. *Progress in Neurobiology*, 7, 1–98.

Wetzel, M. C., Atwater, A. E., Wait, J. V., and Stuart, D. G. (1976). Kinematics of locomotion by cats with a single hindlimb deafferented. *Journal of Neurophysiology*, 39, 667–78.

Wickelgren, W. (1977). Physiological and anatomical characteristics of reticulospinal neurons in lamprey. *Journal of Physiology*, 270, 89–114.

Wiens, T. J. and Gerstein, G. L. (1976). Reflex pathways of the crayfish claw. *Journal of Comparative Physiology*, 107, 309–26.

Wiersma, C. A. G. and Ikeda, K. (1964). Interneurons commanding swimmeret movements in the crayfish, *Procambarus clarkii* (Girard). *Comparative Biochemistry and Physiology*, 12, 509–25.

Wikström, M. and El Manira, A. (1998). Calcium inflax through N- and P/Q-type channels activate apamin-sensitive calcium-dependent potassium channels generating the late afterhyperpolarization in lamprey spinal neurons. *European Journal of Neuroscience*, 10, 1528–32.

Wikström, M., El Manira, A., Zhang, W., Hill, R., and Grillner, S. (1995). Dopamine and 5-HT modulation of synaptic transmission in the lamprey spinal cord. *Society for Neuroscience Abstracts*, 21, p. 1145.

Wikström, M., El Manira, A., and Grillner, S. (1997). N-type Ca^{2+} channels activates apamin-sensitive Ca^{2+} dependent K^+ channels that generate the afterhyperpolarization in lamprey neurons. *International Congress on Physiology*, 33, P012.15.

Willard, A. L. (1981). Effects of serotonin on the generation of the motor program for swimming by the medicinal leech. *Journal of Neuroscience*, 1, 936–44.

Williams, B. J. and Larimer, J. L. (1981). Neural pathways of reflex-evoked behaviours and command systems in the abdomen of the crayfish. *Journal of Comparative Physiology A*, 143, 27–42.

Williams, T. (1989). Locomotion in lamprey and trout: the relative timing of activation and movement. *Journal of Experimental Biology*, 143, 559–66.

Williams, T., Grillner, S., Smoljaninov, V. V., Wallén, P., Kashin, S., and Rossignol, S. (1989). Locomotion in lamprey and trout: the relative timing of activation and movement. *Journal of Experimental Biology*, 143, 559–66.

Wilson, D. M. (1961). The central nervous control of flight in a locust. *Journal of Experimental Biology*, 38, 471–90.

Wilson, D. M. and Waldron, I. (1968). Models for the generation of the motor output pattern in flying locust. *Proceedings of the IEEE*, 56, 1058–64.

Wilson, D. M. and Weis-Fogh, T. (1962). Patterned activity of co-ordinated motor units studied in flying locusts. *Journal of Experimental Biology*, 40, 643–67.

Wilson, D. M. and Wyman, R. J. (1965). Motor output patterns during random and rhythmic stimulation of locust thoracic ganglia. *Biophysical Journal*, 5, 121–43.

Wilson, V. J. (1972). Physiological pathways through the vestibular nuclei. *International Review of Neurobiology*, 15, 27–81.

Winter, D. A. (1991). *The biomechanics and motor control of human gait: normal, elderly and pathological*. University of Waterloo, Waterloo.

Wisleder, D., Zernicke, R. F., and Smith, J. L. (1990). Speed-related changes in hindlimb intersegmental dynamics during the swing phase of cat locomotion. *Experimental Brain Research*, 79, 651–60.

Wolf, H. (1993). The locust tegula: significance for flight rhythm generation, wing movement control and aerodynamic force production. *Journal of Experimental Biology*, 182, 229–53.

Wolf, H. and Burrows, M. (1995). Proprioceptive neurons of a locust leg receive rhythmic presynaptic inhibition during walking. *Journal of Neuroscience*, 15, 5623–36.

Wolf, H. and Büschges, A. (1995). Nonspiking local interneurons in insect leg motor control. II. Role of nonspiking local interneurons in the control of leg swing during walking. *Journal of Neurophysiology*, 73, 1861–75.

Wolf, H. and Pearson, K. G. (1987). Flight motor patterns recorded in surgically isolated sections of the ventral nerve cord of *Locusta migratoria*. *Journal of Comparative Physiology*, 161A, 103–14.

Wolf, H. and Pearson, K. G. (1988) Proprioceptive input patterns elevator activity in the locust flight system. *Journal of Neurophysiology*, 59, 1831–53.

Wolf, H. and Pearson, K. G. (1989). Comparison of motor patterns in the intact and deafferented locust. III. Patterns of interneuronal activity. *Journal of Comparative Physiology*, 165A, 61–74.

Wolstencroft, J. H. (1964). Reticulospinal neurons. *Journal of Physiology*, 174, 91–108.

Wyman, R. J. (1977). Neural generation of the breathing rhythm. *Annual Review of Physiology*, 39, 417–48.

Yagi, N. (1928). Phototropism of *Dixippus morosus*. *Journal of General Physiology*, 11, 297.

Yamaguchi, T. (1991). Cat forelimb stepping generator. In *Neurobiological basis of human locomotion* (eds. M. Shimamura, S. Grillner, and V. R. Edgerton), pp. 103–15. Japan Scientific Societies Press, Tokyo.

Yanagihara, D. and Udo, M. (1994). Climbing fibre responses in cerebellar Purkinje cells during perturbed locomotion in decerebrate cats. *Neuroscience Research*, 19, 245–8.

Yoshino, M., Takahata, M., and Hisada, M. (1980). Statocyst control of the uropod movement in response to body rolling in crayfish. *Journal of Comparative Physiology*, 139, 243–50.

Young, S. R., Dedwylder, R., and Friesen, W. O. (1981). Responses of the medicinal leech to water waves. *Journal of Comparative Physiology*, 114, 111–16.

Zarnack, W. and Möhl, B. (1977). Activity of direct downstroke flight muscle of *Locusta migratoria* (L.) during steering behavior in flight. I. Patterns of time shift. *Journal of Comparative Physiology*, 118, 215–33.

Zelenin, P. V., Ullén, F., Fagerstedt, P., Deliagina, T. G., Orlovsky, G. N., and Grillner, S. (1997). Control of lateral turns in lamprey. *Society for Neuroscience Abstracts*, 23, Part 1, 765.

Zhang, W., Pombal, M.A., Manira, A.E., and Grillner, S. (1996). Rostrocaudal distribution of 5-HT innervation in the lamprey spinal cord and differential effects of 5-HT on fictive locomotion. *Journal of Comparative Neurology*, **374**, 278–90.

Zompa, I. C. and Dubuc, R. A. (1996). A mesencephalic relay for visual inputs to reticulospinal neurons in lampreys. *Brain Research*, **718**, 221–7.

Index

CPSIA information can be obtained at www.ICGtesting.com
Printed in the USA
LVOW071927220212

270011LV00003B/37/A

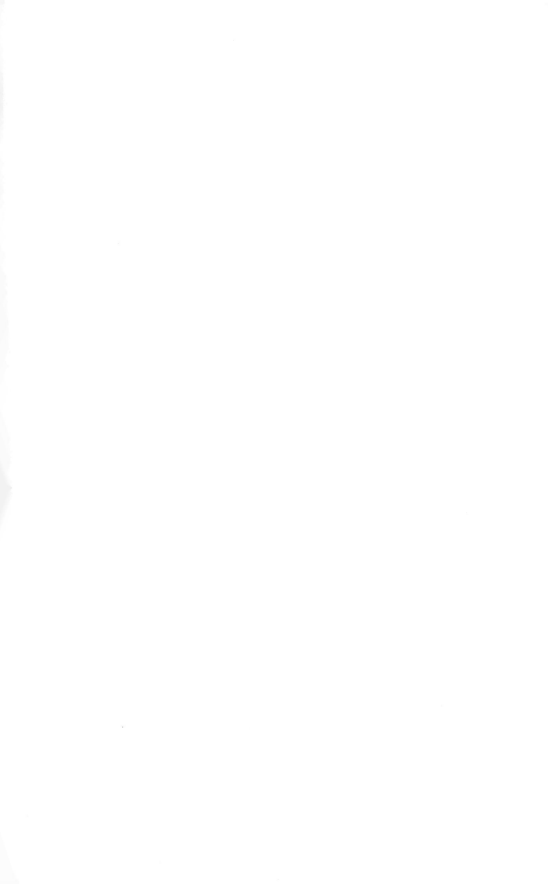